BASIC ELECTROCARDIOGRAPHY

A MODULAR APPROACH

THE METHODIST HOSPITAL

Houston, Texas

EDITED BY

JOAN C. SEIDEL, R.N., M.S., C.C.R.N.

Clinical Specialist, Coronary Care Unit,
The Methodist Hospital,
Houston, Texas

with 319 illustrations

The C. V. Mosby Company

ST. LOUIS • TORONTO • PRINCETON   1986

MOSBY

A TRADITION OF PUBLISHING EXCELLENCE

Editor: Barbara Ellen Norwitz
Developmental editor: Sally Adkisson
Book design: Kay M. Kramer
Cover design: Susan E. Lane
Manuscript editor: Helen C. Hudlin
Production: Jeanne Genz, Florence Fansher, Mary Stueck

Printed in the United States of America

The C.V. Mosby Company
11830 Westline Industrial Drive, St. Louis, Missouri 63146

Library of Congress Cataloging in Publication Data

Main entry under title:

Basic Electrocardiography

Includes bibliographies and index.
1. Arrhythmia—Diagnosis—Programmed instruction.
2. Electrocardiography—Programmed instruction.
I. Methodist Hospital (Houston, Tex.) II. Seidel, Joan C.
[DNLM: 1. Arrhythmia—diagnosis—programmed
instruction. 2. Electrocardiography—programmed instruction. WG 18 B311]
RC685.A65B37 1986   616.1′28′07547   85-13645
ISBN 0-8016-3401-6

T/VH/VH 9 8 7 6 5 4 3 2   01/D/038

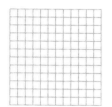

Contributors

MODULE 1

SALLY J. NESS, R.N., M.S.N., C.C.R.N.

Graduate Student, MBA Program in Health Care Administration, The University of Houston, Houston, Texas

MODULES 1, 2 AND 8

JOAN C. SEIDEL, R.N., M.S., C.C.R.N.

Clinical Specialist, Coronary Care Unit, The Methodist Hospital, Houston, Texas

MODULE 3

JOAN M. LOOS, R.N., M.S.

Nurse Clinician, Infectious Disease Service, The Methodist Hospital, Houston, Texas

MODULE 4

KATHI M. WEILER, R.N., B.S.N.

Head Nurse, Cardiology Telemetry Unit, The Methodist Hospital, Houston, Texas

RONDA BRAND STERN, R.N., B.S.N.

Formerly Cardiovascular Nurse Specialist, Medical Nursing Service, The Methodist Hospital, Houston, Texas

MODULES 5 AND 6

SHARON L. VANDERSLICE, R.N.

Director of Diagnostic Testing and Cardiac Rehabilitation, The Institute of Preventive Medicine, The Methodist Hospital, Houston, Texas

MODULE 7

PATRICIA VERBITSKEY, R.N., B.S.N.

Manager, International Affairs Department, The Methodist Hospital, Houston, Texas

MODULE 8

GARY M. GUSICK, R.N., C.C.R.N.

Clinical Practitioner Teacher II, Cardiovascular Surgical Intensive Care Unit, The Methodist Hospital, Houston, Texas

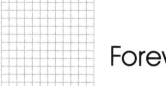

Foreword

As chief executive of one of the largest teaching hospitals in the country, I am constantly emphasizing the importance of high quality medical education and teaching programs to support our hospital's mission of providing the best patient care. As professionals dedicated to the comprehensive care of patients with a variety of health care needs, it is our responsibility to disseminate the knowledge gained through our unique experience so that other health care professionals can benefit, thereby ensuring the continued provision of high quality health care. This book represents an excellent example of health care professionals dedicating themselves to this concept.

Developed over a period of 4 years by a group of nurse practitioners, this book was originally intended to address the need for internally consistent standards of instruction for basic electrocardiographic (ECG) interpretation at The Methodist Hospital. The Methodist Hospital, a 1218 bed major international referral center and teaching hospital recognized as a pioneer in cardiovascular surgery and specialized intensive care units, treats one of the country's largest patient populations at risk for developing cardiac dysrhythmias. In view of the diverse health care team required to care for this population, the authors recognized an increasing need to develop a consistent, basic understanding of ECG interpretation for nonprofessionals as well as professionals. The overwhelmingly successful acceptance of these instructional modules at Methodist clearly has established their usefulness to a wide variety of health care personnel outside the hospital.

This book draws upon the authors' extensive experience in the clinical care of thousands of cardiac dysrhythmia patients and has evolved from numerous hours of teaching ECG interpretation to professionals and nonprofessionals. The Methodist Hospital is proud to be associated with the respected clinicians and teachers who have authored this book; I am confident you will benefit from the knowledge, expertise, and experience they have consolidated in this definitive work.

Larry L. Mathis
President, Chief Executive Officer,
The Methodist Hospital,
Houston, Texas
March, 1985

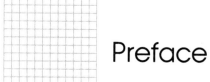

Preface

Basic Electrocardiography: A Modular Approach is comprised of a series of eight modules developed by the authors to provide consistent instructional content about basic electrocardiographic interpretation for a wide variety of learners in a large teaching institution. The text focuses on the recognition of basic cardiac rhythm disturbances, treatment, and nursing management. It is directed toward professionals and nonprofessionals who have little or no background in ECG interpretation but who may be involved in the care of the patient at risk for developing cardiac dysrhythmias. The target population includes medical students, student and graduate nurses, emergency medical technicians, monitoring technicians, and all other members of the health care team interested in learning basic electrocardiographic interpretation.

Each module is complete with a pretest, behavioral objectives, vocabulary, content, posttest, and supplement section for practice. Therefore, it can serve as an independent self-paced instructional unit for an individual learner or as a guideline for a classroom instructor. The field of electrocardiography has been markedly influenced by the advent of electrophysiology laboratories. Research from these areas has provided a plethora of new information on how cardiac dysrhythmias are initiated and propagated. A basic approach to the most current information on rhythm disturbances, pacemakers, and antidysrhythmic drugs is provided in this text. The drug module includes updated information regarding conventional pharmacological agents used in the management of dysrhythmias as well as newer investigational drugs.

Based on our own personal experience in attempting to provide this material to diverse audiences, we have taken this modular approach because we believe it is a concise, comprehensive, and time-efficient means of imparting this knowledge.

The authors wish to acknowledge the following people for their dedication and support of this project: Kathy Kyper, for her illustrations; Margaret L. Woods, Vice President of Patient Services Division, and LaDonna Doud, Administrative Assistant of Patient Services Division, for their administrative support; Jo Ann McBride, Director of Word Processing and her staff: Julianna Williams, Cathy Fitzpatrick, and Theresa Wasilewski for their typing support; Joan Mitchell and Carmella Cinefro for their secretarial support; Johanna Frerichs from Medtronic and Derryl Smith from Intermedics for providing photographs; Dr. Christopher Wyndham and Dr. Jerry Luck for providing rhythm strips; Dr. William H. Spencer III, for providing radiographs; Lydia Ramos, Lina Treleaven, and Tory Schmitz for their critiques, and to all of our colleagues, friends, and families for their unending encouragement and support.

Gary M. Gusick
Joan M. Loos
Sally J. Ness
Joan C. Seidel
Ronda Brand Stern
Sharon L. Vanderslice
Patricia Verbitskey
Kathi M. Weiler

Contents

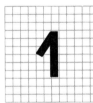
1 Anatomy and electrophysiology of the heart

PRETEST (Answers on pp. 25-26)

A. Label the following structures on Fig. 1-1.
1. Major blood vessels (5)
2. Cardiac chambers (4)
3. Cardiac valves (4)
4. Layers of cardiac muscle (3)

C. Matching: Place the appropriate letter in Column B with the coronary artery in Column A.

Column A Coronary arteries	Column B Areas supplied
___ 1. Right	a. Septal and apical portions of left ventricle
___ 2. Left main	b. Branches of left anterior descending artery
___ 3. Circumflex	c. Right atrium, right ventricle, and inferior left ventricular wall
___ 4. Left anterior descending	d. Branch of the circumflex
___ 5. Obtuse marginal	e. Left atrium and left lateral ventricular wall
___ 6. Diagonals	f. Bifurcation into left anterior descending and circumflex arteries

D. Label the structures of the cardiac conduction system on Fig. 1-3.

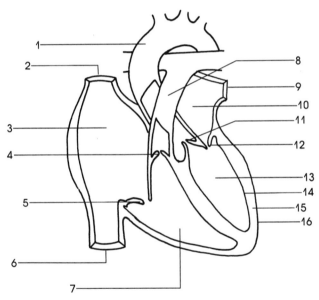

FIG. 1-1

B. Label the coronary arteries on Fig. 1-2.

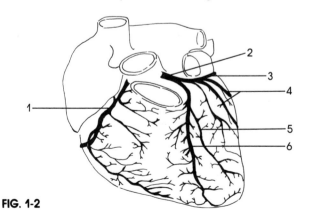

FIG. 1-2

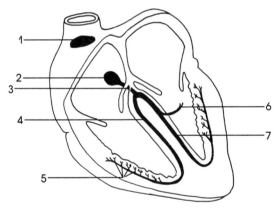

FIG. 1-3

E. Label the following on Fig. 1-4.
1. P wave
2. QRS
3. T wave

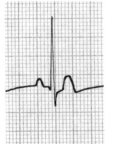

FIG. 1-4

1

F. Fill in the blanks.
   In normal sinus rhythm, the rate is between _____
   and _____ beats per minute, the rhythm is _____,
   and there is a _____ wave for every QRS complex.

G. Identify the positive and negative poles in each of the
   following leads:

   (−pole)   (+pole)
   1. Lead I
   2. Lead II
   3. Lead III

H. On Fig. 1-5, label the placement of the chest leads.

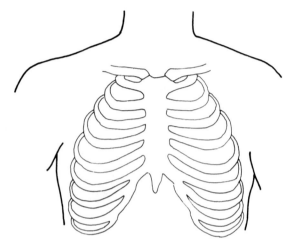

FIG. 1-5

Directions: Circle one answer to each question unless
otherwise indicated.

I. The normal PR interval is between:
   1. 0.06-0.10 second
   2. 0.10-0.16 second
   3. 0.12-0.20 second
   4. 0.16-0.24 second

J. The normal QRS interval is between:
   1. 0.06-0.10 second
   2. 0.12-0.20 second
   3. 0.08-0.12 second
   4. 0.04-0.08 second

K. The P wave on the ECG represents:
   1. Firing of the SA node
   2. Ventricular repolarization
   3. Atrial repolarization
   4. Atrial depolarization

L. The QT interval on the ECG represents:
   1. Ventricular depolarization
   2. Atrial depolarization
   3. Ventricular repolarization
   4. Conduction through the AV node
   5. 1 and 3

M. Parasympathetic stimulation of the heart results in
   (circle all that apply):
   1. Increased heart rate
   2. Increased force of contraction

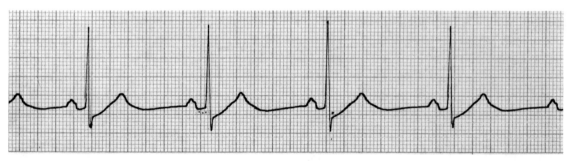

FIG. 1-6   Lead II

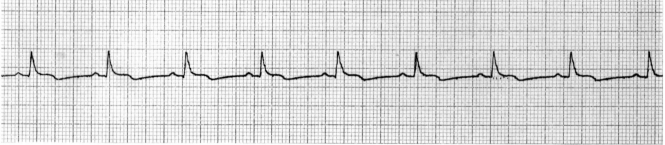

FIG. 1-7   Lead II

3. Decreased heart rate
4. Increased speed of AV conduction
5. Slowed AV conduction

N. Interpret the rhythm strip in Fig. 1-6.
   1. Heart rate:
   2. PR interval:
   3. QRS interval:
   4. QT interval:
   5. Label the P-QRS-T complexes.

O. Interpret the rhythm strip in Fig 1-7.
   1. Heart rate:
   2. PR interval:
   3. QRS interval:
   4. QT interval:

PURPOSE

The purpose of this module is to provide the learner with basic information about the anatomy and physiology of the heart and its conduction system and the principles of electrophysiology.

BEHAVIORAL OBJECTIVES

Upon completion of this module, the learner should be able to:

A. Label a view of the heart including anatomical structures
B. Correctly label the coronary arteries, including the following: left main (LMCA), left anterior descending (LAD), circumflex (LC), diagonals, obtuse marginals (OM), right coronary (RCA), and posterior descending (PDA)
C. List the areas of the myocardium and conduction system that are supplied by each of the principal coronary arteries
D. Correctly label the structures of the cardiac conduction system
E. Identify the layers of the heart
F. State three functions of the pericardial sac
G. Correctly label the four heart valves and briefly describe their function
H. Describe the effects of the sympathetic and the parasympathetic nervous systems on the heart
I. State the locations of the principal pressoreceptors in the neck and chest vessels
J. Describe the rationale, objectives, and nursing responsibilities related to carotid sinus massage
K. Define systole and diastole
L. Define automaticity, contractility, excitability, and conductivity
M. Define depolarization and repolarization

N. Identify the normal vectors of atrial and ventricular depolarization
O. Correctly label the Einthoven triangle
P. List the 12 leads of the standard ECG and describe which are bipolar and unipolar and why
Q. Define ECG standardization
R. State the normal speed of ECG paper
S. Label the P, QRS, and T waves on a diagram
T. State and measure correctly normal PR, QRS, and QT intervals
U. Determine two methods of calculating heart rate from an ECG strip

VOCABULARY

Absolute refractory period An interval of total unexcitability during which a cell cannot respond to a stimulus. This correlates from the beginning of the QRS to the beginning of the T wave on the ECG.

Accessory pathway An "extra" pathway through which impulses may be conducted to bypass the normal delay in the AV junction.

Acetylcholine Parasympathetic neurotransmitter substance.

Annulus Fibrous ring surrounding each atrioventricular valve orifice.

Aortic semilunar valve Consists of three pocket-like cusps through which blood ejected from the left ventricle passes into the aorta. The orifices (openings) of the two principal coronary arteries arise from two of these cusps.

Atrial appendage Irregularly shaped continuation of the atria.

Atrioventricular (AV) node A dense bundle of conduction fibers within the right side of the lower interatrial septum, the function of which is to delay impulse conduction from the atria to the ventricles.

Atrium One of two upper thin-walled receiving chambers of the heart.

Automaticity Electrical property of cells that permits spontaneous initiation of the cardiac impulse.

Bundle of His Compact conduction tissue fibers through which the impulse passes from the AV node into the ventricles. It divides into the right and left bundle branches.

Carotid sinus massage Unilateral pressure over the carotid artery bifurcation in the carotid sinus region causing increased vagal nervous discharge. An ectopic atrial pacemaker may abruptly cease firing while a sinus pacemaker often slows gradually.

Chordae tendineae Fine fibrous threads anchoring the AV valve leaflets to their respective papillary muscles.

Chronotropic Refers to automaticity from the SA node; may be positive (↑ heart rate) or negative (↓ heart rate).

Conductivity The spread of electrical activity from one specialized cell to another.

Contractility A mechanical property characterized by the coordinated shortening of cardiac muscle fibers, resulting in a pumping effect.

Coronary arteries
   left main (LMCA) Originating from the left sinus of Valsalva, it bifurcates after 2 to 3 cm into the left anterior descending and circumflex coronary arteries.
   left anterior descending (LAD) Extension of the LMCA, it continues down the anterior interventricular groove to the apex.
   circumflex (LC) A branch of the LMCA, which runs into the left atrioventricular sulcus with branches to the left atrium and left lateral ventricular wall.

diagonals Of variable size and number, these vessels are branches of the LAD.

obtuse marginals (OM) Branches of the circumflex artery that supply the left lateral ventricular wall.

right (RCA) Arising from the right sinus of Valsalva and continuing in the right atrioventricular sulcus, this vessel supplies the sinoatrial and atrioventricular nodes in the majority of hearts and sends branches to the right atrium and ventricle.

posterior descending (PDA) Supplies the inferior wall of the left ventricle in the majority of hearts as a continuation of the right coronary artery.

Coronary sinus Opening into the right atrium, it drains venous blood from the myocardium into the general circulation.

Crux The point on the posterobasal surface of the heart that forms the junction at which all four chambers meet.

Depolarization The process of activation of automatic, conductile, and contractile elements from the resting or polarized state.[9]

Diastole Relaxation phase of the cardiac cycle during which the ventricles and coronary arteries are filling.

Dromotropic Refers to speed of AV conduction and may be positive or negative.

Einthoven's triangle An equilateral triangle which, when drawn on the chest, plots the axes of the bipolar standard limb leads.

Electrical axis The mean direction of current flow within the heart.

Electrical potential The energy possessed by a cell relative to ionic imbalance across its membrane.

Electrocardiogram (ECG) A graphic recording of the electrical activity of the heart plotted against time.

Endocardium The smooth inner lining of the cardiac chambers, including the papillary muscles, which is composed of epithelial cells.

Epicardium The outer layer of the heart, continuous with the visceral portion of the pericardium overlying the heart and the proximal segments of the great vessels.

Excitability The ability to respond to a stimulus.

Fossa ovalis A shallow, ovoid depression in the interatrial septum, a trace of the embryologic interatrial opening.

Frank-Starling law of the heart The force of contraction is directly proportional to the stretch of myocardial fibrils, up to a point of physiological limits.

Inotropic Refers to force of myocardial contraction. May be positive or negative.

Interatrial septum Fibromuscular wall separating the atria.

Interventricular septum A wall separating the right and left ventricles.

membranous Thinner, upper portion of the septum between the aortic valve cusps and the tricuspid valve.

muscular Major part of the septum that participates in left ventricular contraction.

Junctional Area of conduction tissue, including the AV node and the bundle of His.

Lead Arrangement of electrical conductors through which electrical activity from the body is brought to a recording device.

Lead axis The direct line between the negative and positive poles of a bipolar lead or between the positive pole and reference point of a unipolar lead.[5]

Lead systems
frontal plane
a. Standard limb leads (I, II, III)
b. Augmented vector leads (aV_R, aV_L, aV_F)
horizontal plane
a. Chest, precordial, or V leads
b. V_1, V_2, V_3, V_4, V_5, V_6

Left bundle branch (LBB) Fibers in the subendocardial layer of the left interventricular septum that conduct the impulse from the bundle of His to the Purkinje fibers. There are two divisions: (1) the anterior-superior division or fascicle and (2) the posterior-inferior division or fascicle.

Mitral valve Atrioventricular (AV) valve composed of two leaflets (bicuspid) through which blood passes from the left atrium to the left ventricle.

Myocardium Thick muscular contractile portion of the heart wall.

Norepinephrine Neurotransmitter substance of the sympathetic nervous system.

Papillary muscles Located in the endocardium of the right and left ventricles, they anchor the AV valves via the chordae tendineae and prevent eversion of the valve leaflets into the atria during ventricular systole. There is one papillary muscle for each valve cusp.

Parasympathetic A division of the autonomic nervous system. Stimulation decreases cardiac impulse formation and conduction.

P cells Specialized cells located in the center of the SA node that possess the property of automaticity.

Pericarditis Inflammation of the pericardium.

Pericardium Conical-shaped serous cavity covering the heart and proximal portions of the great vessels.

Polarity Refers to the location of the positive and negative poles of a lead axis or to the difference in electrical potential between the inner and outer surface of the cell membrane.[9]

Precordium Refers to the anterior surface of the lower thorax.

Pressoreceptors Receptors found in the superior vena cava, right atrium, aortic arch, and carotid sinus, which sense stretch and increase or decrease heart rate and blood pressure accordingly.

Pulmonary artery The vessel transporting venous blood from the right ventricle to the lungs.

Pulmonary veins Usually two from each lung transport arterial blood from the lungs to the left atrium.

Pulmonic semilunar valve Consists of three pocket-like cusps through which blood is ejected from the right ventricle to the pulmonary artery.

Purkinje fibers Terminal branches of the right and left bundles bringing the impulse rapidly and directly to the myocardial cells of the septum, ventricular walls, and papillary muscles, depolarizing the ventricles and allowing the mechanical event of ventricular contraction to occur.

Relative refractory period A period corresponding to the beginning of the T wave to almost the end of the T wave on the ECG in which a stronger than normal stimulus may excite and depolarize the cells.

Repolarization The process of restoration, following depolarization, to the normal resting electrical state of the cell.

Right bundle branch (RBB) A long, thin bundle of fibers within the subendocardial layer of the right interventricular septum that conducts impulses from the bundle of His to the Purkinje fibers in the right ventricle.

Sinoatrial (SA) node The node located at the junction of the superior vena cava and right atrium, consisting of specialized automatic cells and known as the natural pacemaker of the heart.

Sinus of Valsalva Pocket-like pouches of the aortic valve cusps in which the openings of the coronary arteries are located.

Sulcus A groove.

Supernormal period A period at the end of the T wave during which depolarization may be initiated by a lesser stimulus than is normally required. Also known as the vulnerable period.

Sympathetic A division of the autonomic nervous system which, when stimulated, increases impulse formation (automaticity), speed of conduction, and force of myocardial contraction.

Systole The contraction phase of the cardiac cycle, related to expelling blood from chambers.

Transitional cells Specialized cells that lie in the periphery of the SA node that conduct impulses from the P cells to the atrial myocardium.

Tricuspid valve Atrioventricular (AV) valve composed of three leaflets through which blood passes from the right atrium to the right ventricle.

U wave A small wave on the ECG following the T wave, which may represent repolarization of the Purkinje fibers.[5]

Vagus The major nerve of the parasympathetic nervous system, the tenth cranial nerve.

Vector A force with direction and magnitude, representing electrical current flow by use of an arrow.

Ventricle One of two lower muscular pumping chambers of the heart.

CONTENT
General anatomy
GROSS HEART STRUCTURE

The heart is a fist-sized, blunt, conical, muscular pumping organ situated in the thoracic cavity posterior to the sternum and lungs, inferior to the trachea and thymus, superior to the diaphragm, and anterior to the vertebral column. At the base are located the great vessels: the aorta, pulmonary artery, and venae cavae. Opposite to the base is the pointed apex, tipped inferiorly and anteriorly to the left at a 60-degree angle.[8]

The heart is composed of four chambers housing two separate circulations (Fig. 1-8).

The venous, on the right side, is under low pressure; the right ventricle pumps blood to the lungs only. The arterial, on the left side, is under high pressure since it must pump blood to all parts of the body. Venous blood returning to the heart enters the right atrium, one of two upper thin-walled receiving chambers, via the large veins or venae cavae. The superior vena cava drains the head, neck, and arms of venous blood, while the inferior vena cava brings venous blood back to the heart from the trunk and legs. The coronary sinus, located in the lower portion of the right side of the atrial septum, is the opening from which venous blood from the heart muscle itself is returned to general circulation in the right atrium.

From the right atrium the blood passes into the right ventricle via the tricuspid valve, which has three leaflets or cusps. Chordae tendineae, small tendon-like cords, are attached to each leaflet and are then anchored to three papillary muscles located in the right ventricular wall. This apparatus controls valve opening and closing, as well as preventing the leaflets from prolapsing into the right atrium during ventricular systolic contraction (Fig. 1-9, p. 6).

The right ventricle, one of the two lower chambers, is a thin-walled, low-pressure pump. Its function is to propel venous blood from the right atrium to the lung for gas exchange. Blood leaves the right ventricle via the pulmonary artery through the pulmonic semilunar valve, comprised of three concave, triangular-shaped cusps.

In the lung, the transfer of oxygen and carbon dioxide between the blood in the pulmonary capillaries and the alveoli* takes place through an extremely thin yet vast membrane by simple diffusion. Pressure differences between these gases across the alveolar-capillary membrane determine the direction of movement: oxygen moves

* The microscopic gas exchange unit of the lung.

FIG. 1-8
Basic anatomy of heart.

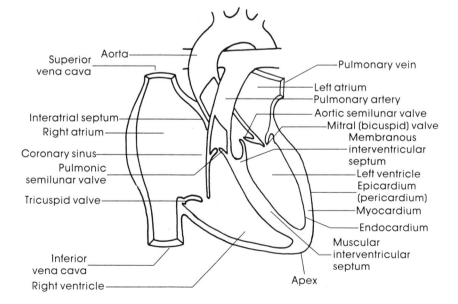

Superior vena cava — Aorta

Pulmonary vein

Left atrium

Pulmonary artery

Aortic semilunar valve

Interatrial septum

Right atrium

Mitral (bicuspid) valve

Membranous interventricular septum

Coronary sinus

Pulmonic semilunar valve

Left ventricle

Epicardium (pericardium)

Tricuspid valve

Myocardium

Endocardium

Inferior vena cava

Muscular interventricular septum

Right ventricle

Apex

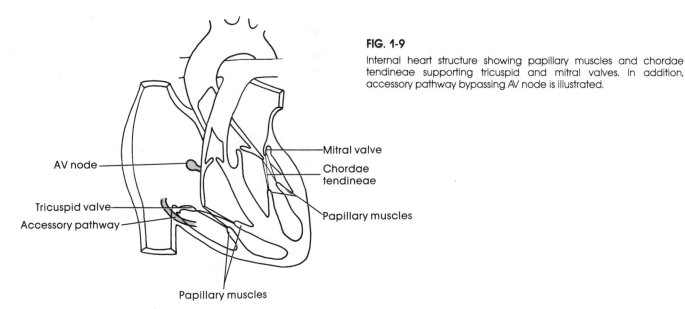

FIG. 1-9

Internal heart structure showing papillary muscles and chordae tendineae supporting tricuspid and mitral valves. In addition, accessory pathway bypassing AV node is illustrated.

AV node

Tricuspid valve

Accessory pathway

Mitral valve

Chordae tendineae

Papillary muscles

Papillary muscles

from alveoli to capillaries and carbon dioxide moves from capillaries to alveoli.

From the lungs, freshly oxygenated blood returns to the left atrium, still under low pressure, via four pulmonary veins, two from each lung. It crosses into the left ventricle, the high-pressure muscular pumping chamber, through the mitral or bicuspid valve. This valve is so named because, when in the open position, it is thought to resemble a bishop's hat, or miter. The mitral valve has two cusps, each attached to chordae tendineae and to a respective papillary muscle in the left ventricular wall (Fig. 1-9). The left ventricle pumps blood under high pressure out the aorta via the aortic semilunar valve to all parts of the body.

Between the left and right atria is the interatrial septum, a fibromuscular wall characterized by a shallow depression, the fossa ovalis, a vestige of the foramen ovale, or the oval window that in fetal life provides communication between the atria. The atrial appendage is an irregularly shaped continuation of the atrium, lined with muscles. It is of no circulatory significance except that in the case of atrial fibrillation blood clots may form there because of stagnation of blood produced by the quivering atria.[8]

The interventricular septum is composed of an upper thin membranous portion, the rest being a much thicker muscular wall. The latter bulges into the right ventricle and participates in left ventricular contraction. On cross section, the thinner right ventricular wall appears to be wrapped part way around the left ventricle.

The aortic semilunar valve at the root of the aorta is shaped similarly to the pulmonic valve, having three pocket-like cusps, here known as sinuses of Valsalva. Located in two of these sinuses are the openings of the coronary arteries, the right (RCA) and the left or left main coronary artery (LMCA).

CORONARY ARTERIES (Figs. 1-10 and 1-11)

The left main coronary artery (LMCA), a short trunk of from 2 to several cm in length, bifurcates into the left anterior descending (LAD) and circumflex (LC) coronary arteries near the base of the left atrial appendage. The LAD enters the anterior interventricular sulcus or groove, between the right and left ventricles anteriorly, and courses to the apex (see Fig. 1-10). It may stop there or continue on to the diaphragmatic (inferior) surface of the left ventricle. It gives off major branches to the left ventricular wall, the interventricular septum, and smaller branches to the right ventricle. Included among these branches are the septal perforators and diagonals. The septal perforators, which number from three to five, come off at right angles to the LAD and supply the anterior two thirds of the interventricular septum, most of the muscular interventricular septum, the majority of the right bundle branch (RBB) and the anterior-superior fascicle of the left bundle branch (LBB). The diagonals, which number from one to three, supply the anterior and part of the lateral surface of the left ventricle and a portion of the posterior-inferior fascicle of the left bundle.[4]

The circumflex (LC) coronary artery arises perpendicularly to the LMCA, coursing beneath the left atrial appendage between the left atrium and left ventricle, and continues around the posterior left ventricle. In most people, it ends in a varying number of small posterior

FIG. 1-10

Anterior view of coronary circulation.

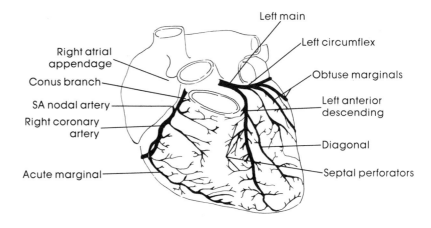

FIG. 1-11

Posterior view of coronary circulation. (Modified from Conner, R.P.: Crit. Care Nurse **3**(3):69, 1983.)

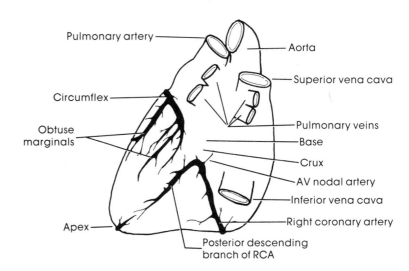

branches; however, in 10% of the population, it continues to the crux (the point at which all four chambers meet posteriorly at the base) and ends as the posterior descending coronary artery (PDA). In this latter group of people, it is described as a left dominant coronary artery system. Branches of the LC are called obtuse marginals (OM) and number between one to three. These are responsible for supplying the left atrium, lateral wall of the left ventricle, and a portion of the posterior wall of the left ventricle with blood. The AV node is supplied by the LC in 10% of individuals (see Fig. 1-11).[4]

The right coronary artery (RCA) arises from the right cusp of the aortic valve and courses beneath the right atrial appendage, continuing in the right atrioventricular groove until it reaches the crux. At this point it makes a 90-degree turn to become the PDA in 80% to 90% of individuals; in this population it is known as a right dominant coronary system. The first branch off the RCA is called the conus branch and supplies the area of the right ventricle below the pulmonic valve. The next branch

becomes the SA nodal branch, which supplies the SA node in 55% to 60% of individuals (see Fig. 1-10). The PDA also has septal perforator branches that supply the posterior one third of the interventricular septum and branches that supply the posterior-inferior fascicle of the left bundle.[4,6]

The coronary arteries receive their blood supply during the diastolic phase of the cardiac cycle or when the ventricular muscle mass is relaxing. They all lie embedded in fat tissue for protection.

LAYERS OF THE HEART

The layers of the heart include the endocardium, myocardium, and epicardium, all enclosed in the pericardium.

The *endocardium* is the smooth, inner lining of the heart, the valves, and papillary muscles. This continuous surface of epithelial cells helps to prevent clot formation, which is promoted by roughened areas. The *myocardium* is the thick, muscular middle layer composed of millions of contractile units providing the force necessary to eject blood from the ventricles. The left ventricular myocardium is three times as thick as that of the right ventricle. The *epicardium* is the outermost covering, which promotes integrity of the organ. It is continuous with the inner or visceral layer of the *pericardium,* the sac-like balloon covering the heart and the proximal portions of the great vessels. The outer portion of the pericardium is the tough, fibrous parietal layer. The functions of both layers of the pericardium include:

1. Anchoring and support for the heart in the thoracic cavity; it attaches to the diaphragm, vertebral column, and xiphoid process
2. Protection from diseases that might otherwise invade the heart, such as malignancies of the thorax and mediastinum
3. Resistance to overfilling, thus limiting right and left ventricular work loads and, as a consequence, protecting the valves[8]

Between the parietal and visceral layers is a potential space called the pericardial space. There are 10 ml to 30 ml of clear pericardial fluid secreted within this space, which acts as a lubricating cushion for the heart in motion.

CONDUCTION SYSTEM

The conduction system of the heart is a group of specialized tissues and cells that possess special electrical and mechanical properties. There are three electrical properties, which include:

1. *Automaticity* or the ability to automatically initiate impulses
2. *Excitability* or the ability to respond to an impulse once received
3. *Conductivity* or the ability to conduct or transmit the impulse from one point to another

The mechanical property of the conduction system is that of *contractility* or the pumping response of the myocardial cells to the electrical impulse. It is important to note that the myocardium cannot contract without *first* receiving a conducted electrical impulse.

The conduction system is capable of automatically initiating impulses independent of outside stimulation or control. The impulses are conducted throughout the entire myocardium, allowing the normal mechanical sequence of atrial and ventricular contraction to occur. This activity requires a proper balance of calcium, sodium, and potassium ions that move across a cell membrane and an energy source in the form of adenosine triphosphate (ATP) (Fig. 1-12).

The sinoatrial (SA) node is a crescent-shaped structure that lies subepicardially at the junction of the superior vena cava and the right atrium. It consists of three distinct cell types: P cells, transitional cells, and Purkinje cells (Fig. 1-13).

The P cells, located in the center of the SA node, close to the SA nodal artery, have the property of automatically initiating impulses at a rate of 60 to 100 per minute. This is faster than any other part of the conduction system; therefore, the SA node is known as the natural pacemaker of the heart.

Once the impulses are initiated by the P cells, they are conducted to the atrial myocardium by the transitional and Purkinje cells to allow the atria to conduct the impulses to the AV node and, ultimately, to allow the atria to contract.[1]

The anatomical location of the SA node is close to the pericardium and is easily affected by such conditions as pericarditis. The SA nodal artery arises from the RCA in 55% to 60% of people and from the LC in 40% to 45%. The artery is large in comparison to the size of the node and pressure influences may alter the heart rate.[1]

Obstruction of the SA nodal artery may cause sinus dysrhythmias from resultant hypoxia and acidosis (see Sinus Dysrhythmias Module).

The atrial muscle tissue conducts the impulses from

FIG. 1-12

Specialized conduction tissue.

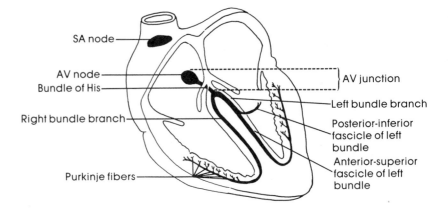

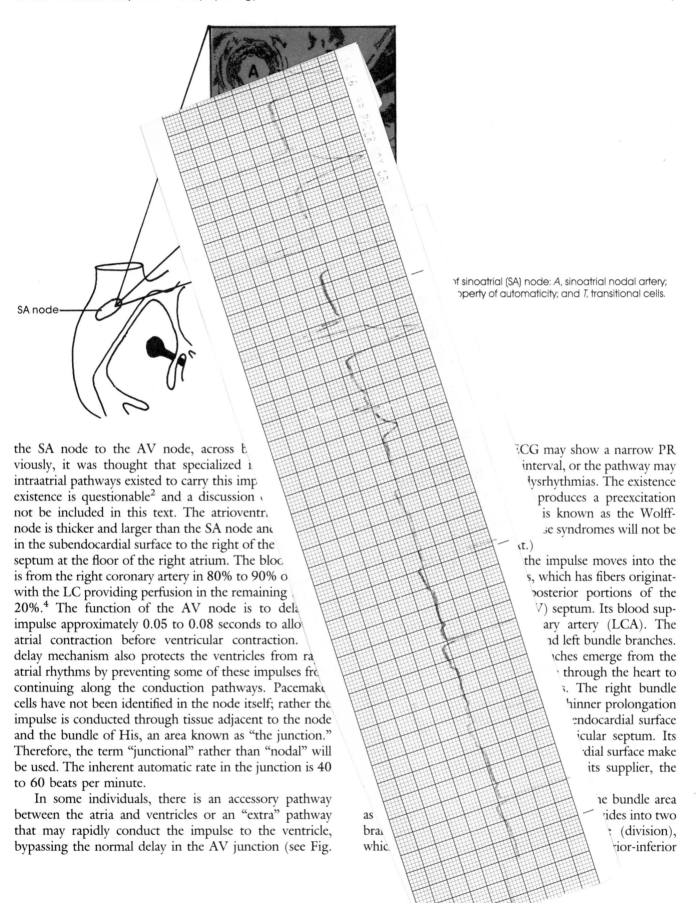

SA node

...f sinoatrial (SA) node: *A*, sinoatrial nodal artery; ...operty of automaticity; and *T*, transitional cells.

the SA node to the AV node, across t... viously, it was thought that specialized i... intraatrial pathways existed to carry this imp... existence is questionable[2] and a discussion ... not be included in this text. The atrioventr... node is thicker and larger than the SA node an... in the subendocardial surface to the right of the ... septum at the floor of the right atrium. The bloo... is from the right coronary artery in 80% to 90% o... with the LC providing perfusion in the remaining ... 20%.[4] The function of the AV node is to dela... impulse approximately 0.05 to 0.08 seconds to allo... atrial contraction before ventricular contraction. ... delay mechanism also protects the ventricles from ra... atrial rhythms by preventing some of these impulses fr... continuing along the conduction pathways. Pacemake... cells have not been identified in the node itself; rather the... impulse is conducted through tissue adjacent to the node... and the bundle of His, an area known as "the junction." Therefore, the term "junctional" rather than "nodal" will be used. The inherent automatic rate in the junction is 40 to 60 beats per minute.

In some individuals, there is an accessory pathway between the atria and ventricles or an "extra" pathway that may rapidly conduct the impulse to the ventricle, bypassing the normal delay in the AV junction (see Fig.

...CG may show a narrow PR interval, or the pathway may ...ysrhythmias. The existence ...produces a preexcitation ...is known as the Wolff- ...se syndromes will not be ...t.)

...the impulse moves into the ...s, which has fibers originat- ...osterior portions of the ...V) septum. Its blood sup- ...ary artery (LCA). The ...d left bundle branches. ...ches emerge from the ...through the heart to ...s. The right bundle ...hinner prolongation ...ndocardial surface ...icular septum. Its ...dial surface make ...its supplier, the

...e bundle area ...ides into two ...e (division), ...ior-inferior

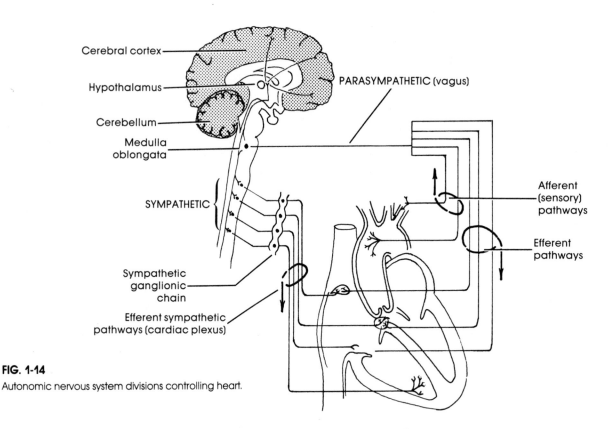

FIG. 1-14
Autonomic nervous system divisions controlling heart.

fascicle (division), which is thick and short. The left anterior-superior fascicle receives its blood supply from the LAD, with the posterior-inferior fascicle possessing the advantage of a dual blood supply, being perfused by the RCA as well as the LAD. This provides additional protection from ischemia related to vessel occlusion. The left bundle branches contact the left subendocardial surface of the interventricular septum deep beneath the aortic valve.

The terminal branches of the right and left bundles bring the impulse to every cell in the ventricular muscle mass, via the Purkinje fibers. These fibers receive their blood supply from the LAD. Their inherent automaticity rate is 15 to 40 beats per minute, the so-called idioventricular rhythm.

Thus, the SA node, AV junction, and Purkinje fibers all have the property of automaticity.

NERVE SUPPLY

The heart is under the control of the sympathetic and parasympathetic divisions of the autonomic nervous system (Fig. 1-14).

The sympathetic fibers originate in the spinal cord between the first thoracic and second lumbar vertebrae and emerge to form the cardiac plexus. These efferent fibers (carrying impulses toward the heart) terminate in the SA node, atrial muscle, AV node, and ventricular muscle. The neurotransmitter hormone for the sympathetic nervous system is norepinephrine.

The parasympathetic neurotransmitter hormone is acetylcholine and it exerts its effects via the tenth cranial nerve, the vagus. The vagus nerve originates in the medulla oblongata of the brain stem and its divisions course bilaterally toward the heart in close proximity to the carotid artery in the neck. These fibers terminate mainly in the SA node, atrial muscle, and AV node with minimal fibers to the ventricular muscle or Purkinje fibers.[5,6,9] It is thought the right vagus has more fibers to the SA node and the left vagus more fibers to the AV node. The effects of cardiac stimulation and inhibition of these two divisions are shown in Table 1-1.

Pressoreceptors that are rich in vagal fibers are located in the carotid bodies at the junction of the common and internal carotid arteries (known as the carotid sinus), in the aortic arch, the atrial muscle, and the eyeballs. These receptors sense pressure or chemical alterations internally and send messages to the medulla via afferent pathways to stimulate or inhibit the cardiac vagal responses via the efferent pathways. The receptor sites will decrease or increase the heart rate and/or blood pressure accordingly.

External stimulation may also be applied, most frequently in the form of carotid sinus message (Fig. 1-15).

TABLE 1-1. Cardiac effects of the autonomic nervous system

	Heart rate	AV conduction time	Force of contraction
STIMULATION			
Sympathetic	Increases	Increases	Increases
Parasympathetic	Decreases	Decreases	No significant effect
INHIBITION			
Sympathetic	Decreases	Decreases	Decreases
Parasympathetic	Increases	Increases	No significant effect

This may produce a slowing of the heart rate, which may be gradual or abrupt.

The physician may perform carotid sinus massage in an attempt to break a rapid supraventricular dysrhythmia. This procedure is never a nursing responsibility; rather, the nurse monitors the patient, runs an ECG strip, and identifies with a pen the point on the rhythm strip occurring at the time the maneuver was performed. The patient's vital signs and reaction to the procedure are documented.

ELECTROPHYSIOLOGY

The electrocardiogram (ECG) is a graphic recording of the electrical activity of the heart plotted against time. It is necessary to have a reference system, or a set of observation points, from which to view the current flow within the heart. This reference system is known as the 12-lead ECG.

DEPOLARIZATION AND REPOLARIZATION

Current flow through the cells of the heart muscle occurs by the following process: As discussed previously, specialized cells within the conduction system of the heart

possess the property of automaticity or the ability to automatically initiate impulses. These automatic cells are known as pacemaker cells and rely on a dynamic flow of ions, particularly sodium (Na^+) and potassium (K^+) across the cell membrane, in order for the impulse to "fire." Calcium (Ca^{++}) ions are also involved. Myocardial cells, both in the atria and ventricles, do not possess this property of automaticity but sit in anticipation of responding to the impulse once it is automatically initiated. These myocardial cells, while in the resting, or polarized, state have an intact cell membrane and have a net difference in polarity across that cell membrane, the inside of the cell being netly negative and the outside of the cell being netly positive. The principal extracellular ion is sodium and the principal intracellular ion is potassium. Since both of these ions carry a positive charge, the net negativity inside the cell results from large negatively charged molecules such as phosphates and proteins that do not easily cross the cell membrane. Thus, in the resting (polarized) state, the cell has what is known as "latent energy," or the property of "waiting" for an event to happen (Fig. 1-16).

Such an event is an electrical impulse. Once the impulse arrives at the cell, the intregrity of the cell membrane is altered, changing its permeability, allowing sodium ions to rush inside the cell, very much like opening a can packaged under a vacuum. As sodium ions continue to enter the cell, potassium ions leave the cell. This causes the inside of the cell to become positive in relation to the outside, which becomes negative—a reversal in polarity. The impulse is propagated from cell to cell, each one repeating the process until all are excited and depolarized, or the entire cell is completely reversed in its polarity (Fig. 1-16, C). It is during this time that the cell is considered to be absolutely refractory, or is totally unexcitable, and cannot respond to a stimulus no matter how strong. In the heart, depolarization occurs from endocardium to epicardium. This electrical stimulus pass-

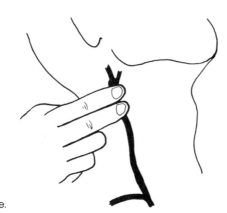

FIG. 1-15
Carotid sinus massage.

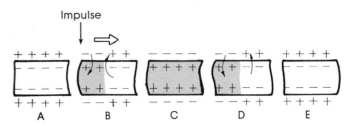

FIG. 1-16
Process of depolarization and repolarization. **A**, resting (polarized) cell. Impulse is received at **B**, which begins the process of depolarization. Arrow above cell **B** illustrates direction of current flow. **C**, totally depolarized cell; **D**, process of repolarization; and **E**, return to resting (polarized) state.

ing through the heart cells causes the entire myocardial muscle fiber mass to contract mechanically as a single coordinated entity, with each microscopic contractile unit shortening against its neighbor.

After depolarization, a recovery process requiring energy occurs, which begins to restore the ionic balance to normal. Sodium ions are pumped out of the cell, while potassium ions are pumped into the cell, returning the cell to its previous resting or polarized state, awaiting the next impulse. This reversal process is called repolarization (see Fig. 1-16). Repolarization occurs from epicardium to endocardium.

Current flow through the heart is illustrated by a net direction and magnitude, which is depicted by an arrow or vector. The vector may be illustrated as a large arrow, having a great magnitude of flow or flowing through a large muscle mass, or as a small arrow, having a smaller magnitude or flowing through a thinner muscle mass (Fig. 1-17).

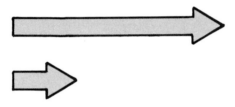

FIG. 1-17
Vectors of current flow illustrating direction and magnitude.

Fig. 1-18 represents the net vectors of electrical current flowing through the heart. The mean vector of ventricular current flow (arrow 5) is called the electrical axis. This current flow occurs in the same direction with each heart beat. It is only the lead, or reference system used, that may alter the complexes seen on the ECG, since each lead monitors the current flow from a different vantage point.

Fig. 1-18 represents ECG complexes viewed from two leads or reference points, lead II and lead aV_R. As viewed from lead II, the SA node automatically initiates an impulse. As the impulse is conducted to the atrial muscle, the net current flow during atrial depolarization is right to left and downward, as represented by arrow 1, producing the first upright wave on the ECG, the P wave. The AV junction delays the impulse approximately 0.05 to 0.08 second (represented by a flat or isoelectric line). The impulse is then conducted toward the left bundle branch first as the short, thick structure of these fibers speed the impulse conduction. Thus, the impulse makes initial contact with the left subendocardial interventricular septum and begins depolarizing the septum from left to right (arrow 2), which is written out as a small negative deflection, or Q wave. The impulse then conducts rapidly through the right and remaining left bundle branches and reaches the Purkinje fibers to begin ventricular depolarization. Since the greatest muscle mass is on the left, the magnitude of current flow is directed leftward (arrows 3, 4, and 5), which produces a positive R wave. The last part of the ventricular myocardium to be depolarized is the posterobasilar portion (arrow 6), which produces a negative S wave on the ECG. The positive wave following the QRS is the T wave and represents ventricular repolarization. From lead II, the current viewed as coming toward the positive electrode produces a positive deflection (above the line), and the current viewed as going away from the positive electrode produces a negative deflection (below the line).

THE LEAD SYSTEMS

In looking at current flow from a single lead, it is necessary to consider how each lead monitors current flow from its respective lead axis. A lead axis is a straight line that connects the positive electrode of that lead to the opposite end of the lead. If the lead is bipolar, it will have a positive and negative end (Fig. 1-19).

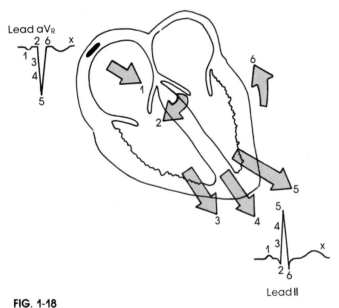

Lead aV_R

Lead II

FIG. 1-18
Normal vectors of electrical current flow through heart. Complexes are viewed from lead II and lead aV_R.

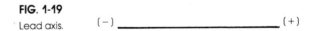

FIG. 1-19
Lead axis. $(-)$ _____ $(+)$

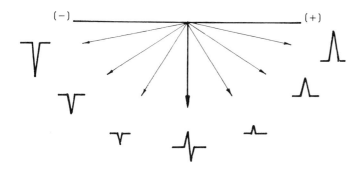

FIG. 1-20

Variations of vectors of current flow along lead axis, illustrating possible resultant complexes. (See text.)

If the lead is unipolar, it will have a positive end and a reference point, which will be the opposite end of its lead axis.

Fig. 1-20 illustrates seven possible vectors of current flow as viewed from a single lead axis. For any given lead axis, a perpendicular line may be drawn to intersect the lead. This divides the lead into four quadrants, two on the positive electrode side and two on negative electrode side. Fig. 1-20 shows only two quadrants, one positive and one negative. Current flowing in a direct perpendicular line to the lead axis will produce either an equiphasic complex (equal above and below the line) or no electrical activity (an isoelectric line). The more directly current flows toward the positive electrode of a lead axis, the more positive the magnitude of the complex. The more directly the current flows away from the positive electrode or the more directly toward the negative electrode, the more negative in magnitude the complex will be. The complex will be upright if current is flowing between the perpendicular line and the positive electrode, but it will vary in its positivity, becoming less positive closer to the perpendicular line. The reverse is true with current flowing between the perpendicular line and the negative electrode of a lead axis. The complex will be negative but will, again, vary in its degree of negativity.

Standard limb leads

Einthoven developed the first set of leads used to record electrical activity of the heart. These three bipolar leads—designated by Roman numerals I, II, III—form a triangle that is known as Einthoven's triangle[5] (Fig. 1-21).

The axis of lead I goes from a negative right arm to a positive left arm, the axis of lead II from a negative right arm to a positive left leg, and the axis of lead III from a negative left arm to a positive left leg.

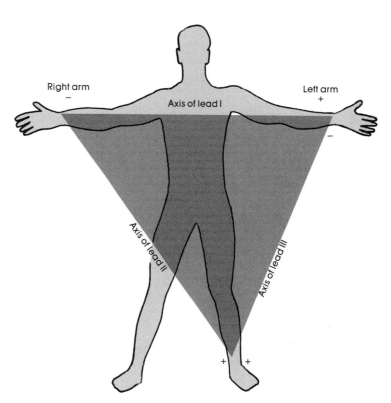

FIG. 1-21

Einthoven's triangle and the three bipolar standard limb leads.

The electrodes of the standard limb leads, which are located in a frontal plane, are placed equidistant from the heart and form a true equilateral triangle. Einthoven's law states that the voltage of the ECG complexes in lead II equals the voltage in lead I plus lead III.[5,6]

Three electrodes are necessary to monitor the standard limb leads: a positive electrode, a negative electrode, and a ground electrode (which may be placed anywhere on the chest).

Augmented leads

A second set of frontal plane leads are known as the augmented vector leads. These leads are termed "augmented" because their electrical currents are so small they need to be increased (augmented) in the ECG machine before they can be seen on a tracing. Since their positive electrodes are at the periphery and their common reference point is at the heart, which has an electrical potential of zero, they are designated as unipolar leads.

These leads are termed: aV_R (augmented vector right) with the positive electrode at the right arm, aV_L (augmented vector left) with the positive electrode at the left arm, and aV_F (augmented vector foot) with the positive electrode at the foot. They may be plotted in the Einthoven triangle (Fig. 1-22). Four electrodes are required on the chest to record the augmented vector leads.

The six frontal plane leads are, therefore, leads I, II, III, aV_R, aV_L, and aV_F. They measure the heart's electrical activity from inferior to superior or right to left only.

However, since the heart is a three-dimensional organ, a method of measuring electrical activity from a horizontal plane is necessary to complete the picture. The precordial leads are the horizontal leads.

Precordial leads

The precordial, chest, or V leads monitor electrical current from a horizontal plane and are described by Arabic numerals: V_1, V_2, V_3, V_4, V_5, and V_6. These leads, like the augmented vector leads, are unipolar, having the positive electrode at the placement position on the chest and the opposite end of the lead axis at a zero reference point, which, again, is the heart.

Fig. 1-23 shows the placement of the leads: V_1 at the fourth intercostal space to the right of the sternum, V_2 at the fourth intercostal space to the left of the sternum, V_3 at the one-half way between V_2 and V_4, V_4 at the fifth intercostal space in the midclavicular line, V_5 at the fifth intercostal space in the anterior axillary line, and V_6 at the fifth intercostal space in the midaxillary line.

The V leads are the best leads to determine ventricular activity, that is, to differentiate between a premature ventricular complex or an aberrantly conducted complex,[7] (see the Ventricular Dysrhythmias Module).

VARIATIONS IN LEAD PLACEMENT

In monitoring systems that only allow for bipolar limb lead selections, it is possible to modify these bipolar leads to clarify information regarding atrial or ventricular activity.

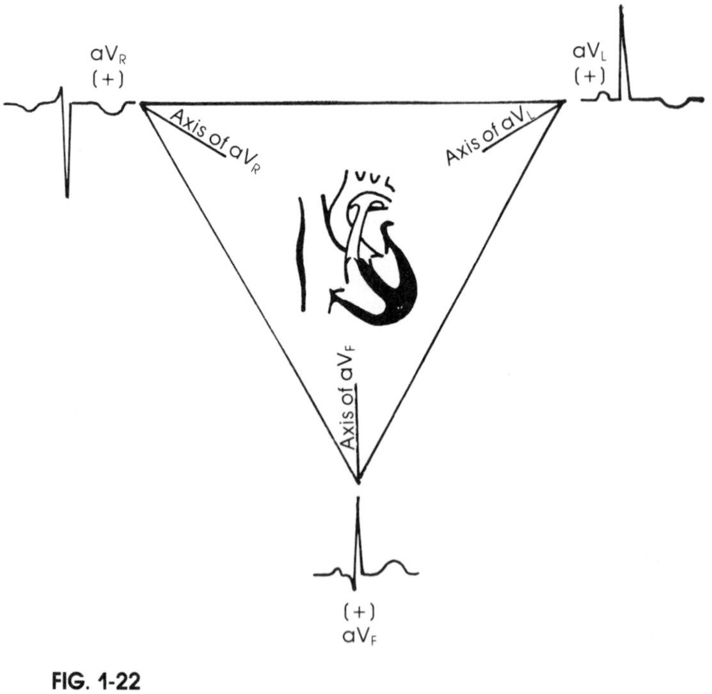

FIG. 1-22
Augmented vector leads with resulting complexes.

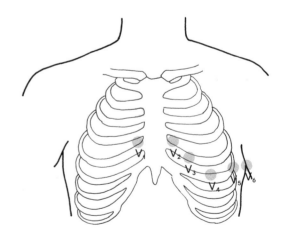

FIG. 1-23
Precordial lead placement.

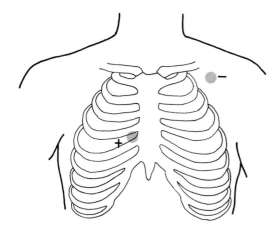

FIG. 1-24
Modified chest lead 1 (MCL₁) placement.

The most frequently used lead, which is a modification of a V_1 unipolar chest lead, is the MCL$_1$, or modified chest lead 1.[7] This lead can closely simulate the ventricular activity seen on a regular V_1 lead by placing the positive electrode in the usual V_1 position (fourth intercostal space to the right of the sternum) and the negative electrode at the left arm. This lead placement is illustrated in Fig. 1-24. A ground electrode may be placed at any location on the chest.

A modified chest lead 6 (MCL$_6$) can also be obtained by placing the positive electrode in the usual V_6 position (fifth intercostal space in the midaxillary line) and the negative electrode at the left arm (Fig. 1-25).

This lead also is helpful in looking closely at ventricular activity, specifically to differentiate between ventricular or supraventricular activity.[7] Again, the ground electrode may be placed in any location.

A third modified lead that is helpful in clarifying atrial electrical activity is known as the Lewis lead. This lead placement consists of placing the positive electrode in the V_1 position (fourth intercostal space to the right of the sternum) and the negative electrode in the second intercostal space to the right of the sternum (Fig. 1-26).[6] This lead is used when it is difficult to determine whether P waves are present or to differentiate between sinus, atrial, or junctional activity.

As one becomes more familiar with the negative and positive electrodes for each lead, it becomes easier to alter lead placement for the variant leads. For example, if a MCL$_1$ lead were needed, it is necessary to switch the lead selector on the ECG unit to lead 1. In lead 1, the right arm electrode is negative and the left arm electrode is positive. To change to a MCL$_1$ lead, the positive, or left arm electrode is placed in the fourth intercostal space to the right of the sternum, and the negative, or right arm electrode, is placed on the left arm. This is also easily done with telemetry (ambulatory monitoring) units, which usually have a positive, a negative, and a ground electrode wire.

ORGANIZATION OF THE ECG

As electrical activity of the heart is recorded on paper, the standard paper speed coming from the recording device is 25 mm or 1 inch per second. The paper is composed of large squares, each of which is divided into five small squares. Time is measured on the horizontal

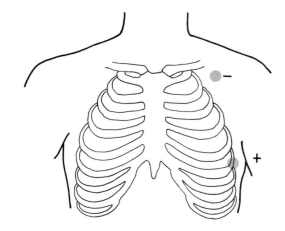

FIG. 1-25
Modified chest lead 6 (MCL₆) placement.

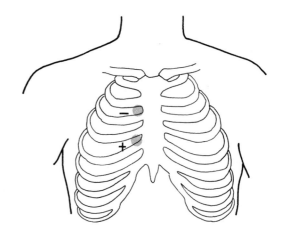

FIG. 1-26
Lewis lead placement.

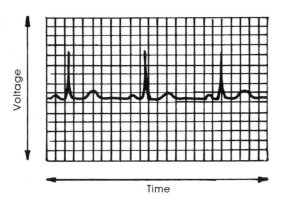

FIG. 1-27

ECG paper representing time measured on horizontal axis and voltage on vertical axis.

axis. Five large squares comprise 25 mm or 1 inch in length and move from the machine over 1 second in time. One large square is therefore equal to 0.2 second in time and is 5 mm in length, while one small square is equal to 0.04 second in time and is 1 mm in length (refer to the upper right hand corner of Fig. 1-29).

Amplitude (voltage) is measured on the vertical axis (Fig. 1-27).

One small square is equal to 0.1 mV or 1 mm and one large square is equal to 0.5 mV or 5 mm in height.

All diagnostic 12-lead ECG machines are standardized internationally in order to accurately compare voltage criteria on ECGs done in different locations throughout the world. Normal ECG standardization is 1 mV. In other words, it takes 1 mV of current to deflect the ECG stylus upward two large squares (10 mm) (Fig. 1-28).

This standardization calibration signal should be on all 12-lead ECGs. If the voltage of the ECG complexes is exceptionally high, the standardization may be reduced

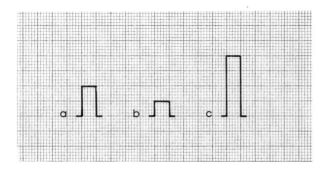

FIG. 1-28

ECG standardization: a, normal standardization; b, one-half standardization (for large voltage complexes); and c, double standardization (for low voltage complexes).

one half, so that the stylus is deflected upward 0.5 mV (5 mm) or one large square. Likewise, if the voltage is exceptionally low, the standardization mark may be doubled, to indicate deflection of the stylus upward four large squares or 2 mV (20 mm). If any alteration in normal standardization is used, it must be clearly marked on the ECG.[3,5]

Waveforms and intervals

The deflections on the ECG are described as upright, inverted, or equiphasic in relation to an isoelectric (straight) baseline. Fig. 1-29 illustrates the common wave forms and intervals seen on the ECG.

P wave

The P wave is the first complex seen on the ECG and represents atrial depolarization, which is an electrical and not a mechanical event. The P wave does not reflect sinus node impulse formation but only reflects depolarization of the atrial muscle tissue once the sinus impulse reaches the atria from the node.[1]

It is generally symmetrical in shape, upright in lead II, and inverted in lead aV_R (see Fig. 1-18). It may be variable in other leads. It should not exceed 2.5 mm in height (two and one-half small squares) nor 0.11 second in length or time (two and three-fourths small squares).

PR interval

The PR interval is calculated from the beginning of the P wave to the beginning of the QRS complex. It represents the time it takes for the impulse to travel from the atria to the ventricles, including the normal physiological delay in the AV junction. The normal delay in the AV junction is represented by the PR segment, or the isoelectric line between the end of the P wave and the beginning of the QRS, and is usually between 0.05 to 0.08 second in length. The PR interval should be within 0.12 to 0.20 second or no longer than one large square.[5,6]

QRS complex

The QRS complex represents ventricular depolarization and is measured from the beginning of the Q wave to the end of the S wave. It is normally 0.06 to 0.10 second in duration or one and one-half to two and one-half small squares. The Q wave is the initial downward deflection of the complex and may not always be present. The Q wave is defined as the first negative deflection after the P wave. The initial upright deflection or R wave is defined as the first upright deflection after the P wave. It should not exceed 20 mm in height in the limb leads or 25 to 30 mm in the precordial leads.[5,6] The first negative deflection after the R wave is the S wave. It should normally return

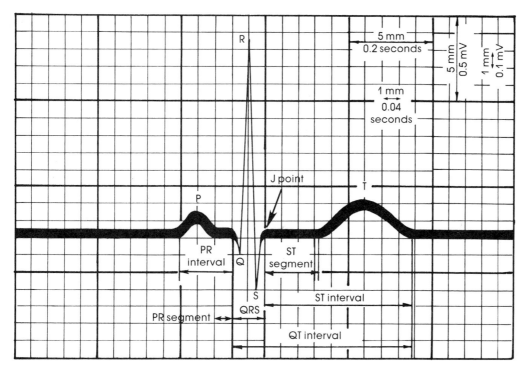

FIG. 1-29

ECG paper grid with normal ECG complexes and intervals. Time and voltage axes are seen in upper right hand corner: PR interval—0.12 second (three small squares); QRS interval—0.08 second, (two small squares), and QT interval—0.43 second (ten and three fourths small squares).

to the baseline (represented as the J point in Fig. 1-29). Various configurations of the QRS complex may occur and the term "QRS complex" is used to describe this complex of ventricular depolarization regardless of the deflections present.[6]

ST segment

The ST segment falls between the end of the QRS complex and the beginning of the T wave and is normally isoelectric, although it may curve slightly into the T wave. The ST segment departs from the QRS at the J point (see Fig. 1-29) and it may be elevated (above the baseline) 2 mm or depressed (below the baseline) 0.5 mm or less and still be considered normal. If the ST segment elevates or is depressed greater than this, it is abnormal.[5,6] ST depression may indicate myocardial ischemia, and ST elevation may indicate infarction or pericarditis.

The period between the beginning of the QRS and the beginning of the T wave (including the ST segment) is known as the absolute (or effective) refractory period of the ventricles. It is during this time that the ventricles have become completely depolarized and are at the early

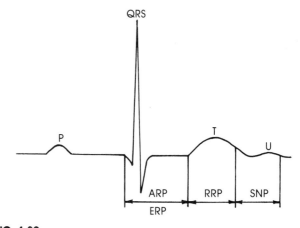

FIG. 1-30

Refractory periods in relation to ECG complexes: *ARP (ERP)*, absolute refractory period; *RRP*, relative refractory period; and *SNP*, supernormal period.

stages of repolarization or recovery. Because of the reversal in ionic balance, the cells are incapable of responding to a stimulus regardless of its strength. This incapacity normally acts as a protection from excitable tissue that may desire to set up a very serious rapid rhythm (Fig. 1-30).

T wave

The T wave represents ventricular repolarization. It is usually asymmetrical in shape, slightly rounded, and should not exceed 5 mm in height in the limb leads nor 10 mm in height in the precordial leads. It is generally inverted in lead aV_R but upright in most other leads. Factors affecting the T wave may be ischemia, infarction, acidosis, exercise, drugs, fever, stroke, and electrolyte imbalances.[6]

The period between the beginning of the T wave and almost to the end of the T wave is known as the relative refractory period (see Fig. 1-30). It is during this time that the ventricular repolarization process is almost complete and a stronger than normal stimulus may excite the cells, resulting in a rapid rhythm.[3,6]

QT interval

This interval is measured from the beginning of the QRS to the end of the T wave and represents both ventricular depolarization and repolarization on the ECG. It varies with age, sex, and heart rate but generally is up to 0.44 second or one half of the preceding RR interval.

It is important to note changes in the QT interval over time rather than its absolute value.[5] The QT interval may be prolonged or shortened with various drug therapies or electrolyte imbalances, and a prolonged QT interval may elicit serious rhythm disturbances (see Ventricular Dysrhythmias Module).

U wave

The U wave is a small deflection following the T wave and is usually in the same direction as the T wave. Little is known regarding its significance, but it may represent slow repolarization in the Purkinje system, stretch of the ventricles in diastole, or "after-depolarizations" (see Antidysrhythmic Drug Module). It is more pronounced in such conditions as hyperthyroidism or hypokalemia.[5,6]

The period between the end of the T wave and the end of the U wave is known as the supernormal period. It is also known as the vulnerable period, whereby a weaker than normal stimulus may elicit a response[5] (see Fig. 1-30).

In the review of lead systems and waveforms, Fig. 1-31 represents the normal vectors of current flow through the heart and the resultant waveforms as viewed from lead II on the ECG. (Remember, lead II is one of the bipolar standard limb leads with the negative electrode at the right arm and the positive electrode at the left leg.)

Since normally the mean atrial and ventricular vectors (arrows) of current flow are directed toward the positive end of the lead II axis, the P and R wave deflections are

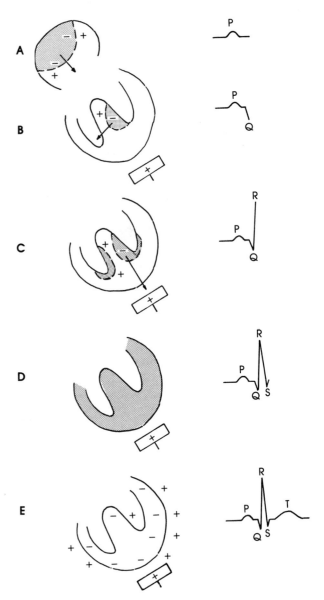

FIG. 1-31

Process of depolarization and repolarization as viewed from lead II with resultant waveforms: **A**, atrial depolarization; **B**, septal depolarization; **C**, mean vector of ventricular depolarization; **D**, ventricles completely depolarized; and **E**, ventricular repolarization.

very positive (upright). This is generally the best lead in which to view atrial activity.

Calculation of heart rate

Many methods may be used to calculate heart rate but only three methods will be discussed in this text:

1. Count the number of cycles (P waves and/or R waves) in a 6-second strip and multiply by 10. This method can be used with a regular or irregular

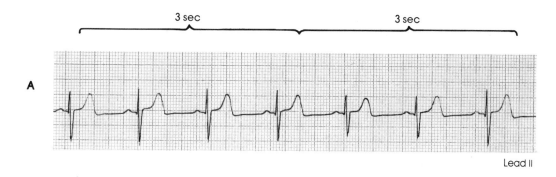

3 sec   3 sec

A

Lead II

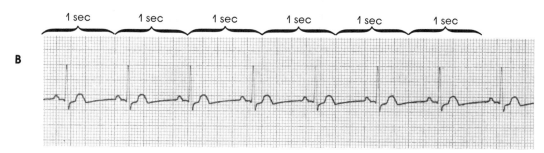

1 sec   1 sec   1 sec   1 sec   1 sec   1 sec

B

FIG. 1-32

Lead II

Calculating rate by six-second strip: **A**, marked in three-second intervals and **B**, marked in one-second intervals.

rhythm, is fast and simple, and provides a close estimation of the actual heart rate.

a. ECG paper from the manufacturer may be marked off in 1-second or 3-second intervals that may be at the top or at the bottom of the paper. There are five large squares in a 1-second interval and 15 large squares in a 3-second interval. Therefore there are 30 large squares within a 6-second interval (in case the paper is not marked or the interval markers have been trimmed).

b. A complete complex (QRS-T) must be within the markers.

In Fig. 1-32 the top strip is marked in 3-second intervals and the number of complete complexes within the 6-second interval is six. Therefore the rate of this strip is 60 intervals per minute (6 × 10 = 60). In the second strip, the paper is marked in 1-second intervals. Therefore, a 6-second interval would incorporate six of these markers. In this case, the number of complete complexes within this interval is seven, which makes the heart rate approximately 70 beats per minute.

2. For regular rhythms, two methods are suggested:

a. Count the number of small (0.04-second) squares between two R waves and divide into

1500. Since there are 25 small squares in a 1-second interval (five large squares), there are 1500 small squares in 1 minute (300 large squares). In Fig. 1-33, there are 22 small squares between two R waves. Thus the heart rate is 68 beats per minute (1500 ÷ 22 = 68).

b. Measure the time interval in seconds between two R waves and divide into 60. For example, if there are four large squares between two R waves, this equals 0.8 second in time. The heart rate here is 75 beats per minute (60 ÷ 0.8 = 75). Fig. 1-33 shows a 0.88-second interval between two R waves (22 small squares). The heart rate in this case is 68 beats per minute (60 ÷ 0.88 = 68).

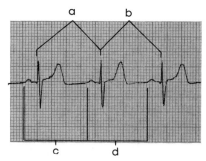

a   b

c   d

FIG. 1-33

Calculating rate for regular rhythms and measuring intervals: *a* and *b* represent measuring R to R and *c* and *d* represent measuring P to P.

Before a rate can be calculated, it is necessary to establish the rhythm of the strip, as the methods of rate calculations vary with regular or irregular rhythms.

Rhythm refers to regular or irregular intervals and is not related to an interpretation of the rhythm strip. In order to establish rhythm, intervals must be measured between two R waves or between two P waves, continuing throughout the strip to assure all intervals are the same or regular. If they are not the same, then the rhythm is irregular. Measuring intervals may be accomplished by marking a card and moving the marks along the strip, or by calipers, if available, which make this step much easier (see Fig. 1-33).

Rhythm is thus described as being regular R to R (meaning the ventricular QRS complexes are regular) or regular P to P (meaning the P wave, or atrial activity, is regular). Under normal conditions, both intervals should be regular; however, with certain rhythm disturbances, referred to as dysrhythmias, they are not. Therefore, it becomes necessary to review each rhythm strip analytically.

The rhythm analysis used in this text is designed to identify each of the following in sequence:

1. Rate:
    Atrial:
    Ventricular:
2. Rhythm:
    Atrial:
    Ventricular:
3. P waves:
    Present? Same morphology (shape)?
4. PR interval: Same or different?
5. Ratio of P/QRS: 1:1 or different?
6. QRS interval: Same morphology?
7. QT interval:
8. Interpretation:

ECG in relation to the cardiac cycle

It has been emphasized that the complexes of the ECG represent electrical and not mechanical activity. It has also been emphasized that electrical activity must *precede* mechanical activity. Fig. 1-34 represents the events in the cardiac cycle in relation to the ECG complexes. Atrial contraction occurs after the P wave (atrial depolarization), ventricular contraction (systole) occurs after the QRS or the wave of ventricular depolarization, and ventricular relaxation (diastole) occurs following the T wave or the wave of ventricular repolarization.

Systole should be one third of the cardiac cycle, while diastole should be two thirds. It is during diastole that the ventricles fill with blood and the coronary arteries receive blood. This is important for providing sufficient stroke volume to maintain a normal cardiac output and for

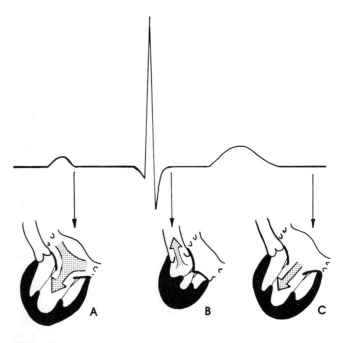

FIG. 1-34

The cardiac cycle in relation to the ECG: **A**, atrial contraction; **B**, ventricular contraction (systole); and **C**, ventricular relaxation (diastole).

providing adequate blood perfusion and oxygenation to the myocardial cells.

Cardiac output is described as the amount of blood pumped from the heart per minute, which is normally between 4 to 8 liters. It depends on two components: stroke volume or the amount of blood pumped from the left ventricle with each stroke or beat and heart rate. The normal stroke volume is approximately 70 ml. If the heart rate is 72 per minute, the cardiac output is equal to 5 liters per minute ($72 \times 70 = 5.040$).

Most rhythm disturbances described in this text will alter either cardiac output or coronary perfusion; these are concepts to be continually kept in mind as each rhythm disturbance is reviewed.

REFERENCES

1. Alpert, M.A., and Flaker, G.C.: Arrhythmias associated with sinus node dysfunction—pathogenesis, recognition and management, JAMA **250**(16):2160, 1983.
2. Anderson, R.H., and Becker, A.E.: Gross anatomy and microscopy of the conducting system. In Mandel, W.J., editor: Cardiac arrhythmias, Philadelphia, 1980, J.B. Lippincott Co.
3. Andreoli, K.G., et al: Comprehensive cardiac care, ed. 5, St. Louis, 1983, The C.V. Mosby Co.
4. Conner, R.P.: Coronary artery anatomy: the electrocardiographic and clinical correlations, Crit. Care Nurse **3**(3):68, 1983.

5. Conover, M.B.: Understanding electrocardiography: arrhythmias and the 12-lead ECG, ed. 4, St. Louis, 1984, The C.V. Mosby Co.
6. Kernicki, J.G., and Weiler, K.M.: Electrocardiography for nurses: physiological correlates, New York, 1981, John Wiley & Sons Inc.
7. Marriott, H.J.L., and Conover, M.B.: Advanced concepts in arrhythmias, St. Louis, 1983, The C.V. Mosby Co.
8. Netter, F.: The CIBA collection of medical illustrations: the heart, vol. 5, Summit, New Jersey, 1969, CIBA Pharmaceutical Company.
9. Phillips, R.E., and Feeney, M.K.: The cardiac rhythms—a systematic approach to interpretation, ed. 2, Philadelphia, 1980, W.B. Saunders Co.

SUGGESTED LEARNING ACTIVITIES AND EXPERIENCES

A. Visit a special care unit that uses hemodynamic monitoring. Find a patient with an arterial blood pressure line and compare the sequencing of the ECG to the blood pressure waveform. You will note that the ECG complex precedes the blood pressure waveform.

B. Obtain several ECG strips and practice calculating rate and measuring intervals. Seek the assistance of experienced peers if necessary.

POSTTEST (Answers on p. 26)

Directions: Circle one answer to each question unless otherwise indicated.

A. The branch of the autonomic nervous system which, when stimulated, increases the heart rate and the force and strength of contraction is called:
   1. Inotropic
   2. Chronotropic
   3. Sympathetic
   4. Parasympathetic

B. The parasympathetic nervous system has fibers in the heart. Which cranial nerve is the mediator of this system?
   1. Vagus
   2. Trigeminal
   3. Hypoglossal
   4. Pharyngeal

C. One of the properties of cardiac tissue is spontaneous initiation of the cardiac impulse. This is known as:
   1. Irritability
   2. Conductivity
   3. Automaticity
   4. Contractility

D. Your patient is in a rapid atrial rhythm and you observe the doctor rubbing one side of the patient's neck. The rationale behind this maneuver is:
   1. Jugular venous compression causes a reflex lowering of the blood pressure
   2. Having the patient swallow rapidly increases intrathoracic pressure
   3. Stimulation of vagus nerve fibers in the carotid body slows the heart rate
   4. Palpation of the tracheal rings produces altered respiratory function

E. The process of activation of automatic, conductile, and contractile elements from the resting or polarized state is known as:
   1. Repolarization
   2. Depolarization
   3. Depolarized
   4. Polarized

F. Inflammation of the pericardium is known as:
   1. Epicarditis
   2. Endocarditis
   3. Myocarditis
   4. Pericarditis

G. The principal ions involved in the propagation of the impulse from cell to cell in the myocardium are (circle all that apply):
   1. Magnesium
   2. Calcium
   3. Potassium
   4. Phosphates
   5. Sodium

H. Fine fibrous threads anchoring the AV valve leaflets to their respective papillary muscles are the:
   1. Pectinates
   2. Trabeculae carnae
   3. Conduction fibers
   4. Chordae tendineae

I. The smooth inner lining of the cardiac chambers, valves, and papillary muscles is known as the:
   1. Myocardium
   2. Endocardium
   3. Pericardium
   4. Epicardium

J. A graphic record of cardiac voltage variations plotted against time is called _____.

K. Which of the following are functions of the pericardium? (Circle all that apply.)
   1. Prevention of ventricular overfilling
   2. Equilibration of pericardial fluid pressure through the so-called pericardial window.
   3. Anchoring of the heart in the mediastinal cavity
   4. Protection of the heart from invasive disease processes

L. A 10-mm upward deflection of the ECG stylus in response to 1 mV of electrical current is known as:
1. Depolarization
2. Polarity
3. Standardization
4. Conductivity

M. The three augmented leads are:
_____, _____, and _____

N. The augmented leads are considered to be:
1. Bipolar
2. Unipolar

O. The bundle of His divides into the _____,
_____, and
_____.

P. ECG paper normally travels at a speed of:
1. 20 mm per second
2. 25 mm per second
3. 30 mm per second
4. 35 mm per second

Q. Label the site of the negative and positive electrodes in the following:
– electrode   + electrode
1. Lead I:
2. Lead II:
3. Lead III:

R. The precordial leads view electrical activity from which plane?
1. Frontal
2. Horizontal

S. Describe the electrode placement for a MCL₁ lead:
1. Negative electrode: _____
2. Positive electrode: _____
3. Ground electrode: _____

T. The coronary arteries receive their blood supply during:
1. Systole
2. Diastole

U. T F The QRS complex correlates directly with ventricular systole.

V. T F The P wave represents SA node impulse formation.

W. The QT interval represents (circle all that apply):
1. Atrial repolarization
2. Ventricular depolarization
3. Normal delay in the AV junction
4. Ventricular repolarization

X. Matching: Place the appropriate letter in Column B with the number in Column A.

Column A Coronary arteries	Column B Areas supplied
___ 1. Right	a. Interventricular septum
___ 2. Posterior descending	b. Right bundle branch
___ 3. Left main	c. Lateral wall of left ventricle
___ 4. Obtuse marginals	d. Branches off the LAD
___ 5. Septal perforators	e. Supplies AV node in 10% of people
___ 6. Left anterior descending	f. Divides into LAD and LC
___ 7. Diagonals	g. Supplies AV node in 80% to 90% of people
___ 8. Left circumflex	h. Supplies SA node in 55% to 60% of people

SUPPLEMENTS

This is a work section. A work space is provided beneath each strip to the left. The answers are to the right. It is suggested you cover the answer section with a card or paper while you work the strips. Check your answers on the right.

A.

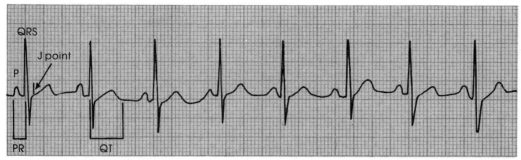

FIG. 1-35

Lead II

1. Rate: 83-85
2. PR interval: 0.14 second
3. QRS interval: 0.08 second
4. QT interval: 0.34 second

B.

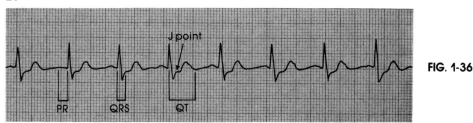

FIG. 1-36

Lead II
1. Rate: 85
2. PR interval: 0.14 second
3. QRS interval: 0.08-0.10 second
4. QT interval: 0.36 second (NOTE: The P wave is flat; the ST segment is depressed 1 mm below baseline)

C.

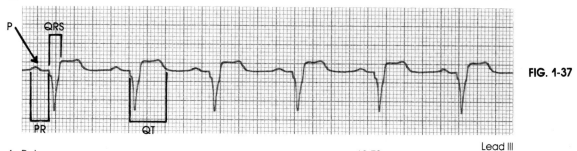

FIG. 1-37

Lead III
1. Rate: 69-70
2. PR interval: 0.20 second
3. QRS interval: 0.13 second
4. QT interval: 0.40 second (NOTE: The QRS is not upright in lead II, which is abnormal; the QRS is also wider than normal; this is officially known as a QS wave (all negative deflection) but will still be called the QRS complex; the measurement intervals are marked off for your convenience; the ST segment is elevated 2 mm above the baseline)

D.

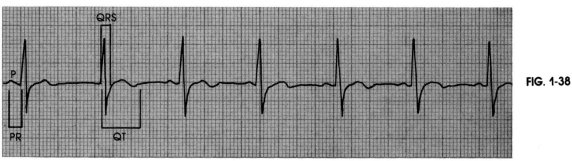

FIG. 1-38

Lead II
1. Rate: 70
2. PR interval: 0.14 second
3. QRS interval: 0.10 second
4. QT internal: 0.44 second (NOTE: The P wave is flat; there is some slight artifact (60-cycle interference) at the beginning of the strip (wavy baseline); there are no markers so you may count off 30 large squares and count the QRS complexes in between, or, since the rhythm is regular, you may count rate for a regular rhythm)

E.

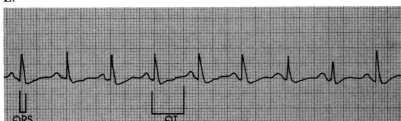

FIG. 1-39

Lead II

1. Rate: 100
2. PR interval: 0.16 second
3. QRS interval: 0.08 second
4. QT interval: 0.40 second (NOTE: The third QRS complex from the end of the strip has a lower voltage than the rest [see Ventricular Dysrhythmias Module])

F.

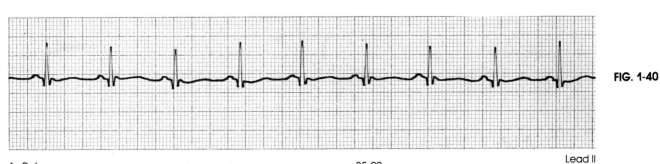

FIG. 1-40

Lead II

1. Rate: 85-90
2. PR interval: 0.12 second
3. QRS interval: 0.08 second
4. QT interval: 0.44 second

G.

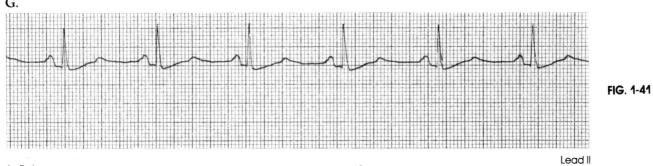

FIG. 1-41

Lead II

1. Rate: 60
2. PR interval: 0.18 second
3. QRS interval: 0.08 second
4. QT interval: 0.52 second

H.

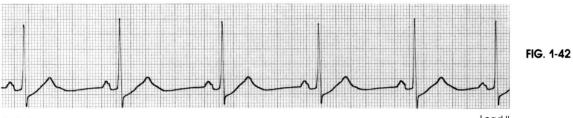

FIG. 1-42

Lead II

1. Rate: 50
2. PR interval: 0.22 second
3. QRS interval: 0.08 second
4. QT interval: 0.60 second (NOTE: The rhythm is slightly irregular)

ANSWERS TO PRETEST AND POSTTEST
Pretest

A. Fig. 1-1.
  1. Aorta   9. Pulmonary vein (left)
  2. Superior vena cava   10. Left atrium
  3. Right atrium   11. Aortic valve
  4. Pulmonic valve   12. Mitral valve
  5. Tricuspid valve   13. Left ventricle
  6. Inferior vena cava   14. Endocardium
  7. Right ventricle   15. Myocardium
  8. Pulmonary artery   16. Epicardium (pericar-
                              dium)

B. Fig. 1-2.
  1. Right coronary artery (RCA)
  2. Left main coronary artery (LMCA)
  3. Left circumflex (LC)
  4. Obtuse marginals (OM)
  5. Diagonals
  6. Left anterior descending (LAD)

C. Matching:
  1. c
  2. f
  3. e
  4. a
  5. d
  6. b

D. Fig. 1-3.
  1. SA node
  2. AV node
  3. Bundle of His
  4. Right bundle branch
  5. Purkinje fibers
  6. Posterior-inferior fascicle of left bundle branch
  7. Anterior-superior fascicle of left bundle branch

E.

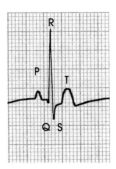

F. Normal sinus rhythm.
   Rate: 60-100
   Rhythm: Regular
   a P wave for every QRS complex

G.   (⁻ pole)   (⁺ pole)
  1. Lead I   right arm   left arm
  2. Lead II   right arm   left leg
  3. Lead III   left arm   left leg

H.

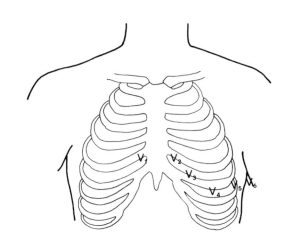

I. 3

J. 1

K. 4

L. 5

M. 3, 5

N. Fig. 1-6.
1. Heart rate: 40
2. PR interval: 0.20 second
3. QRS interval: 0.08 second
4. QT interval: 0.56 second

O. Fig. 1-7.
1. Heart rate: 70-72
2. PR interval: 0.14 second
3. QRS interval: 0.08 second
4. QT interval: 0.32 second

Posttest

A. 3

B. 1

C. 3

D. 3

E. 2

F. 4

G. 2, 3, 5

H. 4

I. 2

J. electrocardiogram (ECG)

K. 1, 3, 4

L. 3

M. aV_R, aV_L, aV_F

N. 2

O. right bundle branch, posterior-inferior fascicle of the left bundle, and anterior-superior fascicle of the left bundle branch

P. 2

Q. 1. Lead I   right arm ($^-$)   left arm ($^+$)
2. Lead II   right arm ($^-$)   left leg ($^+$)
3. Lead III   left arm ($^-$)   left leg ($^+$)

R. 2

S. 1. Negative: left arm
2. Positive: fourth intercostal space to the right of the sternum
3. Ground: any location

T. 2

U. F

V. F

W. 2, 4

X. Matching:
1. h
2. g
3. f
4. c
5. a
6. b
7. d
8. e

Sinus dysrhythmias

PRETEST (Answers on pp. 57-58)

Directions: Circle one answer to each question unless otherwise indicated.

A. The intrinsic rate of the sinoatrial (SA) node is:
1. 60-80 per minute
2. 40-60 per minute
3. 100-150 per minute
4. 60-100 per minute

B. The intrinsic rate of the atrioventricular (AV) node is:
1. 60-80 per minute
2. 40-60 per minute
3. 100-150 per minute
4. 60-100 per minute

C. The normal PR interval is:
1. 0.06-0.10 second
2. 0.10-0.16 second
3. 0.12-0.20 second
4. 0.04-0.06 second

D. The normal QRS interval is:
1. 0.06-0.10 second
2. 0.10-0.16 second
3. 0.12-0.20 second
4. 0.04-0.06 second

E. The normal QT interval (circle all that apply):
1. May be up to 0.38 second
2. May be up to 0.56 second
3. May vary with age, sex, and rate
4. May be one half of previous RR interval
5. May be up to 0.44 second

F. The sinotrial (SA) node is called the natural pacemaker of the heart because it:
1. Is the only portion of the conduction system that automatically initiates impulses
2. Initiates impulses more slowly than other parts of the conduction system
3. Initiates impulses at a faster rate than other parts of the conduction system

G. Automaticity is:
1. The ability of pacemaker cells to automatically initiate impulses

2. An automated ECG simulator
3. An external power source that has the ability to initiate electrical impulses

H. Label the following waveforms on Fig. 2-1.
1. P wave
2. QRS
3. T wave

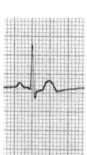

FIG. 2-1

I. Identify the following intervals on Fig. 2-2.
1. PR
2. QRS
3. QT

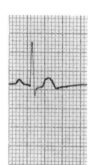

FIG. 2-2

J. On the ECG paper in Fig. 2-3, p. 28:
1. Label accurately, on one *small* square, the amplitude and time it represents
2. Label accurately, on one *large* square, the amplitude and time it represents
3. Mark the normal ECG standardization

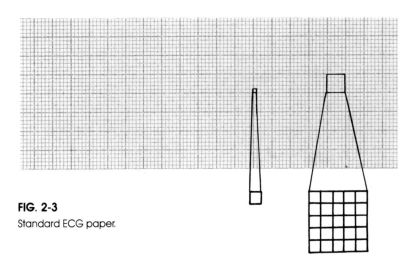

FIG. 2-3
Standard ECG paper.

K. An escape complex refers to a complex that:
   1. Comes before it should
   2. Comes after it should
   3. Comes right on time

L. When the parasympathetic nervous system is stimulated, the following occur (circle all that apply):
   1. Heart rate increases
   2. Conduction through the AV node is decreased
   3. Force of contraction increases
   4. Heart rate decreases

M. The P wave on the ECG represents:
   1. Firing of the sinus node
   2. Ventricular repolarization
   3. Atrial repolarization
   4. Atrial depolarization

N. The QRS on the ECG represents:
   1. Atrial depolarization
   2. Ventricular repolarization
   3. Ventricular depolarization
   4. 2 and 3

O. Sinus tachycardia is treated by:
   1. Drugs that will slow the heart rate
   2. Drugs that will speed the heart rate
   3. Identifying and treating the cause
   4. Rest and sedation

P. When the sympathetic nervous system is stimulated, the following occur (circle all that apply):
   1. Heart rate increases
   2. Speed of AV conduction decreases
   3. Force of contraction decreases
   4. Heart rate decreases
   5. Speed of AV conduction increases
   6. Force of contraction increases

Q. Interpret the rhythm strip in Fig. 2-4.
   1. Rate:
      Atrial:
      Ventricular:
   2. Rhythm:
      Atrial:
      Ventricular:
   3. P waves:
   4. PR interval:
   5. Ratio of P/QRS:
   6. QRS interval:
   7. QT interval:
   8. Interpretation:

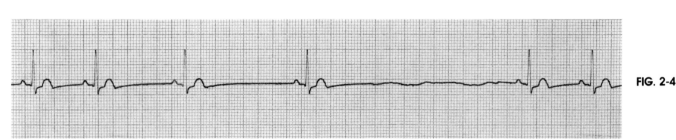

FIG. 2-4

Lead II

R. Interpret the rhythm strip in Fig. 2-5.
  1. Rate:
       Atrial:
       Ventricular:
  2. Rhythm:
       Atrial:
       Ventricular:
  3. P waves:
  4. PR interval:
  5. Ratio of P/QRS:
  6. QRS interval:
  7. QT interval:
  8. Interpretation:
S. Interpret the rhythm strip in Fig. 2-6.
  1. Rate:
       Atrial:
       Ventricular:
  2. Rhythm:
       Atrial:
       Ventricular:

  3. P waves:
  4. PR interval:
  5. Ratio of P/QRS:
  6. QRS interval:
  7. QT interval:
  8. Interpretation:
T. Interpret the rhythm strip in Fig. 2-7.
  1. Rate:
       Atrial:
       Ventricular:
  2. Rhythm:
       Atrial:
       Ventricular:
  3. P waves:
  4. PR interval:
  5. Ratio of P/QRS:
  6. QRS interval:
  7. QT interval:
  8. Interpretation:

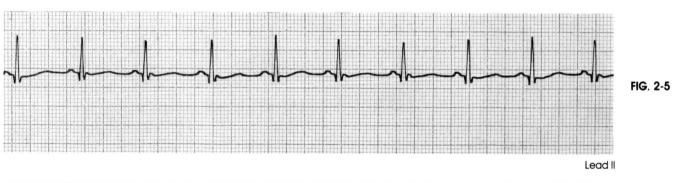

FIG. 2-5

Lead II

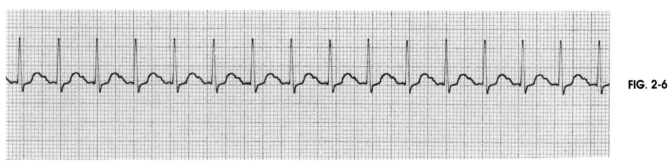

FIG. 2-6

Lead II

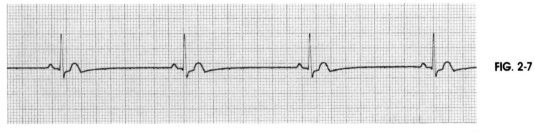

FIG. 2-7

Lead II

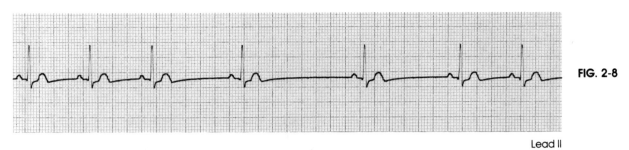

FIG. 2-8

Lead II

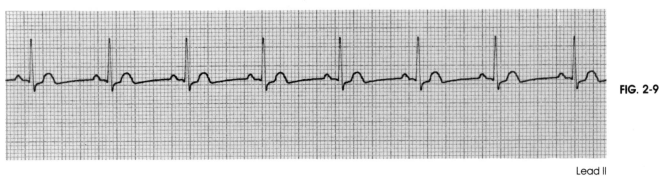

FIG. 2-9

Lead II

U. Interpret the rhythm strip in Fig. 2-8.
1. Rate:
    Atrial:
    Ventricular:
2. Rhythm:
    Atrial:
    Ventricular:
3. P waves:
4. PR interval:
5. Ratio of P/QRS:
6. QRS interval:
7. QT interval:
8. Interpretation:

V. Interpret the rhythm strip in Fig. 2-9.
1. Rate:
    Atrial:
    Ventricular:
2. Rhythm:
    Atrial:
    Ventricular:
3. P waves:
4. PR interval:
5. Ratio of P/QRS:
6. QRS interval:
7. QT interval:
8. Interpretation:

PURPOSE

The purpose of this module is to provide a guideline of instruction for health care professionals and nonprofes-sionals with limited ECG interpretation skills, to facilitate successful recognition of normal sinoatrial (SA) node function and conduction, and to identify and interpret those rhythm disturbances arising from the SA node and the common treatment measures associated with each.

BEHAVIORAL OBJECTIVES

Upon completion of this module, the learner should be able to:
A. List possible etiological factors of, define and identify criteria for, recognize on rhythm strips, state the clinical features of, and discuss modes of treatment and nursing management for the following rhythms and dysrhythmias:
    1. Normal sinus rhythm
    2. Sinus bradycardia
    3. Sinus tachycardia
    4. Sinus arrhythmia
    5. Sinus pause or sinus arrest
    6. Sinoatrial block (sinus exit block)
B. Discuss the syndrome of sinus node dysfunction (sick sinus syndrome)

VOCABULARY

Automaticity Electrical property of cells that permits spontaneous initiation of the cardiac impulse.
Carotid sinus sensitivity An exaggerated vagal response to slight pressure on the carotid sinus (a point on the neck where the internal and external carotid arteries divide). The SA and AV nodes are richly endowed with parasympathetic nerve fibers and a mild

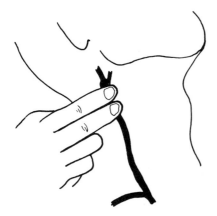

FIG. 2-10

Right carotid artery showing pressure applied to carotid sinus.

pressure on the carotid sinus (which stimulates the vagus nerve) can result in profound slowing of the sinus node impulse and may even result in sinus arrest (Fig. 2-10). These attacks may result from wearing a slightly snug collar, turning the head to look while driving a car, extreme rotation of the head or neck, or lifting heavy objects.[9]

Escape complex/rhythm An escape complex/rhythm is initiated by a lower pacemaker when the sinus node slows or fails. It is usually preceded by a pause in the normal heart rhythm. Also known as a passive rhythm or a rhythm by default.

P cells Specialized cells located in the center of the SA node that possess the property of automaticity (see Fig. 2-12, p. 32).

PP interval The interval of distance between two sinus P waves, measured from the beginning of one P wave to the beginning of the next P wave. The PP interval is normally regular in rhythm (Fig. 2-11).

Purkinje cells Cells located at the junction of the SA node and atrial muscle tissue. The cells conduct impulses from the transitional cells to the atrial myocardial cells to depolarize the atria (see Fig. 2-12, p. 32).

Purkinje fibers Terminal branches of the right and left bundles bringing the impulse rapidly and directly to the myocardial cells of the septum, ventricular walls, and papillary muscle, depolarizing the ventricles and allowing the mechanical event of ventricular contraction to occur (see Fig. 1-12, p. 8).

Surface ECG The usual 12-lead ECG that is performed with electrodes placed on the skin. This differs from an electrode wire that is placed inside the heart to obtain a more precise picture of electrical activity.

Transitional cells Specialized cells that lie in the periphery of the SA node, which conduct impulses from the P cells to the Purkinje cells and then to the atrial myocardium (see Fig. 2-12, p. 32).

Valsalva maneuver A maneuver whereby an individual takes a quick inspiratory breath followed by forced expiratory straining against a closed glottis. An example would be straining at stool. This maneuver elevates venous pressure by obstructing blood flow into the chest; this results from stimulation of the parasympathetic nervous system and may decrease the heart rate.[3]

Vasovagal reaction A reaction resulting in slowing of heart rate and lowering of blood pressure. Any large volume of blood or mechanical or chemical stimulation of pressure sensors or receptors located in the carotid artery and arch of the aorta convey impulses to the vagus (parasympathetic) nerve at its origin in the medulla of the brain. This stimulates receptors that affect parasympathetic fibers in the heart, which reflexly slow heart rate and decrease contractility of the myocardium. This is known as a vasovagal reflex and can occur from strong emotional stress as well.[9]

CONTENT
Suggested review

Before beginning this module on sinus dysrhythmias, it is recommended that the learner review the following:

1. Anatomy of the conduction system
2. Basic principles of electrophysiology
3. Nervous innervation of the sinoatrial (SA) and atrioventricular (AV) nodes
4. Anatomical blood supply to the sinoatrial (SA) and atrioventricular (AV) nodes
5. Calculation of rate on ECG paper
6. Normal intervals
7. Analytical approach to interpretation of the ECG strip

General anatomy and physiology related to the sinoatrial node

Anatomically, the sinoatrial (SA) node is cresent shaped and lies subepicardially in the posterior atrial wall at the junction of the superior vena cava and the right atrium. It consists of three distinct cell types: P cells, transitional cells, and Purkinje cells (Fig. 2-12, p. 32).[1,6]

The P cells, located in the center of the SA node, have the property of automaticity, at a rate of 60 to 100

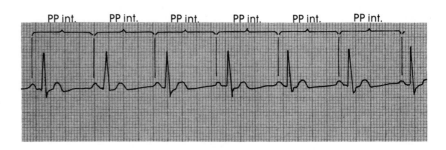

FIG. 2-11

Measurement of PP intervals.

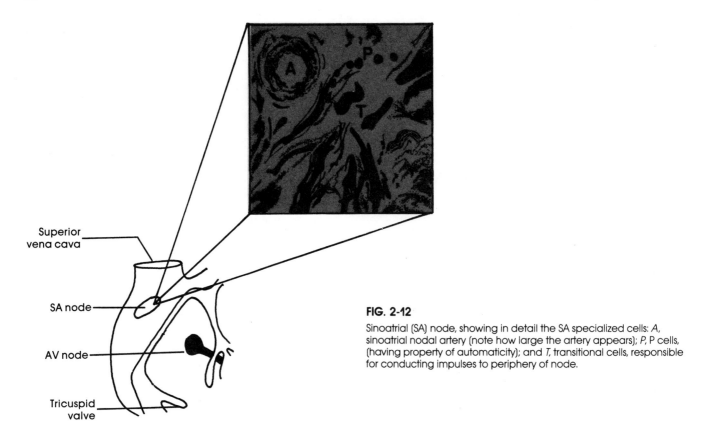

FIG. 2-12

Sinoatrial (SA) node, showing in detail the SA specialized cells: *A*, sinoatrial nodal artery (note how large the artery appears); *P*, P cells, (having property of automaticity); and *T*, transitional cells, responsible for conducting impulses to periphery of node.

impulses per minute, which is faster than any other cells in the conduction system. Therefore, the SA node is known as the natural pacemaker of the heart.

The transitional cells lie in the periphery of the SA node and transmit the impulse from the P cells to the Purkinje cells. The Purkinje cells lie on the margins of the node; these margins lie between the node and the atrial muscle and are responsible for ultimately conducting the impulse to the atrial muscle tissue. The impulse then stimulates the adjacent atrial muscle cells and allows the atria to be depolarized, followed by atrial contraction.

Contrary to popular belief, current evidence[2] suggests specialized internodal pathways do not exist, and the impulse from the SA node is conducted rapidly through the atrial muscle cells themselves, creating the P wave on the ECG. To reemphasize, there is no recorded evidence of sinus impulse formation on the ECG; only when the impulse conducts to the atrial muscle and the atria are depolarized is there a P wave on the ECG.

As the impulse invades the AV node from the atria, there is a delay of approximately 0.08 second to allow the atria to completely empty their blood into the ventricles. The impulse then enters the bundle of His and quickly conducts to the right and left bundle branches and the

Purkinje system. This activates and depolarizes the ventricular myocardium, creating the QRS complex on the ECG, followed by the mechanical response of ventricular contraction.

Abundant nerve fibers of both the parasympathetic (vagus) and sympathetic nervous systems invade both the SA and AV nodes. The rate of impulse formation (automaticity) varies with influences from these nerve endings.[6]

As the SA node lies close to the epicardial surface of the right atrium, it is subjected to any inflammation or disease states that may invade the pericardium such as pericarditis or invasive malignant tumors.[6]

If the SA node slows its rate of automaticity or fails to initiate an impulse, lower conduction system pacemaker cells may take over the function of the heart until the sinus node recovers. They may do so by actively taking over pacemaker control (initiating impulses faster than the SA node) or by passively "kicking-in" to initiate impulses to allow the ventricular myocardium to depolarize and contract, even if at a slower rate.[5]

NOTE: Electrical activity *always* precedes the mechanical activity of contraction. The ECG records *only* electrical activity.

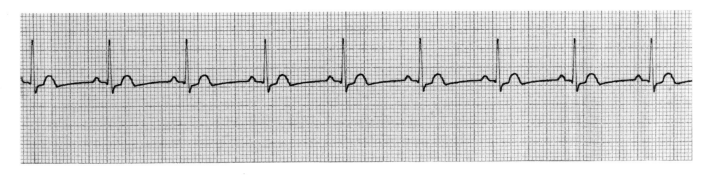

FIG. 2-13

Normal sinus rhythm.

Sinus rhythms and rhythm disturbances

NORMAL SINUS RHYTHM (FIG. 2-13)

Definition

Normal sinus rhythm is the inherent mechanism of heart function whereby the sinus node automatically initiates impulses at a rate of 60 to 100 per minute and each impulse is transmitted in a predictable sequence to the ventricles, creating coordinated contraction of the upper (atrial) and lower (ventricular) chambers.[9]

Etiology

Normal mechanism

Characteristics of rhythm

1. Rate: 60-100 per minute (atrial and ventricular the same)
2. Rhythm: Regular to slightly irregular (atrial and ventricular the same); the rhythm may vary up to 0.06 second between the shortest and longest PP interval
3. P waves: Present; all with same morphology; the P wave is upright in lead II and inverted in lead AVR; however, in other leads, the sinus P wave may be upright, isoelectric, or biphasic[3]
4. PR interval: Between 0.12-0.20 second; may vary slightly with rhythm and/or rate changes
5. Ratio of P/QRS: 1:1
6. QRS interval: 0.06-0.10 second; all with the same morphology
7. QT interval: Up to 0.44 second or one half of preceding RR interval; this varies with heart rate, age, and sex

Clinical features

None

Treatment measures

None required

Nursing management

None required

Special considerations

None

SINUS BRADYCARDIA (FIG. 2-14, p. 34)

Definition

1. The pacemaker is the SA node and it initiates impulses at a rate less than 60 per minute in the adult; sinus bradycardia is said to exist in the infant at a rate less than 100 and at a rate less than 80 per minute in young children[6]
2. This may be a normal rhythm during sleep and in trained athletes or in physically conditioned individuals; in trained hearts, the ventricular myocardium can eject a larger volume of blood with each contraction (complex), thereby maintaining a normal cardiac output at a slower heart rate[2,5,6,11]
3. This may be an abnormal rhythm in individuals with heart disease, acute myocardial infarction (usually involving the inferior or posterior wall), or those on certain drug regimens (digoxin, propranolol, verapamil); or with carotid sinus sensitivity, obstructive jaundice, eye surgery, meningitis, intracranial tumors or bleeding, cervical and mediastinal tumors, myxedema, or hypopituitrism[3,6]

Etiology

1. Sinus bradycardia results from a decrease in rate of impulse formation (automaticity) within the P cells of the SA node, which may be caused by intrinsic disease of the sinus node itself or a variety of extracardiac factors[1]
2. Sinus bradycardia may result from excessive vagal or decreased sympathetic tone in such situations as vomit-

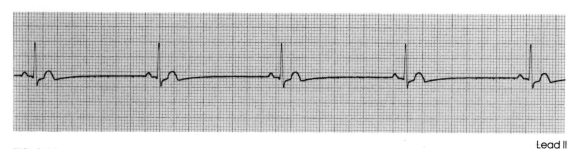

FIG. 2-14
Sinus bradycardia.

ing, forced voiding, straining at stool (all forms of the Valsalva maneuver), pharyngeal suctioning, or vasovagal syncope; these all stimulate the parasympathetic nervous system, causing the sinus discharge rate to slow[6,9]

3. In obstructive jaundice, sinus bradycardia may be related to depressant effects of bile salts on the SA node[6]
4. In hypopituitrism, myxedema, or sleep, the mechanism is related to decreased sympathetic stimulation caused by decreased metabolic activity[6]
5. Increased intracranial pressure may cause an abnormally slow pulse by stimulation of the parasympathetic center in the brain

Characteristics of rhythm

1. Rate: Less than 60 per minute (atrial and ventricular the same)
2. Rhythm: Regular to irregular; may be associated with sinus arrhythmia[3,6]
3. P waves: Present; all with the same morphology
4. PR interval: 0.12-0.20 second
5. Ratio of P/QRS: 1 : 1
6. QRS interval: 0.06-0.10 second; all with the same morphology
7. QT interval: May be prolonged because of slower rate

Clinical features

1. Normal individuals tolerate sinus bradycardia without symptoms
2. If the patient has heart disease and the heart rate is too slow to maintain an adequate cardiac output (usually at 40 or below per minute), the following may occur:
   a. Hypotension
   b. Angina
   c. Weakness
   d. Dizziness
   e. Diaphoresis
3. In patients with acute myocardial infarction:

a. Sinus bradycardia may be dangerous if the patient is symptomatic:
   (1) With unusually slow rates, dizziness (syncope) may occur
   (2) The slow rate may allow an irritable focus to take over the pacemaker function and may lead to a more serious dysrhythmia, such as ventricular tachycardia and/or fibrillation
   (3) Other risks include slow heart rates that may affect a patient's coronary and cerebral blood flow, resulting in such symptoms as:
      (a) Weakness
      (b) Syncope, dizziness, or even loss of consciousness
      (c) Altered level of consciousness and mentation (restlessness, disorientation, confusion)
      (d) Decrease in urine output
      (e) Chest pain
b. May be beneficial if the patient is asymptomatic (without symptoms) because of:
   (1) Decreased oxygen demands of the myocardium
   (2) Possibility of minimizing infarct size
   (3) Decrease in the frequency of more serious dysrhythmias[3]

Treatment measures

1. Usually no treatment is required if the patient is asymptomatic
2. If further slowing of the heart rate occurs, the patient may be stimulated to increase the sinus rate by:
   a. Increasing activity
   b. Awakening from sleep
   c. Changing position
3. If the patient is symptomatic:
   a. Atropine sulfate is the drug of choice; atropine is known as a vagolytic (vago = vagus; lytic = "to lyse" or interfere with) drug that interferes with the parasympathetic neurotransmitter substance, acetyl-

choline, at the nerve endings and allows more sympathetic activity to occur; the sinus discharge rate should then increase; atropine is administered as a 0.5- to 1.0-mg bolus by I.V. push

b. Isoproterenol (Isuprel) 1 to 2 μg per minute I.V. may be an alternative drug

c. A temporary pacemaker may be employed if the sinus rate is extremely slow and congestive heart failure is evident; ideally, an atrial ventricular (AV) sequential pacemaker is preferred since this type of pacemaker maintains the normal sequencing of atrial and ventricular contraction (see Pacemaker Module)[3,6]

Nursing management

1. Assess the patient and immediately:
   a. Record vital signs
   b. Assess neurovital signs (orientation, altered mentation, level of consciousness, restlessness) and record
   c. Observe for other symptoms as described in the "Clinical features" section
2. Document the rhythm by ECG strip; make sure the slow rate is not caused by a more serious dysrhythmia such as heart block or junctional rhythm; examine the P waves carefully
3. Monitor the patient's ECG closely for ectopic (irritable) activity, such as premature ventricular complexes
4. Observe, measure, and record intake and output
5. Observe for any changes in skin color, temperature, or diaphoresis
6. Monitor electrolytes, especially serum potassium (K^+), as an increased serum K^+ can cause bradycardia
7. Always be aware and knowledgeable of medications your patient is taking and know their actions (some medications slow sinus rate)

Special considerations

1. As above
2. Continue to monitor patient as described in Nursing management section

SINUS TACHYCARDIA (FIG. 2-15)
Definition

1. The pacemaker is the SA node and the impulses travel in the usual sequence to the ventricles; therefore, the P-QRS-T complexes appear the same as normal sinus rhythm
2. The rate is over 100 per minute; the usual rate of sinus tachycardia in the adult is 100 to 160 but may be faster; sinus tachycardia is said to exist in the child at a rate greater than 150 and in the infant at up to 300 per minute[6]
3. As the rate becomes faster, the P waves become closer to the previous T waves and it may be difficult to differentiate sinus tachycardia from other supraventricular (above the ventricle) tachycardias such as atrial or junctional
4. The rhythm is usually regular but may be very slightly irregular

Etiology

1. Sinus tachycardia occurs from vagal inhibition or sympathetic stimulation and is a response to a variety of situations or conditions:
   a. A physiological response to an increase in metabolic activity requiring increased oxygen demand caused by:
      (1) Exercise
      (2) Fever (for every degree of body temperature elevation, the rate may increase 8 to 10 beats per minute[6])
      (3) Emotion

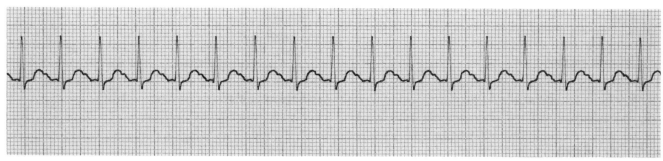

Lead II

FIG. 2-15
Sinus tachycardia.

(4) Pain
(5) Stimulants:
   (a) Alcohol
   (b) Coffee
   (c) Cigarette smoking
(6) Hyperthyroidism
b. A compensatory mechanism of the body to increase cardiac output in response to:
  (1) Anemia
  (2) Anxiety
  (3) Hypoxia (altitude or respiratory depression)
  (4) Hypovolemia
  (5) Hypotension
c. A pharmacological response to:
  (1) Isoproterenol
  (2) Atropine
  (3) Quinidine
  (4) Epinephrine
  (5) Aminophylline
  (6) Any "over-the-counter" drug preparations, including atropine
  (7) Eyedrop preparations with atropine or epinephrine (especially in elderly populations)
d. A response to an underlying pathological state:
  (1) Pericarditis
  (2) Shock (hypovolemic, septic, cardiogenic, or neurogenic)
  (3) Pulmonary emboli
  (4) Pulmonary edema
  (5) Hypoxemia (related to pulmonary or lung disease)
  (6) Myocardial infarction (MI) associated with heart failure (usually more frequent with anterior wall MI)
  (7) Congestive heart failure
2. Carotid sinus massage, which stimulates the parasympathetic nervous system (vagus), may or may not slow the rate of sinus tachycardia; if it does, the rate returns to the previous rate as soon as carotid sinus pressure is released

Characteristics of rhythm

1. Rate: 100-160 per minute (atrial and ventricular the same)
2. Rhythm: Regular to very slightly irregular (atrial and ventricular the same)
3. P waves: Present, with same morphology; if the rate is rapid, the P wave may encroach on or merge with the preceding T wave
4. PR interval: Within normal limits; tends to shorten with faster rates
5. Ratio of P/QRS: 1:1

6. QRS interval: Within normal limits
7. QT interval: Up to 0.44 second or one half preceding RR interval; may shorten with faster rates

Clinical features

1. The patient may be unaware of the rapid heart beat or may feel palpitations ("racing of the heart") within the chest
2. In the presence of acute myocardial infarction, sinus tachycardia may be one of the first signs of congestive heart failure, cardiogenic shock, pulmonary embolism, or extension of the infarct; symptoms may be:
  a. Palpitations
  b. Dyspnea (the feeling of shortness of breath)
  c. Dizziness
  d. Hypotension
  e. Diaphoresis
  f. Altered mental status
3. Sinus tachycardia is distinguished from other tachycardias by careful examination of the P waves, which usually occur with regular rhythm and rate
4. Sinus tachycardia starts *gradually* and terminates *gradually* (*not* an abrupt slowing), as the cause of the tachycardia is corrected or alleviated
5. Dangers in patients with coronary artery disease include:
  a. Angina
  b. Congestive heart failure
  c. Myocardial infarction
6. Dangers in patients with myocardial infarction include:
  a. Increased oxygen demands of the myocardium
  b. Extension of the infarct size
  c. Precipitation of congestive heart failure because of shortening of diastole, or filling time, in the cardiac cycle

Treatment measures

Treatment is *always* related to the underlying cause, such as:
1. Fever
2. Exercise
3. Emotion
4. Stimulants (coffee, alcohol, cigarettes)
5. Pain
6. Hypoxemia
7. Hyperthyroidism
8. Heart failure
9. Shock
10. Anemia
11. Secondary response to myocardial infarction

Nursing management

1. Assess the patient for possible causes of tachycardia
2. Notify the physician
3. Monitor vital signs: blood pressure, heart rate, respiratory rate and rhythm, temperature, skin color and warmth, altered mental status; document and note any changes
4. Treat the cause
5. Document the rate and rhythm by ECG strip; examine P waves carefully to differentiate between sinus, atrial, or junctional tachycardia
6. Monitor the ECG closely for any change in rate or rhythm
7. Assess adequacy of oxygenation (measure arterial blood gasses, if indicated)
8. Observe, measure, and record intake and output
9. Always be aware of your patient's diagnosis and be knowledgeable of the medications your patient is receiving and their actions (some medications can speed sinus rate)

Special considerations

Observe patients with acute myocardial infarction closely and record vital signs and neurovital signs every 30 minutes to 1 hour or as condition warrants

SINUS ARRHYTHMIA (FIG. 2-16)
Definition

1. The pacemaker is the sinus node but impulses are not generated in a regular fashion; impulses are released at alternating faster and slower rates
2. There are two types of sinus arrhythmia:
   a. Respiratory
      (1) There is a cyclic speeding and slowing of sinus impulses correlated to the respiratory cycle
      (2) The sinus rate speeds with inspiration and slows with exhalation
      (3) The degree of speeding and slowing of rate is exaggerated by extremes in respiratory effort and by breath holding
   b. Nonrespiratory
      The cyclic variations in rate are unrelated to the respiratory cycle
3. Sinus arrhythmia exists when the difference between the shortest and longest PP interval is 0.16 second or longer[3,6,9]
4. Conduction is normal through the ventricles, unless the interval with exhalation becomes exceedingly slow; then a lower pacemaker may take over as an escape rhythm

Etiology

1. Respiratory:
   a. With inspiration, the venous return increases to the right atrium and to the lung, decreasing the stretch in the right atrial wall; this allows the parasympathetic nervous system to be inhibited and the rate increases; with exhalation, pressures in the right heart increase and heart rate decreases
   b. Sinus arrhythmia of the respiratory type is considered to be a normal physiological variant in young children, in some healthy adults, and less frequently in the elderly population
2. Nonrespiratory:
   a. May be the result of medications that influence vagal tone, such as morphine sulfate or digoxin
   b. May be more common in individuals with heart disease[3,5,6]

Characteristics of rhythm

1. Rate: 60-100 per minute (atrial and ventricular the same); may be bradycardic
2. Rhythm: Irregular (both atrial and ventricular); this irregularity is usually caused by respiratory variations or may have no relationship to the respiratory cycle

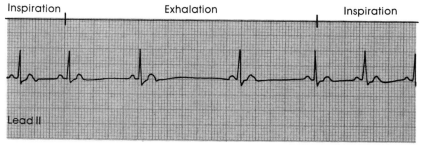

Inspiration   Exhalation   Inspiration

Lead II

FIG. 2-16
Sinus arrhythmia.

Lead II

3. P waves: Present; all with the same morphology
4. PR interval: Within normal limits; may vary with rate changes
5. Ratio of P/QRS: 1 : 1
6. QRS interval: Within normal limits; if a lower pacemaker takes over during slow rates, the interval may be widened
7. QT interval: Within normal limits

Clinical features

1. The individual is usually unaware of the irregularity
2. The diagnosis can be made by documenting with ECG strip or by taking the pulse and observing the speeding and slowing of rate with respirations
3. If the rate is extremely slow, the individual may describe:
   a. Palpitations
   b. Dizziness
   c. Angina (especially if heart disease is present)

Treatment measures

1. Generally, no treatment is needed
2. If the individual is symptomatic because of a slow heart rate, treatment is directed toward increasing the heart rate by:
   a. Exercise
   b. Atropine
   c. Isoproterenol for excessively slow rates (see Antidysrhythmic Drug Module)

Nursing management

1. Observe the degree of slowing of heart rate with exhalation and observe the patient for signs and symptoms of bradycardia
2. Document the rhythm on the patient record

Special considerations

1. Sinus arrhythmia should be treated like sinus bradycardia *only* if the patient is symptomatic
2. The risk in patients with heart disease or myocardial infarction is usually minimal; however, this group should be monitored closely for development of more serious dysrhythmias
3. Sinus arrhythmia should not be confused with serious causes of irregular rhythm

SINUS PAUSE OR SINUS ARREST
(Figs. 2-17, 2-18, and 2-19)

Definition

1. Sinus pause and sinus arrest have been used interchangeably to describe a rhythm characterized by failure of the sinus node to initiate an impulse at the expected time for one or more cycles; thus, the atria are not depolarized and normal conduction to the ventricles does not occur; the conduction from the sinus node to the atrial muscle remains intact; the problem is one of failure of the SA node to initiate, or generate, an impulse[7]
2. If the sinus node or a lower pacemaker does not escape and assume pacemaker function, a long pause, or arrest, may occur
3. Since the sinus node fails to initiate an impulse, one or more cardiac cycles are missed, as evidenced by the absence of the corresponding P-QRS-T complex on the ECG; this transient absence of P waves may last less than 2 seconds (10 large squares) to several minutes[7]
4. The PP interval of the pause is *not* a multiple of the regular PP interval
5. The duration of the resulting pause as well as the ability of a lower (escape) pacemaker to assume temporary control of the heart determines the seriousness of the dysrhythmia[1,3,9,11]

Etiology

1. Sinus pause or arrest may occur in normal individuals as a result of excessive vagal stimulation, such as the Valsalva maneuver (gagging, vomiting, straining at stool), carotid sinus sensitivity, or extreme emotional stress
2. Reversible or self-limiting causes are ischemia of the SA node (from coronary artery disease or myocardial infarction), surgical injury to the SA node, and infectious processes such as myocarditis and acute pericarditis, hypothermia, or hyperkalemia
3. Pharmacological agents causing slowing of the sinus node include:
   a. At toxic serum levels:
      (1) Digoxin
      (2) Quinidine sulfate or gluconate
      (3) Lidocaine hydrochloride
      (4) Atropine sulfate
   b. As an expected pharmacological response:
      (1) Beta-blocking agents
      (2) Reserpine
      (3) Guanethidine sulfate
      (4) Clonidine hydrochloride
   c. Lithium carbonate (used in manic-depressive states)

Characteristics of rhythm

1. Rate: 60-100 per minute; may be bradycardic
2. Rhythm: Regular when the SA node is the normal pacemaker; becomes irregular with missed complexes
3. P waves: Present with sinus beats; all P waves have the

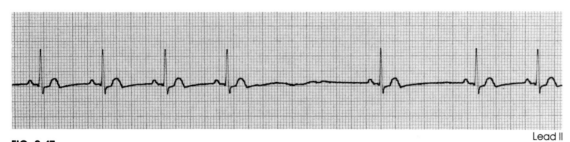

FIG. 2-17

Sinus pause or arrest.

Lead II

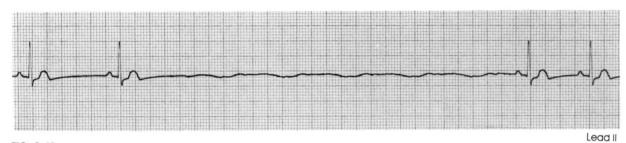

FIG. 2-18

Sinus pause or arrest. Figure illustrates a 5.5-second pause, which is not a direct multiple of regular PP interval.

Lead II

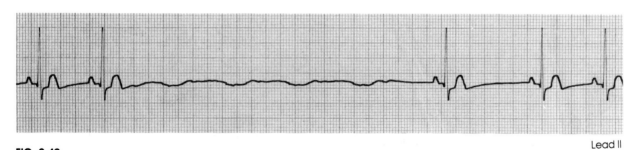

FIG. 2-19

Sinus pause or arrest. Figure illustrates a 4.5-second pause, which is not a direct multiple of regular PP interval.

Lead II

same morphology, even when the sinus node "kicks in" following the pause or arrest

4. PR interval: 0.12-0.20 second with sinus-conducted beats; normally constant

5. Ratio of P/QRS: 1:1 with normal sinus complexes; may be altered if a junctional or ventricular escape rhythm takes over

6. QRS interval: 0.06-0.10 second with sinus-conducted beats; the QRS is absent during sinus arrest because of failure of the SA node to conduct to the ventricle and the QRS morphology is the same with sinus beats but

may change if a lower pacemaker escapes for one or more complexes

7. QT interval: Within normal limits

Clinical features

1. Sinus arrest may cause no symptoms; however, faintness, dizziness, syncope, or convulsions may result from prolonged asystole

2. Unexpected (sudden) death may occur from ventricular standstill if a lower pacemaker fails to take over

3. The diagnosis of sinus arrest should be suspected when

palpation of the pulse or auscultation of the heart discloses a pause in the normal sequence
4. An ECG is necessary to distinguish sinus arrest from other dysrhythmias such as nonconducted atrial premature complexes
5. More serious dysrhythmias may occur as a result of slow rates

Treatment measures

1. Drug therapy:
   a. Goal: to increase the rate of the SA node
   b. Sympathomimetic agents:
      Isoproterenol: 1 to 2 μg/minute
   c. Vagolytic agent:
      Atropine sulfate: 0.5 to 1.0 mg I.V.; may be repeated if necessary up to 2 mg total
2. Pacemaker therapy (see Pacemaker Module):
   a. This dysrhythmia may produce no symptoms; however, a temporary pacemaker should be available for insertion or may be inserted if a lower pacemaker fails to escape or the sinus node remains excessively depressed
   b. Patients with acute myocardial infarction who require large doses of myocardial depressant drugs, such as quinidine, procainamide, lidocaine, or digoxin to control dysrhythmias, are susceptible to sinus arrest; a temporary pacemaker allows continuation of drug therapy while assuring stimulation of the myocardium if a lower pacemaker fails to escape
   c. Insertion of a permanent pacemaker may be necessary if sinus arrest is a symptom of sinus node dysfunction (see p. 44)

Nursing management

1. Assess the patient for symptoms related to the dysrhythmia:
   a. Hypotension
   b. Dizziness
   c. Syncope
2. Document the dysrhythmia:
   a. Examine the P waves carefully
   b. Determine that the slow rate is not caused by heart block or junctional rhythm
3. When sinus arrest is transient, no other nursing action may be indicated except to notify the physician of the dysrhythmia; he/she may want to insert a temporary pacemaker
4. If the arrest is prolonged and the patient is symptomatic, emergency measures must be carried out:
   a. Prepare for cardiopulmonary resuscitation
   b. Notify the physician "STAT"
   c. Bring the emergency cart to the bedside or outside the patient's room
   d. If a pacemaker is already in place, make sure it is turned "on" and pacing adequately
   e. Prepare an isoproterenol drip; dose: usually 1 mg in 250 ml D_5W to run at 1 to 2 μg/min I.V.
   f. Prepare for insertion of a temporary pacemaker

Special considerations

In patients with acute myocardial infarction, drugs used to increase heart rate may:
1. Increase the workload of the heart and, thus, increase oxygen requirements of the myocardium
2. Increase angina
3. Extend the size of the infarct

SINOATRIAL BLOCK (SINUS EXIT BLOCK) (Fig. 2-20)
Definition

1. Sinoatrial (SA) block or sinus exit block differs from sinus pause or arrest in that the P cells in the sinus node continue to initiate impulses in a regular sequence, but the impulses generated are prevented from depolarizing the atrial muscle tissue because of a block in the transitional and/or Purkinje cells on the edges of

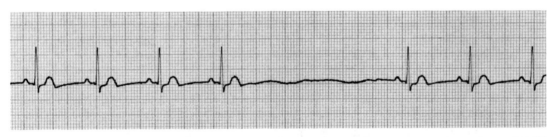

Lead II

FIG. 2-20
Second-degree sinoatrial (SA) block, type II. There is a 3:1 direct multiple from P wave before the pause to P wave interrupting the pause.

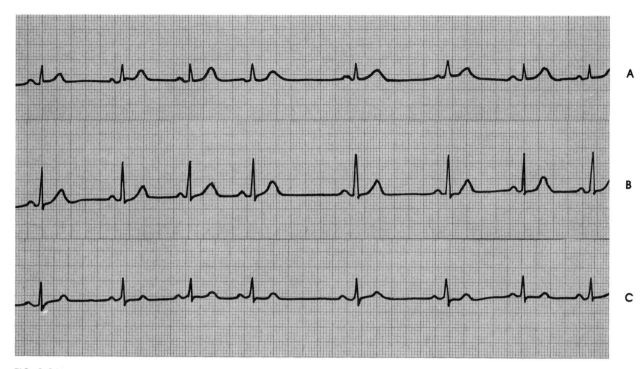

FIG. 2-21
Second-degree SA block, type I. **A,** Lead I; **B,** lead II; **C,** lead III. Simultaneous tracing.

the SA node or in the atrial muscle itself; this results in an interference (block) in the actual conduction of the impulses
2. There are three identified types of sinoatrial block:
   a. First-degree SA block
   In this type of block, there is a consistently delayed entry of each sinus impulse into the atrial myocardium; since the sinus impulse is not seen on the ECG until it activates the atrial muscle, first-degree SA block cannot be differentiated from normal sinus rhythm on the surface ECG

   b. Second-degree SA block
   (1) Type I (Wenckebach) (Fig. 2-21)
   The sinus impulse is automatically initiated from the SA node in a regular sequence; however, there is a progressive delay in impulse transmission to the atrial muscle until the impulse is not conducted; in some cases it may be difficult to distinguish type I second-degree SA block from sinus arrhythmia
   (2) Type II (Fig. 2-22)
   There is failure of the sinus impulse to appear

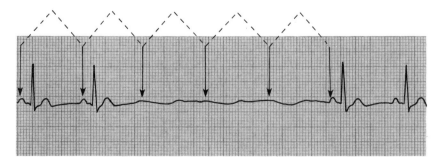

FIG. 2-22
Second-degree SA block, type II. There is a 4:1 direct multiple from P wave before the pause to P wave interrupting the pause, suggesting a problem with SA nodal impulse conduction. (See text.)

at the appropriate time; the length of the pause between two PP intervals is a direct multiple of the basic PP interval (the multiple may be 2 : 1, 3 : 1, 4 : 1, or longer); as with sinus arrest, the pause may be terminated by a lower pacemaker complex or rhythm (atrial, junctional, or ventricular); in such cases it is difficult to differentiate type II second-degree SA block from sinus arrest

c. Third-degree SA block
This type of SA block is consistent with atrial arrest (failure of the atrial muscle to conduct the impulse) and cannot be distinguished from sinus arrest on the surface ECG

Etiology

1. Sinoatrial block may be caused by transitional cell dysfunction, resulting in conduction delay within the SA node
2. Reversible causes are related to:
   a. Excessive vagal stimuli
   b. Acute infectious process such as diphtheria and rheumatic carditis, myocarditis, and pericarditis
   c. Ischemia caused by coronary artery disease or acute myocardial infarction, including atrial infarction
   d. Certain drug therapy that may depress sinus node function:
      (1) Digoxin
      (2) Quinidine, procainamide
      (3) Acetylcholine (neurotransmitter substance for the parasympathetic nervous system)
   e. Other:
      (1) Hyperkalemia ($\uparrow K^+$)
      (2) Thyrotoxicosis
      (3) Hypothyroidism

      (4) Elevated carbon dioxide levels
      (5) Carotid sinus sensitivity[1,3,5]
3. Irreversible causes may include:
   a. Surgical trauma
      (1) Repair of congenital defects
      (2) Placing cannulas for heart-lung bypass
   b. Sclerodegenerative diseases of the SA node
   c. Amyloidosis
   d. Hemochromatosis
   e. Duchenne and myotonic muscular dystrophy
   f. Friedreich's ataxia
   g. Systemic lupus erythematosus
   h. Familial disease of the SA node
   i. Metastatic cancer (lymphomas)
   j. Systemic embolism to SA nodal artery
   k. Possible mitral valve prolapse[1,6]
4. Type II second-degree SA block is usually more serious and may be associated with sinus node dysfunction (see p. 44)[5]

Characteristics of rhythm

1. In first-degree SA block, it is difficult to determine from normal sinus rhythm or sinus bradycardia on the surface ECG. Second-degree SA block, type I (Wenckebach) (Fig. 2-23) can be distinguished by:
   a. Rate: 60-100 per minute (atrial and ventricular the same; may be bradycardic)
   b. Rhythm: Irregular with pauses (atrial and ventricular the same):
      (1) The PP (and RR) intervals become progressively shorter until a pause occurs
      (2) The PP interval including the pause is less than twice the shortest PP interval
      (3) The PP interval after the pause is longer than the PP interval preceding the pause

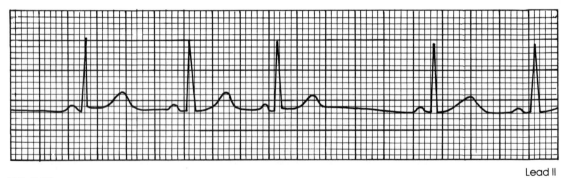

Lead II

FIG. 2-23
Second-degree SA block, type I. PP interval shortens before the pause. PP interval after the pause is longer than PP interval before the pause. (See text.)

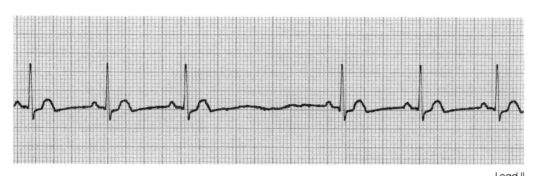

FIG. 2-24   Lead II

Second-degree SA block, type II. There is one P-QRS-T cycle missing in the regular PP cycle.

c. P waves: Present before each QRS with the same morphology
d. PR interval: 0.12-0.20 second; may be greater than 0.20 second but all PR intervals will be the same (e.g., if PR interval is 0.24 second, all PR intervals will be 0.24 second)
e. Ratio of P/QRS: 1:1
f. QRS interval: 0.06-0.10 second; all with the same morphology
g. QT interval: One half the preceding RR interval or may be prolonged (NOTE: It may be difficult in some cases to distinguish from sinus arrhythmia)[1,5,9]

2. Second-degree SA block, type II (Fig. 2-24) has the following characteristics:
   a. Rate: 60-100 per minute (atrial and ventricular usually the same); may be bradycardic or tachycardic
   b. Rhythm: Basically regular; becomes irregular with pauses:
      (1) PP intervals are regular until a pause results, showing no atrial activity
      (2) The P-QRS-T complex interrupting the pause will be a direct multiple of the regular PP interval: 2:1, 3:1, 4:1, or more
   c. P waves: Present; all with the same morphology
   d. PR interval: 0.12-0.20 second; may be prolonged but will be consistent
   e. Ratio of P/QRS: 1:1 usually, unless a lower pacemaker escapes
   f. QRS interval: 0.06-0.10 second; with all the same morphology unless a lower pacemaker escapes, then may be widened
   g. QT interval: One half the preceding RR interval of regular complexes or may be prolonged (NOTE: If the pause is prolonged, it may be interrupted by a lower pacemaker such as junctional or ventricular)

3. Third-degree SA block is difficult to distinguish from sinus arrest in some cases (see p. 38)[1,3,5]

Clinical features

1. Symptoms produced by SA block will depend on the number of sinus impulses blocked (the duration of the pause) and the ability of a substitute pacemaker to initiate impulses
2. The patient may experience any of the following:
   a. Irregular heart beats
   b. Dizziness
   c. Faintness
   d. Attacks of syncope
   e. Seizures
3. Palpation of the pulse or auscultation of the heart reveals a slow, regular rhythm or recurring cycles of irregularity
4. An ECG is necessary to confirm the diagnosis

Treatment measures

1. Usually sinoatrial block is transient and the clinical importance relates to identifying the underlying cause; if the block is prolonged and a lower pacemaker fails to escape, syncope may result
2. Digoxin toxicity may manifest itself with type I second-degree SA block (Wenckebach) and not type II; in this case digoxin is withheld or the dose decreased until the block resolves
3. Drugs used to increase sympathetic tone or decrease parasympathetic tone may be used, such as isoproterenol or atropine (see Antidysrhythmic Drug Module for specific dosages)
4. If the SA block is prolonged without an escape pacemaker and drug therapy is not effective, a ventricular or AV sequential pacemaker may be necessary (see Pacemaker Module)

Nursing management

1. Document the rhythm with a rhythm strip
2. Observe duration of pauses
3. Assess the patient by monitoring vital signs and neurovital signs
4. Be aware of the patient's diagnosis, laboratory values, medications, and possible side effects
5. Notify the physician of the rhythm disturbance
6. Continue to monitor the patient closely for signs of further blocking
7. Review the nursing management for sinus arrest, p. 40

Special considerations

As above (see Sinus Pause or Sinus Arrest), p. 40

SINUS NODE DYSFUNCTION (SICK SINUS SYNDROME)

The identification and interpretation of sinus node dysfunction are beyond the scope of the beginning learner in ECG interpretation. However, because of the significance of this syndrome in relation to mortality and morbidity, it is necessary to introduce the concept at this level by presenting a definition, etiology, clinical features, diagnostic techniques, and treatment measures. The interested learner is referred to specific references[1,4,7] for additional information.

Definition

1. Sinus node dysfunction (sick sinus syndrome) results from failure of the specialized cells in the sinus node to initiate and/or conduct impulses in a normal fashion
2. The syndrome may also result from failure of lower pacemakers to take over control of the heart when the sinus node fails
3. This syndrome tends to be progressive over a period of time and can be related to one or more of the following dysrhythmias, which usually appear intermittently:
   a. Persistent, unexplained sinus bradycardia
   b. Sinus pause or arrest with or without the appearance of a lower (escape) pacemaker
   c. Sinoatrial block

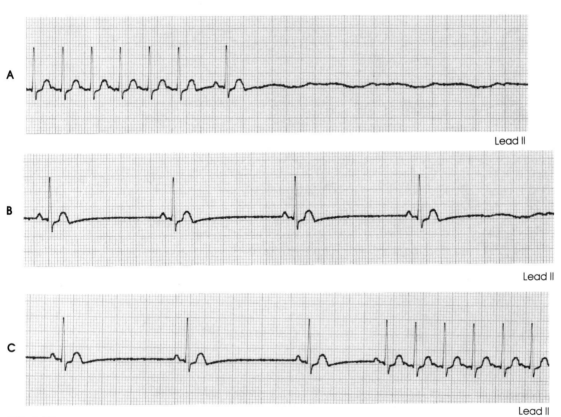

A   Lead II

B   Lead II

C   Lead II

FIG. 2-25

Tachycardia-bradycardia syndrome. Strip shows supraventricular tachycardia with rate of 150 per minute, slowing to profound sinus bradycardia after a 4.5-second pause. Rate eventually speeds again toward end of strip. (Note: **A, B,** and **C** sections are one continuous strip.)

d. Chronic atrial fibrillation with a slow ventricular response (rate) in an individual who is not on drugs to slow sinus rate or AV conduction (see Atrial Module)

e. Failure of the heart to return to a sinus rhythm after electrical cardioversion for atrial fibrillation or after a premature atrial complex (PAC) (see Atrial Dysrhythmias Module)

f. The bradycardia-tachycardia syndrome: sudden appearance of supraventricular tachycardia that alternates with sinus bradycardia, usually with excessively slow rates

4. In addition, many individuals with sinus node dysfunction may have abnormalities of conduction through the AV node and in the bundle branches[1,7,8]

5. Examples of sinus node dysfunction are demonstrated in Figs. 2-25, 2-26, and 2-27

Etiology

1. The cause may be disease of the node itself (intrinsic) or may be compounded by influencing factors on the node such as drugs, nervous or endocrine system influences, or blood supply (extrinsic)

2. Usually the syndrome is found in the elderly but may be seen in young children and adolescents

3. Intrinsic causes:
   a. Coronary atherosclerosis
   b. Hypertension
   c. Atrial amyloidosis
   d. Diffuse fibrosis
   e. Collagen vascular disease
   f. Surgical trauma to the SA node and/or atrial muscle (a common cause in the younger age group)
   g. Infectious and infiltrative disease
   h. See "Irreversible causes of sinoatrial block," p. 42

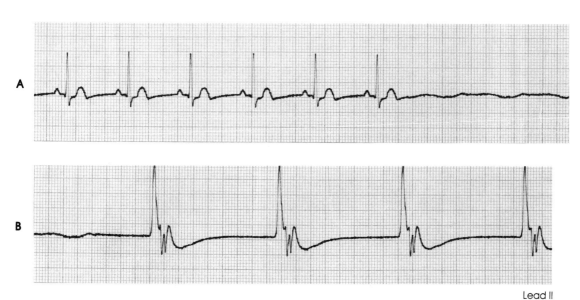

Lead II

FIG. 2-26
Sinus pause or arrest with ventricular escape rhythm.
(Note: **A** and **B** sections are one continuous strip.)

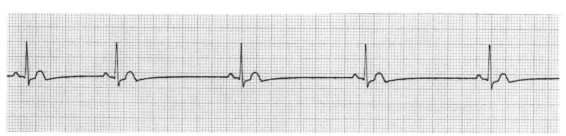

Lead II

FIG. 2-27
Persistent unexplained sinus bradycardia.

4. Extrinsic causes:
   a. Coronary artery disease
   b. Acute myocardial infarction, especially involving the inferior, posterior, or lateral wall
   c. Carotid sinus sensitivity
   d. Drugs that depress sinus node automaticity and/or conduction:
      (1) Beta-blocking agents
      (2) Verapamil
      (3) Digoxin
      (4) Quinidine, procainamide, disopyramide
      (5) Guanethidine
      (6) Reserpine
      (7) Clonidine
      (8) Methyldopa[1,7]

Clinical features

1. The symptoms of sinus node dysfunction depend on the following:
   a. Severity of the sinus node disease
   b. Condition of the lower pacemaker sites
   c. State of myocardial contractility
   d. State or condition of the primary organs: heart, brain, and kidney
2. Over 100,000 Americans experience the dysrhythmias of sinus node dysfunction[1]
3. Symptoms vary widely from no symptoms (for persons who have normal functioning lower pacemakers) to those related to decreased cardiac and/or cerebral blood flow as a result of slow rates; symptoms produced by the following dysrhythmias include:
   a. Sinus bradycardia:
      (1) Marked decrease in exercise tolerance
      (2) Fatigue
      (3) Lightheadedness
   b. Sinus pause or arrest or sinoatrial block (associated with higher mortality rates):
      (1) Dizziness
      (2) Syncope
      (3) Seizures
   c. Supraventricular tachycardia:
      (1) Palpitations
      (2) Congestive heart failure
      (3) Systemic embolism (in 16% to 24% of individuals)[1,4]
      (4) Generalized weakness
      (5) Lassitude
      (6) Altered mental status (may be confused with senility in the elderly)
   d. In the elderly population, symptoms may be associated with other health problems:
      (1) Hypertension

      (2) Cerebrovascular disease
         (a) Confusion
         (b) Transient ischemic attacks (TIAs)
         (c) Stroke
      (3) Coronary artery disease
         (a) Angina
         (b) Congestive heart failure
4. Drugs used to treat cardiac disorders may intensify the severity of the underlying sinus node disease

Diagnostic techniques

1. Most individuals seek treatment at the onset of neurological symptoms; therefore, evaluation is necessary to identify the underlying disorder and attempt to differentiate reversible causes from nonreversible causes
2. Ambulatory monitoring:
   a. A 24-hour (Holter) monitor may be worn in an effort to document the rhythm disturbance at the time symptoms appear; it may be necessary to repeat frequently because of the intermittent nature of the syndrome
   b. A 12-lead ECG will rarely document the causative rhythm
3. A depressed heart rate response to exercise and/or isoproterenol administration may be seen in individuals with sinus node dysfunction
4. Invasive studies, known as electrophysiological studies (EPS), are more diagnostic but beyond the scope of this module; the interested learner is referred to the noted references for more specific information[1,7]

Treatment measures

1. Treatment should be directed toward the control of symptoms
2. Measures should identify causative factors and follow closely to document resolution of dysrhythmias
3. Asymptomatic individuals are managed with close follow-ups without pacemaker insertion and avoidance of drugs known to depress sinus node function
4. Permanent pacemaker insertion is recommended for individuals whose symptoms clearly relate to profound sinus bradycardia, sinoatrial block, sinus arrest, or the bradycardia-tachycardia syndrome
5. A combination of pacemaker and drug therapy is used in the bradycardia-tachycardia syndrome to control the tachy component as well as maintain a suitable rate during the brady episodes
6. With hypertension, drugs depressing sinus node function should be discontinued; hydralazine (Apresoline) and diuretics are shown to be well tolerated and even to improve sinus node function[4]

REFERENCES

1. Alpert, M.A., and Flaker, G.C.: Arrhythmias associated with sinus node dysfunction, JAMA 250(16):2160, 1983.
2. Anderson, R.H., and Becker, A.E.: Gross anatomy and microscopy of the conducting system. In Mandel, W.J., editor: Cardiac arrhythmias, Philadelphia, 1980, J.B. Lippincott Co.
3. Andreoli, K.G., et al.: Comprehensive cardiac care, ed. 5, St. Louis, 1983, The C.V. Mosby Co.
4. Benditt, D.G., et al.: Drug therapy in sinus node dysfunction. In Rapaport, E., editor: Cardiology update, New York, 1984, Elsevier Science Publishing Co. Inc.
5. Conover, M.B.: Understanding electrocardiography: arrhythmias and the 12-lead ECG, ed. 4, St. Louis, 1984, The C.V. Mosby Co.
6 Kernicki, J.G., and Weiler, K.M.: Electrocardiography for nurses: physiological correlates, New York, 1981, John Wiley & Sons Inc.
7. Kerr, C.R., et al.: Sinus node dysfunction. In Zipes, D.P., editor: Symposium on arrhythmias, II. Cardiology clinics, vol. 1 (2), Philadelphia, 1983, W.B. Saunders Co.
8 Marriott, H.J.L., and Conover, M.B.: Advanced concepts in arrhythmias, St. Louis, 1983, The C.V. Mosby Co.
9. Phillips, R.E., and Feeney, M.K.: The cardiac rhythms: a systematic approach to interpretation, ed. 2, Philadelphia, 1980, W.B. Saunders Co.
10. Rossi, L.: The pathologic basis of cardiac arrhythmias. In Zipes, D.P., editor: Symposium on arrhythmias, I. Cardiology clinics, vol. 1 (1), Philadelphia, 1983, W.B. Saunders Co.
11. Sweetwood, H.M.: Clinical electrocardiography for nurses, Rockville, Md., 1983, Aspen Systems Corporation.

SUGGESTED LEARNING ACTIVITIES AND EXPERIENCES

A. Find patients in any of the intensive care units who demonstrate the rhythm disturbances related to the sinus node:
   1. You may ask any ICU nurse for assistance in identifying such patients
   2. Once a rhythm disturbance is identified, review the patient's record, including:
      a. History
      b. Physical examination findings
      c. Diagnosis
      d. Medications (both scheduled and p.r.n.)
      e. Vital signs
   3. Attempt to identify a possible etiology (or cause) of the rhythm disturbance
   4. Identify treatment measures and nursing observations and/or management that relate to the particular rhythm disturbance
   5. Write patient care objectives on the nursing care plan in relation to the dysrhythmia

B. Practice interpreting sinus dysrhythmias by obtaining as many strips as possible; analyze each strip according to the format listed on the practice strips in the Supplements section of this module
C. If one has access to an electrophysiology laboratory, this is an excellent resource to identify sinoatrial blocks and sinus node dysfunction

POSTTEST (Answers on pp. 58-59)

Directions: Circle one answer to each question unless otherwise indicated.

A. Automaticity is best defined as:
   1. An external power source that has the ability to initiate electrical impulses
   2. The ability of a cell to conduct impulses
   3. The ability of pacemaker cells to automatically initiate impulses
B. The primary treatment of choice for sinus tachycardia would most probably be:
   1. Digoxin and/or propranolol
   2. Isoproterenol
   3. Dilantin
   4. All of the above
   5. None of the above
C. Which of the following are true concerning sinus bradycardia? (Circle all that apply.)
   1. Most people tolerate this rhythm without symptoms
   2. It can be normal in trained athletes and during sleep
   3. Propranolol (Inderal) is the drug of choice in symptomatic individuals
   4. Other irritable foci (ventricular) are more apt to break through
D. A rhythm characterized by normal P waves, PR intervals, QRS intervals, rate of 125 beats per minute, and a regular rhythm is called:
   1. Sinus arrhythmia
   2. Normal sinus rhythm
   3. Sinus bradycardia
   4. Sinoatrial block
   5. Sinus tachycardia
E. A rhythm characterized by a slowing and speeding of rate related to respirations is known as:
   1. Sinus arrhythmia
   2. Normal sinus rhythm
   3. Sinus bradycardia
   4. Sinoatrial block
   5. Sinus tachycardia

F. The *first* nursing action in relation to a rhythm disturbance is to:
1. Order a 12-lead ECG
2. Check the patient and assess vital signs and level of consciousness
3. Run a rhythm strip

G. Matching: Match the term in Column A with the definition in Column B.

Column A Term	Column B Definition	
___ 1. Sinoatrial (SA) node	a. Small specialized fibers that carry impulses directly to the myocardial cells	l. Specialized cells within the SA node capable of automaticity
___ 2. Valsalva maneuver	b. A rhythm characterized by irregularity related to the respiratory cycle	m. An irregular rhythm interrupted by a pause; the characteristics are: the PP interval progressively shortens before the pause, the length of the pause is less than twice the shortest PP interval, and the PP interval after the pause is longer than the PP interval prior to the pause
___ 3. Sinus tachycardia		
___ 4. Surface ECG		
___ 5. Automaticity	c. A regular rhythm interrupted by a pause; when the rhythm continues, the length of the pause is a direct multiple of the regular rhythm interval	
___ 6. PP interval		
___ 7. Normal sinus rhythm		
___ 8. Carotid sinus sensitivity	d. A complex initiated by a lower pacemaker when the sinus node fails	n. An interval measured from the beginning of the wave of atrial depolarization to the beginning of the next wave of atrial depolarization
___ 9. P cells		
___ 10. Escape complex	e. This interval includes atrial depolarization plus the physiological delay in the AV node	
___ 11. Sinus pause or arrest		
___ 12. Transitional cells		o. A rhythm characterized by a rate of 100 to 160 per minute with a gradual onset and gradual decline after the underlying cause is identified and treated
___ 13. Second-degree sinoatrial block, type I	f. A rhythm characterized by a decreased rate of automaticity; the rhythm is regular and does not require treatment unless the patient is symptomatic	
___ 14. Vasovagal reaction		
___ 15. Purkinje cells		
___ 16. Sinus bradycardia		p. Decreasing blood pressure and heart rate by rotating the head while wearing a snug collar
___ 17. Purkinje fibers	g. Specialized cells that ultimately conduct impulses from the SA node to the atrial muscle	
___ 18. Sinus arrhythmia		
___ 19. Second-degree sinoatrial block, type II		q. The ability to spontaneously initiate an impulse
___ 20. PR interval	h. A normal 12-lead ECG	
	i. A rhythm characterized by a problem of impulse formation	r. The node consisting of specialized cells capable of automaticity at a rate of 60 to 100 per minute
	j. A reflex reaction of decreased blood pressure and heart rate, sometimes caused by strong emotional stress	
		s. The process of taking a deep breath in and forcing down against a closed glottis, elevating the venous pressure
	k. Specialized cells that conduct impulses initiated in the center of the SA node to the outer portion of the node	
		t. A rhythm most of us would like to enjoy

T F H. Sinus arrhythmia is dangerous and requires immediate treatment.

T F I. The treatment of sinus tachycardia is related to its cause.

T F J. Most patients with sinus bradycardia must be treated.

T F K. If a patient with acute myocardial infarction demonstrates sinus pause on the ECG, a temporary pacemaker must be prepared for insertion.

T F L. Atropine is the drug of choice to increase heart rate in a patient with sinus tachycardia who is symptomatic.

T F M. Sinus arrest is considered to be a benign rhythm disturbance and requires minimal observation.

N. Interpret the rhythm strip in Fig. 2-28.
1. Rate:
   Atrial:
   Ventricular:
2. Rhythm:
   Atrial:
   Ventricular:
3. P waves:
4. PR interval:
5. Ratio of P/QRS:
6. QRS interval:
7. QT interval:
8. Interpretation:

O. Interpret the rhythm strip in Fig. 2-29.
1. Rate:
   Atrial:
   Ventricular:
2. Rhythm:
   Atrial:
   Ventricular:
3. P waves:
4. PR interval:
5. Ratio of P/QRS:
6. QRS interval:
7. QT interval:
8. Interpretation:

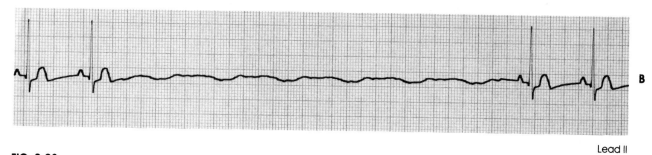

A

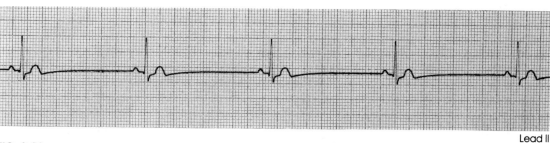

B

Lead II

FIG. 2-28

A and B sections are one continuous strip.

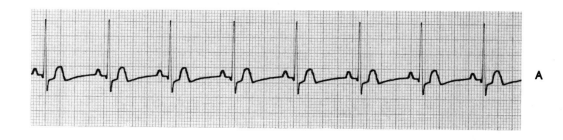

Lead II

FIG. 2-29

P. Interpret the rhythm strip in Fig. 2-30.
    1. Rate:
        Atrial:
        Ventricular:
    2. Rhythm:
        Atrial:
        Ventricular:
    3. P waves:
    4. PR interval:
    5. Ratio of P/QRS:
    6. QRS interval:
    7. QT interval:
    8. Interpretation:
Q. Interpret the rhythm strip in Fig. 2-31.
    1. Rate:
        Atrial:
        Ventricular:
    2. Rhythm:
        Atrial:
        Ventricular:

    3. P waves:
    4. PR interval:
    5. Ratio of P/QRS:
    6. QRS interval:
    7. QT interval:
    8. Interpretation:
R. Interpret the rhythm strip in Fig. 2-32.
    1. Rate:
        Atrial:
        Ventricular:
    2. Rhythm:
        Atrial:
        Ventricular:
    3. P waves:
    4. PR interval:
    5. Ratio of P/QRS:
    6. QRS interval:
    7. QT interval:
    8. Interpretation:

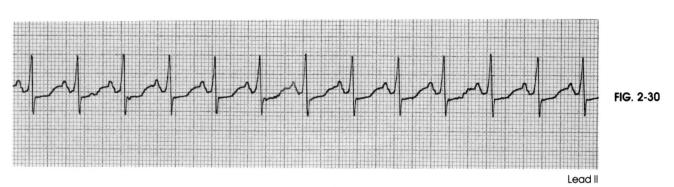

FIG. 2-30

Lead II

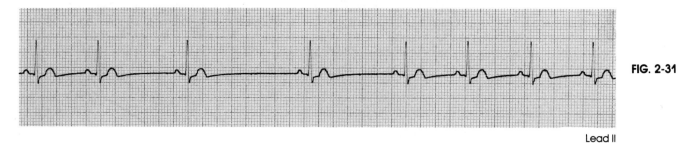

FIG. 2-31

Lead II

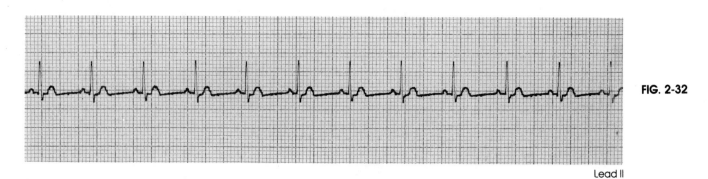

FIG. 2-32

Lead II

S. Interpret the rhythm strip in Fig. 2-33.
   1. Rate:
      Atrial:
      Ventricular:
   2. Rhythm:
      Atrial:
      Ventricular:
   3. P waves:
   4. PR interval:
   5. Ratio of P/QRS:
   6. QRS interval:
   7. QT interval:
   8. Interpretation:

T. Interpret the rhythm strip in Fig. 2-34.
   1. Rate:
      Atrial:
      Ventricular:
   2. Rhythm:
      Atrial:
      Ventricular:
   3. P waves:
   4. PR interval:
   5. Ratio of P/QRS:
   6. QRS interval:
   7. QT interval:
   8. Interpretation:

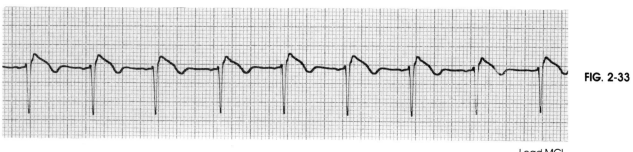

FIG. 2-33

Lead MCL₁

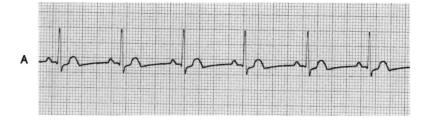

A

FIG. 2-34

A, B, and **C** sections are one continuous strip.

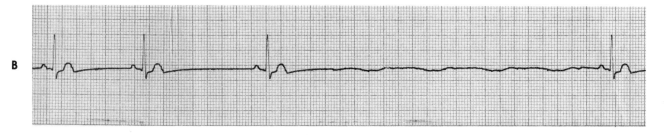

B

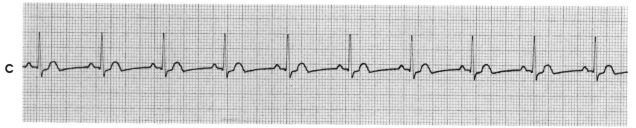

C

Lead II

SUPPLEMENTS

This is a work section. A work space is provided beneath each strip to the left. The answers are to the right. It is suggested you cover the answer section with a card or paper while you work the strips. Check your answers on the right.

A.

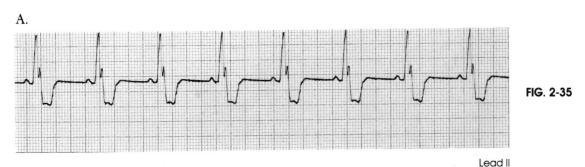

FIG. 2-35

Lead II

1. Rate:	
Atrial:	72
Ventricular:	72
2. Rhythm:	
Atrial:	Regular
Ventricular:	Regular
3. P waves:	Present; all with the same morphology
4. PR interval:	0.12 second
5. Ratio of P/QRS:	1:1
6. QRS interval:	0.14 second (wide and notched)
7. QT interval:	0.40 second
8. Interpretation:	Normal sinus rhythm with wide and notched QRS

B.

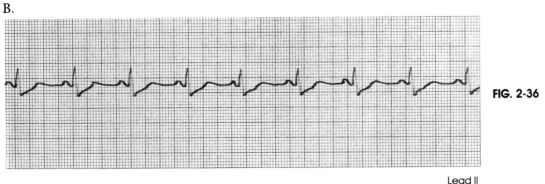

FIG. 2-36

Lead II

1. Rate:	
Atrial:	80
Ventricular:	80
2. Rhythm:	
Atrial:	Regular
Ventricular:	Regular
3. P waves:	Present; all with the same morphology
4. PR interval:	0.16 second
5. Ratio of P/QRS:	1:1
6. QRS interval:	0.10 second
7. QT interval:	0.44 second
8. Interpretation:	Normal sinus rhythm; (ST segment is depressed)

C.

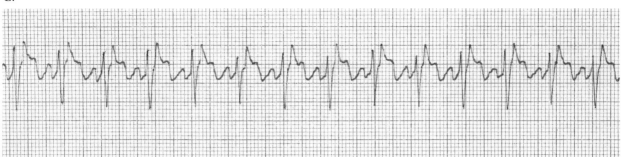

FIG. 2-37

Lead III

1. Rate:
    Atrial: 125
    Ventricular: 125
2. Rhythm:
    Atrial: Regular
    Ventricular: Regular
3. P waves: Present; all with the same morphology
4. PR interval: 0.18 second
5. Ratio of P/QRS: 1:1
6. QRS interval: 0.12 second
7. QT interval: 0.28 second
8. Interpretation: Sinus tachycardia with widened QRS

D.

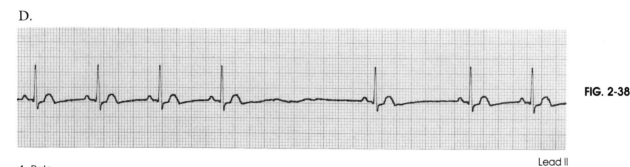

FIG. 2-38

Lead II

1. Rate:
    Atrial: 50
    Ventricular: 50
2. Rhythm:
    Atrial: Irregular
    Ventricular: Irregular
3. P waves: Present; all with the same morphology
4. PR interval: 0.12 second
5. Ratio of P/QRS: 1:1
6. QRS interval: 0.08 second
7. QT interval: 0.32 second
8. Interpretation: Sinus pause/arrest; the fifth sinus beat does not return on schedule

E.

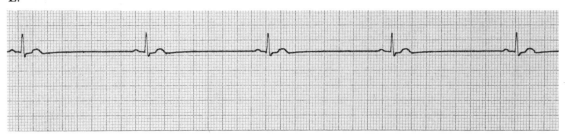

FIG. 2-39

Lead II

1. Rate:	
Atrial:	40
Ventricular:	40
2. Rhythm:	
Atrial:	Regular
Ventricular:	Regular
3. P waves:	Present; all with the same morphology
4. PR interval:	0.14 second
5. Ratio of P/QRS:	1:1
6. QRS interval:	0.06 second
7. QT interval:	0.30 second
8. Interpretation:	Sinus bradycardia

F.

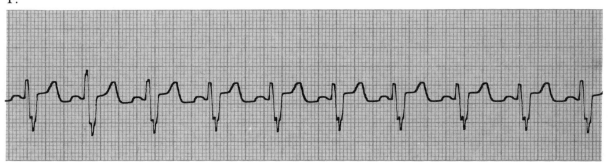

FIG. 2-40

Lead II

1. Rate:	
Atrial:	90
Ventricular:	90
2. Rhythm:	
Atrial:	Regular
Ventricular:	Regular
3. P waves:	Present; all with the same morphology
4. PR interval:	0.14 second
5. Ratio of P/QRS:	1:1
6. QRS interval:	0.16 second
7. QT interval:	0.40 second
8. Interpretation:	Normal sinus rhythm with wide; notched QRS

G.

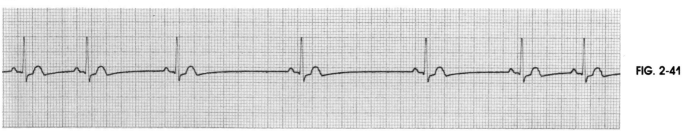

FIG. 2-41

Lead II

1. Rate:	
Atrial:	50
Ventricular:	50
2. Rhythm:	
Atrial:	Irregular
Ventricular:	Irregular
3. P waves:	Present; all with the same morphology
4. PR interval:	0.12 second
5. Ratio of P/QRS:	1:1
6. QRS interval:	0.08 second
7. QT interval:	0.32 second
8. Interpretation:	Sinus arrhythmia; rate speeds with inspiration and slows with exhalation

H.

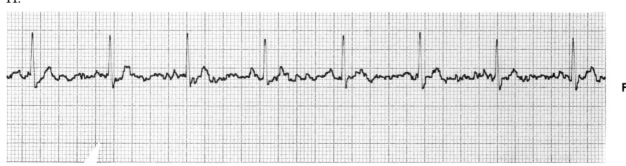

FIG. 2-42

Lead II

1. Rate:	
Atrial:	72
Ventricular:	72
2. Rhythm:	
Atrial:	Regular
Ventricular:	Regular
3. P waves:	Present; difficult to see because of interference
4. PR interval:	Approximately 0.14 second
5. Ratio of P/QRS:	1:1
6. QRS interval:	0.08 second
7. QT interval:	Difficult to determine, approximately 0.30 second
8. Interpretation:	Appears to be normal sinus rhythm with 60-cycle interference

I.

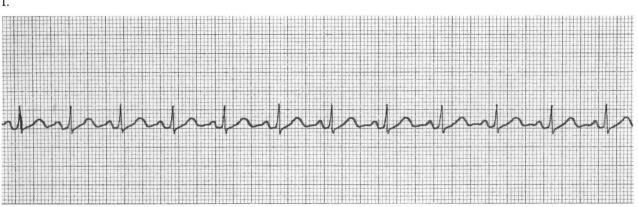

FIG. 2-43

Lead II

1. Rate:	
Atrial:	105
Ventricular:	105
2. Rhythm:	
Atrial:	Regular
Ventricular:	Regular
3. P waves:	Present; all with the same morphology
4. PR interval:	0.14 second
5. Ratio of P/QRS:	1:1
6. QRS interval:	0.06 second
7. QT interval:	0.32 second
8. Interpretation:	Sinus tachycardia

J.

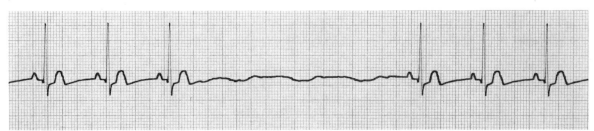

FIG. 2-44

Lead II

1. Rate:	
Atrial:	40
Ventricular:	40
2. Rhythm:	
Atrial:	Regular-irregular with pause
Ventricular:	Regular-irregular with pause
3. P waves:	Present; all with the same morphology
4. PR interval:	0.12 second
5. Ratio of P/QRS:	1:1
6. QRS interval:	0.08 second
7. QT interval:	0.30 second
8. Interpretation:	Second-degree SA block, type II; rhythm begins as regular with a pause; when sinus P wave returns it is a multiple of 4 from the original PP interval

ANSWERS TO PRETEST AND POSTTEST
Pretest

A. 4
B. 2
C. 3
D. 1
E. 3, 4, 5
F. 3
G. 1
H.

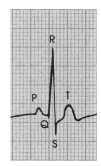

I.

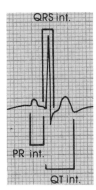

J.

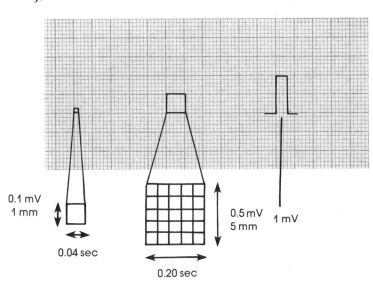

K. 2
L. 2, 4
M. 4
N. 3
O. 3
P. 1, 5, 6
Q. Fig. 2-4.
   1. Rate:
         Atrial: 40
         Ventricular: 40
   2. Rhythm:
         Atrial: Irregular
         Ventricular: Irregular
   3. P waves: Present; all with the same morphology
   4. PR interval: 0.14 second; consistent
   5. Ratio of P/QRS: 1:1
   6. QRS interval: 0.08 second
   7. QT interval: 0.32 second
   8. Interpretation: Combination of sinus pause/arrest and sinoatrial block; the first two and last two complexes have the same PP interval; on the third and fourth complexes, the sinus impulse slows but the fifth complex is a direct multiple of the PP interval from the first and second complexes, suggesting second-degree sinoatrial block, type II
R. Fig. 2-5.
   1. Rate:
         Atrial: 85-90
         Ventricular: 85-90
   2. Rhythm:
         Atrial: Basically regular
         Ventricular: Basically regular
   3. P waves: Present; all with the same morphology
   4. PR interval: 0.12 second
   5. Ratio of P/QRS: 1:1
   6. QRS interval: 0.08 second
   7. QT interval: 0.42 second
   8. Interpretation: Normal sinus rhythm
S. Fig. 2-6.
   1. Rate:
         Atrial: 140
         Ventricular: 140
   2. Rhythm:
         Atrial: Regular
         Ventricular: Regular
   3. P waves: Present; all with the same morphology
   4. PR interval: 0.14 second
   5. Ratio of P/QRS: 1:1
   6. QRS interval: 0.08 second
   7. QT interval: 0.28 second
   8. Interpretation: Sinus tachycardia

T. Fig. 2-7.
   1. Rate:
         Atrial: 40
         Ventricular: 40
   2. Rhythm:
         Atrial: Regular
         Ventricular: Regular
   3. P waves: Present; all with the same morphology
   4. PR interval: 0.14 second
   5. Ratio of P/QRS: 1 : 1
   6. QRS interval: 0.08 second
   7. QT interval: 0.32 second
   8. Interpretation: Sinus bradycardia
U. Fig. 2-8.
   1. Rate:
         Atrial: 50
         Ventricular: 50
   2. Rhythm:
         Atrial: Irregular
         Ventricular: Irregular
   3. P waves: Present; all with the same morphology
   4. PR interval: 0.14 second
   5. Ratio of P/QRS: 1 : 1
   6. QRS interval: 0.08 second
   7. QT interval: 0.32 second
   8. Interpretation: Sinus arrhythmia; rate speeds with inhalation and slows with exhalation
V. Fig. 2-9.
   1. Rate:
         Atrial: 70-72
         Ventricular: 70-72
   2. Rhythm:
         Atrial: Regular
         Ventricular: Regular
   3. P waves: Present; all with the same morphology
   4. PR interval: 0.14 second
   5. Ratio of P/QRS: 1 : 1
   6. QRS interval: 0.08 second
   7. QT interval: 0.30 second
   8. Interpretation: Normal sinus rhythm

Posttest

A. 3
B. 5
C. 1, 2, 4
D. 5
E. 1
F. 2
G. Matching:
      1. r   2. s   3. o

4. h	10. d	16. f
5. q	11. i	17. a
6. n	12. k	18. b
7. t	13. m	19. c
8. p	14. j	20. e
9. l	15. g	

H. F
I. T
J. F
K. F
L. F
M. F
N. Fig. 2-28.
   1. Rate:
         Atrial: 72
         Ventricular: 72
   2. Rhythm:
         Atrial: Regular, irregular with long pause
         Ventricular: Regular, irregular with long pause
   3. P waves: Present; all with the same morphology
   4. PR interval: 0.12 second
   5. Ratio of P/QRS: 1 : 1
   6. QRS interval: 0.08 second
   7. QT interval: 0.30 second
   8. Interpretation: Normal sinus rhythm with second-degree sinoatrial block, type II; there is a 6-second interruption in the sinus cycle; when the P wave returns, it is a 7 : 1 multiple of the regular PP cycle
O. Fig. 2-29.
   1. Rate:
         Atrial: 40
         Ventricular: 40
   2. Rhythm:
         Atrial: Regular
         Ventricular: Regular
   3. P waves: Present; all with the same morphology
   4. PR interval: 0.14 second
   5. Ratio of P/QRS: 1 : 1
   6. QRS interval: 0.08 second
   7. QT interval: 0.30 second
   8. Interpretation: Sinus bradycardia
P. Fig. 2-30.
   1. Rate:
         Atrial: 120
         Ventricular: 120
   2. Rhythm:
         Atrial: Regular
         Ventricular: Regular
   3. P waves: Present; all with the same morphology
   4. PR interval: 0.14 second

5. Ratio of P/QRS: 1:1
6. QRS interval: 0.08 second
7. QT interval: 0.28 second
8. Interpretation: Sinus tachycardia; the S-T segment is depressed

Q. Fig. 2-31.
  1. Rate:
     Atrial: 60
     Ventricular: 60
  2. Rhythm:
     Atrial: Irregular
     Ventricular: Irregular
  3. P waves: Present; all with the same morphology
  4. PR interval: 0.14 second
  5. Ratio of P/QRS: 1:1
  6. QRS interval: 0.08 second
  7. QT interval: 0.30 second
  8. Interpretation: Sinus arrhythmia; the rate speeds with inspiration and slows with exhalation

R. Fig. 2-32.
  1. Rate:
     Atrial: 110
     Ventricular: 110
  2. Rhythm:
     Atrial: Regular
     Ventricular: Regular
  3. P waves: Present; all with the same morphology
  4. PR interval: 0.10 second
  5. Ratio of P/QRS: 1:1
  6. QRS interval: 0.06 second
  7. QT interval: 0.20 second
  8. Interpretation: Sinus tachycardia; the PR interval and QT interval are short; there is 60-cycle interference present (wavy baseline)

S. Fig. 2-33.
  1. Rate:
     Atrial: 90
     Ventricular: 90
  2. Rhythm:
     Atrial: Regular
     Ventricular: Regular
  3. P waves: Present; flat and biphasic but all with the same morphology
  4. PR interval: 0.14 second
  5. Ratio of P/QRS: 1:1
  6. QRS interval: 0.06 second
  7. QT interval: 0.40 second
  8. Interpretation: Normal sinus rhythm

T. Fig. 2-34.
  1. Rate:
     Atrial: 72/slows to 20 during pause
     Ventricular: 72/slows to 20 during pause
  2. Rhythm:
     Atrial: Regular-irregular wth pause
     Ventricular: Regular-irregular with pause
  3. P waves: Present; all with the same morphology
  4. PR interval: 0.14 second
  5. Ratio of P/QRS: 1:1
  6. QRS interval: 0.08 second
  7. QT interval: 0.30 second
  8. Interpretation: Normal sinus rhythm evolving to sinus pause or arrest, returning to normal sinus rhythm; sinus impulse slows and does not fire for almost 5 seconds; when the P wave returns, it is not a direct multiple of the regular PP interval

Atrial dysrhythmias

PRETEST (Answers on p. 82)

Directions: Circle one answer to each question unless otherwise indicated.

A. Premature atrial complexes can be caused by (circle all that apply):
1. Myocardial ischemia
2. Tobacco and caffeine
3. Digitalis therapy
4. Hypoxia

B. Premature atrial complexes are:
1. Dangerous because they compromise cardiac output
2. Significant because they may precede a more serious dysrhythmia
3. Significant only in that they cause anxiety in the patient
4. Insignificant and never require treatment

C. A dysrhythmia that occurs most frequently in paroxysms is atrial:
1. Premature complex
2. Tachycardia
3. Flutter
4. Fibrillation

D. Drugs most commonly used in the treatment of atrial dysrhythmias include:
1. Digitalis, procainamide, lidocaine
2. Disopyramide, procainamide, propranolol
3. Propranolol, verapamil, ethmozine
4. Verapamil, propranolol, digitalis

E. A serious complication of chronic atrial fibrillation is:
1. Heart failure
2. Pulmonary edema
3. Systemic or pulmonary emboli
4. Renal ischemia

F. Symptoms that may be experienced by a patient who suddenly develops atrial fibrillation with a ventricular rate of 160 include (circle all that apply):
1. Palpitations
2. Dyspnea
3. Hypotension
4. Angina

G. DC cardioversion is a term that refers to:
1. Conversion of a dysrhythmia to normal sinus rhythm using antidysrhythmic drugs
2. Termination of ventricular fibrillation with electric shock
3. Conversion of a dysrhythmia to normal sinus rhythm using electric shock
4. Pacing the atria at a rapid rate to terminate a dysrhythmia

H. Individuals with prosthetic heart valves:
1. Are at no greater risk for complications associated with tachydysrhythmias
2. Do not tolerate tachydysrhythmias well and tend to deteriorate rapidly
3. Tolerate tachydysrhythmias as well as other patients
4. Do not frequently experience atrial tachydysrhythmias

I. The rate and rhythm in Fig. 3-1 can best be described as:
1. Approximately 60 and regular
2. Approximately 60 and regularly irregular
3. Approximately 60 and irregularly irregular
4. Approximately 80 and irregular

J. P waves in Fig. 3-1:
1. Are present before every QRS complex
2. Are not identifiable
3. Vary in size and shape
4. Are not consistently present before each QRS complex

K. The rhythm in Fig. 3-1 is:
1. Sinus arrhythmia
2. Wandering atrial pacemaker (atrial escape complex)
3. Atrial flutter
4. Atrial fibrillation

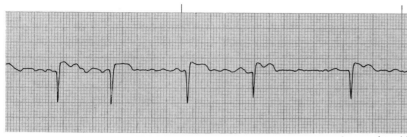

FIG. 3-1　　　　　　　　　　　　　　　　　　　Lead II

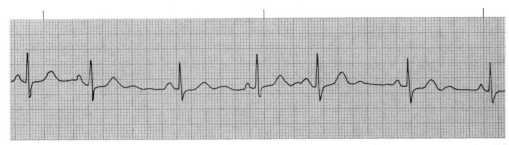

FIG. 3-2　　　　　　　　　　　　　　　　　　　Lead II

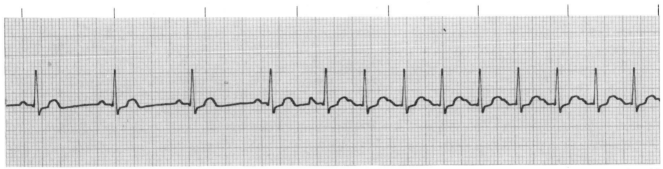

FIG. 3-3　　　　　　　　　　　　　　　　　　　Lead II

L. The rhythm in Fig. 3-2 is:
  1. Normal sinus rhythm
  2. Sinus arrhythmia
  3. Sinus rhythm with premature atrial complexes
  4. Wandering atrial pacemaker (atrial escape complex)

M. The distance between the R waves of the first and third complexes in Fig. 3-2 is called:
  1. Compensatory pause
  2. Noncompensatory pause

N. Drug therapy for the dysrhythmia in Fig. 3-2 may include (circle all that apply):
  1. Disopyramide
  2. Verapamil
  3. Quinidine
  4. Propranolol

O. The rhythm in Fig. 3-3 is:
  1. Sinus rhythm with paroxysmal atrial tachycardia
  2. Sinus arrhythmia
  3. Sinus rhythm with premature atrial complexes
  4. Wandering atrial pacemaker (atrial escape complex)

P. The rhythm in Fig. 3-3:
  1. Can occur as a normal phenomenon in young adults
  2. Is common in athletes with slow heart rates
  3. Often occurs as the result of increased catecholamines
  4. Usually is undetected because the individual is asymptomatic

Q. Matching: Complete the statement in Column A with the correct term in Column B.

Column A	Column B
___ 1. The fastest atrial rate occurs in	a. Atrial paroxysmal tachycardia
___ 2. Noncompensatory pause occurs with	b. Atrial fibrillation
___ 3. A common dysrhythmia in athletes	c. Wandering atrial pacemaker
___ 4. Carotid sinus massage is indicated as treatment in	d. Premature atrial complex

PURPOSE

The purpose of this module is to assist the learner in identifying the atrial dysrhythmias, recognizing signs and symptoms presented by the patient, and planning nursing approaches for patients experiencing these dysrhythmias.

BEHAVIORAL OBJECTIVES

Upon completion of this module, the learner should be able to:
A. List possible etiological factors of, define and identify criteria for, recognize on rhythm strips, state clinical features of, and discuss modes of treatment and nursing management for the following dysrhythmias:
1. Premature atrial complex
2. Atrial tachycardia
3. Atrial flutter
4. Atrial fibrillation
5. Wandering atrial pacemaker (atrial escape complex/rhythm)

VOCABULARY

Active rhythm A rhythm initiated by a premature complex (one occurring early in the regular cycle) that continues at a rate faster than the normal pacemaker and usurps control of the heart rhythm.

Automaticity An electrical property that permits spontaneous initiation of the cardiac impulse.

Bigeminy A term used to describe two successive complexes, one normal and one ectopic, which repetitively occur as couplets.

Cadence The flow or beat of a rhythm as in music or dancing.

Cardioversion Direct electrical current that is synchronized to be delivered on the R wave of the ECG by paddles applied to the chest; used in order to terminate a tachydysrhythmia.

Compensatory pause A type of pause that occurs after a premature beat. If the interval measured between the R wave of the beat *preceding* the premature beat and the R wave of the beat *following* it is *equal to twice* that of the RR interval between the two normal beats, then the pause is fully compensatory. This occurs when the premature beat does not interrupt the sinus node cycle.

Ectopic Refers to an impulse that originates outside the sinus node.

Escape complex/rhythm A rhythm that is initiated by a lower pacemaker when the sinus node slows or fails. Usually preceded by a pause, it is also termed a *passive* rhythm or a rhythm by *default.*

Extrasystole A premature complex arising from a ectopic focus.

"f" waves Fine, undulating fibrillatory waves seen on the ECG in atrial fibrillation.

"F" waves Coarse flutter waves with a distinct sawtooth configuration seen on the ECG in atrial flutter.

Fibrillation Rapid, chaotic, unsynchronized quivering or twitching of the myocardium in which no effective pumping occurs.

Multifocal A term referring to ectopic impulses that originate in different foci.

Noncompensatory pause A delay in ventricular systole, following a premature contraction, which resets the sinus cadence. If the interval measured between the R wave of the beat *preceding* the premature beat and the R wave of the beat *following* it is *less than twice* that of the RR interval between two normal beats, the pause is noncompensatory. This occurs when the premature beat interrupts the sinus node cycle.

Overdrive pacing The use of a pacemaker for the purpose of artifically stimulating the heart at a rate faster than its intrinsic rate in order to suppress an abnormal tachydysrhythmia.

Paroxysmal A term referring to a dysrhythmia with sudden onset and termination that recurs periodically.

P' (P prime) wave A term used to describe a P wave that differs in shape from the sinus P wave because the impulse originates outside the sinus node.

Refractory A period during which fibers are unresponsive to a stimulus.

Retrograde conduction Impulse conduction that occurs in a backward direction.

Sympathomimetic Mimicking the effects of sympathetic nerve stimulation.

Trigeminy A term used to describe three successive complexes, normal and ectopic, which repetitively occur in triplets.

Unifocal A term referring to ectopic impulses that originate in the same pacemaker site.

CONTENT
Suggested review

Before beginning this module on atrial dysrhythmias, it is recommended that the learner review the following:
1. Gross anatomy of the heart and conduction system with specific attention to the atria, SA node, and AV junction
2. Nervous innervation of the SA node, atria, and AV junction
3. Calculation of heart rate on ECG paper
4. Calculation of waveforms
5. Normal duration of PR, QRS, and QT intervals
6. Analytical approach to interpretation of an ECG strip

Rhythm disturbances
PREMATURE ATRIAL COMPLEX (PAC)
Definition

PAC is an atrial complex occurring: 1) early in relation to the basic sinus rate and 2) as a result of an ectopic stimulus originating anywhere in the atria other than the SA node.[3,13]

Etiology

PACs frequently occur in individuals with normal hearts as a result of emotions, stress, and the consumption of alcohol, caffeine, or tobacco. Stimulation of the sympathetic nervous system increases the automaticity of atrial tissue.[3,5]

PACs are frequently associated with rheumatic valvular heart disease and atrial hypertrophy, coronary artery disease and/or myocardial infarction with resulting ischemia, congestive heart failure with increased atrial pressure, toxic states such as sepsis and thyrotoxicosis, electrolyte imbalances, and hypoxia.[14]

PACs may also result from various pharmacological agents. Digitalis and antidysrhythmics such as quinidine and procainamide prolong the refractory period of the SA node, thereby allowing opportunity for premature atrial complexes.[5] Diuretics causing potassium depletion may enhance atrial irritability.

Characteristics of rhythm

1. Rate: The atrial rate is determined by the basic sinus rate and the number of PACs occurring each minute; the atrial and ventricular rates are equal (Fig. 3-4)
2. Rhythm: Irregular; degree of irregularity depends upon the number of PACs; if the PACs occur in a bigeminal (every other complex) (Fig. 3-5) or trigeminal pattern (every third complex) (Fig. 3-6), the

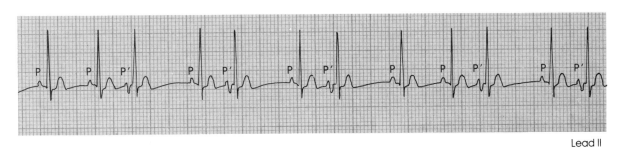

Lead II

FIG. 3-4

Premature atrial complexes (PACs). *P* indicates sinus node impulse.
P' indicates the premature atrial complex.

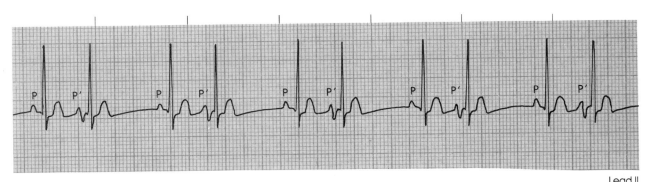

Lead II

FIG. 3-5

Premature atrial complexes in bigeminy.

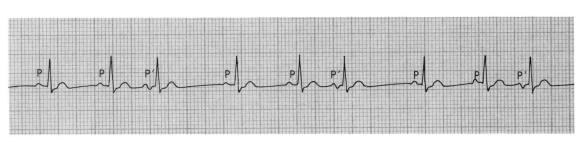

Lead II

FIG. 3-6

Premature atrial complexes in trigeminy.

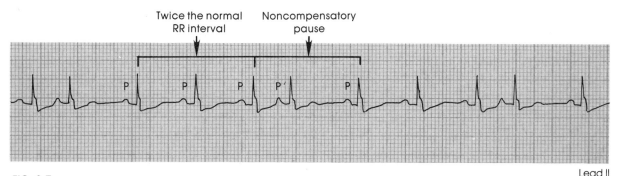

Twice the normal
RR interval

Noncompensatory
pause

Lead II

FIG. 3-7

Noncompensatory pause. RR interval between two sinus complexes
flanking premature atrial complex is less than twice normal RR
interval.

rhythm will be regularly irregular (NOTE: A hallmark
of this dysrhythmia is the presence of a *noncompensatory pause* after the PAC; the RR interval between the
two sinus complexes flanking the PAC is *less* than twice
the normal RR interval; this pause occurs when the SA
node is prematurely depolarized by the PAC resetting
its cycle[20] [Fig. 3-7])

3. P waves: The morphology of the P' wave in the PAC
   will differ from the sinus P wave because the P' wave is
   initiated by an ectopic focus; the P' can be upright,
   biphasic, or inverted depending on its location in the
   atria (Fig. 3-8):
   a. If it is upright, it may be difficult to distinguish it
      from the sinus P wave
   b. If it is inverted, it may be impossible to distinguish
      it from a premature junctional complex (PJC) (see
      the Junctional Dysrhythmias Module)
   c. If the premature complex occurs very early, the P'
      wave will be superimposed on the T wave of the
      preceding complex, thereby distorting its shape,
      rather than being seen as a separate wave[14,15]
4. PR interval: P'R interval of the PAC is usually within
   normal limits; however, it can vary:
   a. If the AV junction is partially refractory when the
      impulse reaches it, conduction will be delayed and
      the P'R interval will be prolonged
   b. If the ectopic focus is located low in the atria close
      to the AV junction, transmission will occur faster
      than normal and the P'R interval will be shorter
      than the PR interval of the sinus complex[15]
5. Ratio of P/QRS: 1:1
6. QRS interval: Within normal limits; the morphology
   of the QRS resembles that of the sinus complexes
   because conduction through the ventricles is usually
   not altered
7. QT interval: Within normal limits

Clinical features

Patients are generally unaware of infrequent PACs. As
the frequency increases, the patient may sense palpitations
but usually remains asymptomatic.

Treatment measures

1. Infrequent PACs usually require no treatment
2. In the absence of heart disease, frequent PACs that are
   disturbing to the patient may be treated by eliminating
   the cause; tranquilizers and/or the omission of all
   stimulants (caffeine, alcohol, and tobacco) can be
   adequate

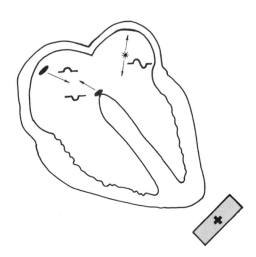

FIG. 3-8

P wave morphology depends on location of the ectopic focus. Impulses arising near SA node are conducted through atria in relatively
normal fashion, producing a P' wave that closely resembles sinus P
wave. Ectopic foci in other areas of atria can produce biphasic P'
waves because the impulse is conducted in opposite directions simultaneously. When an ectopic focus is located in or near AV junction, retrograde conduction occurs, producing inverted P' in leads II,
III, aV$_F$.

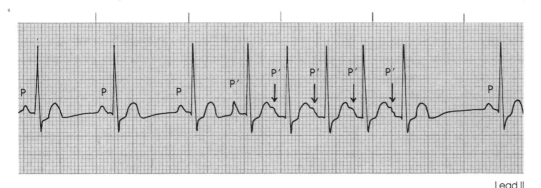

Lead II

FIG. 3-9
Paroxysmal atrial tachycardia (PAT). Burst of atrial tachycardia begins abruptly with premature atrial complex, continues for only a few seconds, and ends abruptly. Ventricular rate during this short paroxysm is approximately 150.

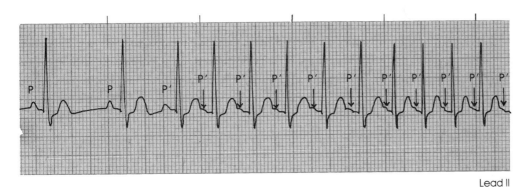

Lead II

FIG. 3-10
Atrial tachycardia beginning with premature atrial complex and continuing at a rate of 180. P' waves can be seen on downslope of T waves.

3. In the presence of heart disease or in symptomatic patients, excessive PACs may be treated with quinidine or procainamide, which prolong atrial refractoriness; propranolol and verapamil may also be used[20]

Nursing management

Assess any symptoms related to the dysrhythmia.

ATRIAL TACHYCARDIA (Figs. 3-9 and 3-10)
Definition

This atrial dysrhythmia is characterized by a minimum of three or more successive ectopic atrial complexes occurring at a rate of 160 to 250 per minute.[13,15] There is usually 1 : 1 conduction of the ectopic impulse, producing a ventricular rate equal to the atrial rate.

The rhythm begins abruptly with a premature atrial complex, continues for a variable length of time (seconds, hours, or days), and ends abruptly. Because of these characteristics and its tendency to recur at intervals, it is commonly termed *paroxysmal atrial tachycardia* (PAT).

There are two mechanisms thought to be responsible for generating atrial tachycardia: (1) an *extrasystolic* or *automatic* mechanism that results from enhanced automaticity of an ectopic atrial focus and (2) a *reentry* mechanism that is caused by the repetitive circus movement of a single ectopic impulse through the conduction system.[6,10,14] Although electrophysiological studies reveal reentry as the more common cause of atrial tachycardia, discussion of reentry phenomenon is reserved for the more advanced learner.

Extrasystolic atrial tachycardia occurs when an ectopic focus situated anywhere in the atria discharges repeatedly at a rate faster than that of the sinus node. Because of its inherent rate (160 to 250), the atrial focus suppresses the sinus node and becomes the pacemaker, resulting in tachycardia.[14]

Etiology

Extrasystolic atrial tachycardia can be seen in all age groups and is generally thought to be associated with disease or drugs. Hypoxia, alkalosis, stretch of the atria, increased catecholamines (endogenous or exogenous), hypokalemia, and digitalis intoxication may all be precipitating factors in the onset of this dysrhythmia. Clinically it can be seen in patients after myocardial infarction, with cardiomyopathies and congenital heart disease (particularly atrial septal defects), as well as secondary to chronic lung disease (especially with acute infection), hyperthyroidism, systemic hypertension, and acute alcohol ingestion.[10,20]

Characteristics of rhythm

1. Rate: The atrial rate ranges from 160 to 250 per minute with 180 to 200 being most common; there may be gradual acceleration of the rate after the onset of the tachycardia; there is usually 1:1 AV conduction producing a ventricular rate equal to the atrial rate[8]
2. Rhythm: At the onset of the tachycardia, the rhythm may be irregular because of gradual acceleration of the rate; however, the rhythm is usually perfectly regular throughout the paroxysm; the rhythm may again become irregular at the termination of the tachycardia as the sinus node attempts to regain pacemaker function
3. P waves: Because the atrial focus is ectopic, the P' wave of the initial complex in the paroxysm differs in shape from the sinus P wave; the initial and subsequent P' waves all have the same abnormal configuration because they are generated by the same focus;[10] however, when the rate is rapid, subsequent P' waves usually merge with the preceding T waves and cannot be identified; without a visible P' wave, atrial tachycardia cannot be distinguished from junctional tachycardia (see the Junctional Dysrhythmias Module) and is then called *supraventricular tachycardia*[13]
4. PR interval: The P'R interval can be normal, short, or prolonged, depending on the rate and the refractoriness of the AV node; the P'R interval is constant throughout the paroxysm but cannot be measured when the P' waves are merged with the T waves of the preceding complex
5. Ratio of P/QRS: 1:1, but may not be seen
6. QRS interval: Within normal limits; the morphology of the QRS resembles that of the sinus complex
7. QT interval: Within normal limits

Clinical features

Symptoms depend on the heart rate during the attack, the duration of the dysrhythmia, and the presence or absence of organic heart disease. Generally, the individual is aware of the sudden onset of palpitations, which evokes nervousness and anxiety. Weakness, dizziness, diaphoresis, sweating, pallor, shortness of breath, and hypotension may rapidly develop because of decreased cardiac output related to the rapid ventricular rate.

Coronary artery blood flow is reduced approximately 25% during atrial tachycardia[1]; therefore, individuals with coronary artery or myocardial disease may rapidly develop angina and/or congestive heart failure. Individuals without cardiac disease may also develop congestive heart failure if the tachycardia persists for a prolonged period of time.[3] Therefore, efforts should be made to promptly terminate the dysrhythmia.

Treatment measures

The urgency of treatment measures depends on a history of the frequency and duration of attacks, the presence of circulatory collapse, congestive heart failure or angina, and the presence of heart disease. In some individuals the attack may be terminated with physical rest, reassurance, and/or sedation. Many attacks terminate spontaneously.

It is important to distinguish atrial tachycardia according to its mechanism of origin (extrasystolic vs. reentry) in order to treat it effectively. Physiological vagal maneuvers (carotid sinus massage, Valsalva, eyeball pressure) and pharmacological vagomimetic agents (pressor drugs), which have historically been the hallmark of treatment, more recently have been found to be ineffective in terminating extrasystolic atrial tachycardia because there is a lack of vagal influence on atrial tissue.[10] In a clinically emergent situation, however, this differentiation may not be possible. A practical approach to terminating the dysrhythmia is as follows (Fig. 3-11):

1. Vagal maneuvers (unilateral carotid sinus massage, Valsalva, gagging, and coughing) can initially be tried if the patient is monitored and a physician is present. Although eyeball pressure is often recommended, the danger of ophthalmic injury must be considered.

   Extrasystolic atrial tachycardia will usually not be affected by vagal maneuvers. Therefore, if the tachycardia persists, other treatment measures should be employed.
2. Verapamil, a calcium-channel blocking agent, is currently the I.V. pharmacological agent of choice for paroxysmal atrial tachycardia.[11] It has been found to be effective in terminating 66% of atrial tachycardias caused by the extrasystolic mechanism[17] and 90% to 100% of those caused by the reentry phenomenon.[16,18]

   By inhibiting the influx of calcium ions into cells

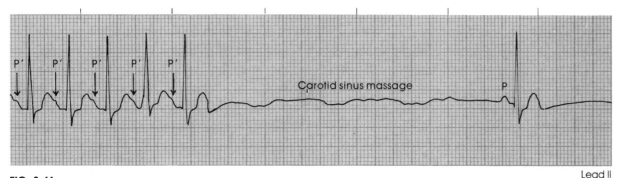

FIG. 3-11

Atrial tachycardia terminated by carotid sinus massage with restoration of normal sinus rhythm.

Lead II

during depolarization, the refractory period of the SA node and AV junction is prolonged and conduction of impulses is slowed. If verapamil fails to terminate the tachycardia, it may at least be successful in slowing the ventricular rate.

If vagal maneuvers and verapamil are unsuccessful in terminating the tachycardia, the mechanism of origin is most likely to be extrasystolic. In this case, the following treatment plan should be considered:

3. At this point, the clinical status of the patient should be assessed and cardioversion considered before the administration of digitalis or propranolol.

4. Propranolol is effective in inhibiting the effect of circulating catecholamines at beta-adrenergic receptor sites, resulting in decreased automaticity of ectopic foci and increased AV block. It is useful in treating atrial tachycardia associated with hyperthyroidism, anxiety states, and digitalis intoxication.[2]

    The patient must be attached to a monitor during I.V. administration of propranolol in order to observe for bradycardia, conduction disturbances, and asystole. Atropine should be readily available to counteract bradycardia.

5. In the absence of digitalis intoxication, I.V. digitalis is indicated. Its vagal properties decrease the automaticity of the ectopic atrial focus and increase the refractory period of the AV junction resulting in slowing of the ventricular response. Once AV block is induced, drugs that primarily decrease atrial automaticity such as quinidine, procainamide, and disopyramide can be given in attempt to convert to sinus rhythm.[10,20]

6. If atrial tachycardia develops in the patient on digitalis, it should be considered the causative factor and discontinued.[20] Withdrawal of the drug and correction of hypokalemia with I.V. or oral potassium supplements are often adequate if the tachycardia rate is not excessive and the patient is asymptomatic. If the patient is symptomatic and rapid termination of the tachycardia is necessary, I.V. administration of phenytoin and propranolol can be very effective in abolishing digitalis-induced automaticity.[20]

7. Overdrive pacing in attempt to suppress the ectopic focus has not been reported to be successful in termining extrasystolic atrial tachycardia.[20]

8. Prevention of extrasystolic atrial tachycardia is difficult. Initially, attempts should be made to control extracardiac factors suspected of contributing to the dysrhythmia. If the frequency and severity of episodes warrant prophylaxis, digitalis alone or in combination with quinidine, procainamide, or propranolol may be used.

Nursing management

Nursing interventions depend on the severity of the patient's symptoms. The following should be considered:

1. Maintain bedrest with the head of the bed flat if tolerated; this position enhances venous return and thereby assists in increasing cardiac output; symptoms of lightheadedness, dizziness, and syncope can be decreased

2. Record vital signs and continue to monitor at 15-minute intervals or more frequently if indicated; neurovital signs are important indicators of cerebral function and should be recorded after an attack as well as pre- and postcardioversion

3. Attach the patient to a cardiac monitor, document the rhythm on a rhythm strip, and record pertinent information in the nurse's notes

4. Do not leave the patient alone if possible; depending on the symptoms that occur during this dysrhythmia, the patient may become extremely anxious; explanations and reassurance are important

5. Continue to observe for hypotension, signs of congestive heart failure, and angina

6. Administer oxygen if indicated
7. If blood pressure begins to drop, start an I.V. of D5W at a keep-open rate in order to maintain venous access for pharmacological agents
8. Have emergency drugs immediately available
9. Maintain a quiet environment; eliminate stimuli such as television and visitors
10. If the attack persists, consider changing the patient's diet order to liquids to prevent nausea and vomiting

Special considerations

1. Patients with prosthetic heart valves tolerate tachydysrhythmias poorly and may quickly develop congestive heart failure following the onset of the dysrhythmia. Patients with a recent myocardial infarction may experience angina, extend the infarct, or develop congestive heart failure. These patients must be observed continuously and all measures must be employed to quickly terminate the dysrhythmia.
2. During a tachycardia, diastole is shortened and coronary blood flow is reduced. Depression of the ST segment and inversion of the T wave may occur during and after the tachycardia as a result of myocardial ischemia. This is known as *posttachycardia syndrome*. A sustained tachycardia can produce this syndrome, which, depending on the extent of existing cardiac disease, may last for hours or days.[3,13]

ATRIAL FLUTTER (Fig. 3-12)
Definition

Atrial flutter is a supraventricular dysrhythmia characterized by rapid, regular depolarization of the atria at a rate of 250 to 350 per minute,[20] producing sawtooth configurations on the ECG known as "F" (flutter) waves.

Like atrial tachycardia, there are two mechanisms thought to be responsible for generating atrial flutter: 1) enhanced *automaticity* of an ectopic atrial focus (similar to extrasystolic atrial tachycardia but at a faster rate) and 2) *reentry* caused by circus movement of the impulse through the atrial myocardium.[3,15]

Atrial flutter tends to be an unstable rhythm and converts to normal sinus rhythm or progresses to atrial fibrillation within a relatively short period of time.[20]

Etiology

Atrial flutter usually occurs in the presence of acute or chronic heart disease. Pathological causes include coronary artery disease, myocardial infarction, pulmonary embolism, pericarditis, infective endocarditis, chronic pulmonary disease or infection, rheumatic heart disease (particularly mitral stenosis), and hyperthyroidism. The dysrhythmia may also develop as a result of digitalis intoxication or be seen as a transitory rhythm when atrial fibrillation is treated with antidysrhythmic drugs. As the atrial rate in fibrillation slows, it may convert to atrial flutter.

Characteristics of rhythm

1. Rate: The atrial rate is 250 to 350 per minute with 300 being the most common[20]; because the refractory time of the AV junction is longer than that of the atria, 1:1 conduction of the atrial impulses to the ventricles is generally impossible; therefore, the ventricular rate directly depends on the degree of AV conduction
2. Rhythm: Regularity of the ventricular rhythm depends on the degree of conduction through the AV junction
   a. If the ratio of atrial flutter waves to ventricular conduction is constant (i.e., 4:1, 3:1, 2:1), the ventricular rhythm will be regular (see Fig. 3-12)

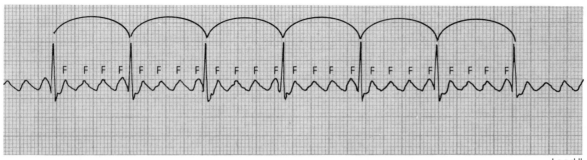

Lead II

FIG. 3-12
Atrial flutter. Distinct sawtooth flutter ("F") waves are readily visible. In this rhythm strip, ratio of "F" waves to QRS is constant and ventricular rhythm is regular.

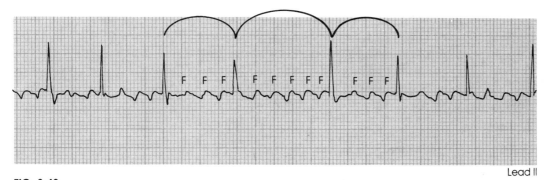

Lead II

FIG. 3-13

Atrial flutter. Distinct "F" waves are visible. Ratio of "F" waves to QRS varies from 3:1 to 5:1, producing irregular ventricular rhythm.

b. However, if the ratio of conduction varies (i.e., from 4:1 to 2:1 to 6:1), the ventricular rhythm will be irregular[15] (Fig. 3-13)

3. P waves: Sinus P waves are replaced by atrial flutter waves or "F" waves, which are the hallmark of this dysrhythmia; "F" waves are distinct, regular, sawtooth waves that can be peaked, rounded, or notched in shape; they are usually best visualized in leads II, III, aV_f and V_1[15,20]

4. PR interval: Unable to determine

5. Ratio of P/QRS: The ratio of "F" waves to QRS can be determined and varies according to the refractoriness of the AV junction; even ratios (2:1, 4:1, 6:1) are more common than odd ratios (3:1, 5:1); often the ratio varies[15] (see Fig. 3-13)

6. QRS interval: Within normal limits

7. QT interval: Unable to determine because T waves are lost in the "F" waves

Clinical features

Clinical symptoms depend on the ventricular rate. If the rate is slow (less than 100), the patient will probably be asymptomatic and unaware of the dysrhythmia. Rapid ventricular rates may be accompanied by a sensation of palpitations and anxiety. In the presence of cardiac disease, the patient may experience shortness of breath, diaphoresis, hypotension, angina, and/or congestive heart failure.

Treatment measures

1. The initial treatment for atrial flutter, particularly when the ventricular rate is rapid and the patient is symptomatic, is cardioversion. Atrial flutter often can be terminated by delivering a low-energy stimulus (<50 joules)[20] to the myocardium that interrupts the circus movement of the ectopic focus in the atria and allows the sinus node to regain pacemaker function. With cardioversion, however, the possibility of converting the atrial flutter to atrial fibrillation always exists. Fibrillation can then be converted to normal sinus rhythm with subsequent shocks at a higher energy level or treated pharmacologically.

2. In a nonemergent situation, rapid atrial pacing has been found to be very successful in terminating atrial flutter.[19]

3. If electrical cardioversion is unsuccessful or contraindicated, drug therapy is instituted. The primary goal of therapy is to slow the ventricular rate by increasing the refractory period of the AV junction. Historically, I.V. digitalis preparations have been used successfully. Currently I.V. verapamil is recommended; however, its effects are short-lived and continuous infusion is required.[17] Occasionally, atrial flutter of recent onset will convert to sinus rhythm with the administration of verapamil alone.[20] The beta-blocking effect of propranolol is also effective in prolonging AV conduction and slowing the ventricular rate. Like verapamil, propranolol has not been observed to have any effect on the flutter rate.[17,20]

4. Once the ventricular response is controlled, the second goal of drug therapy is to abolish the ectopic atrial focus and restore normal sinus rhythm. Treatment of the underlying disorder is necessary in addition to drugs that increase the refractory period of atrial fibers. Quinidine is most commonly used but procainamide and disopyramide are also effective. However, these drugs facilitate AV conduction and can produce 1:1 conduction if the patient has not received adequate doses of verapamil, digitalis, or propranolol.

5. Because atrial flutter tends to be an unstable rhythm, prophylaxis is usually not practical.

Totally irregular ventricular rhythm

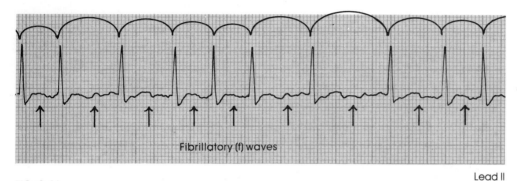

Fibrillatory (f) waves

Lead II

FIG. 3-14

Atrial fibrillation. P waves are replaced by fine fibrillatory ("f") waves. Totally irregular ventricular response is characteristic of this dysrhythmia.

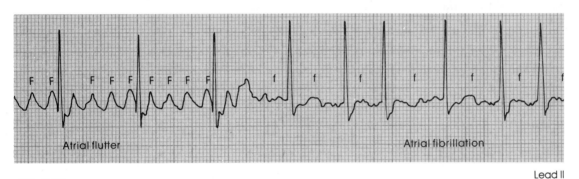

Atrial flutter   Atrial fibrillation

Lead II

FIG. 3-15

Distinct sawtooth "F" waves of atrial flutter seen at beginning of this strip progress to fine fibrillatory "f" waves of atrial fibrillation as atrial rate increases.

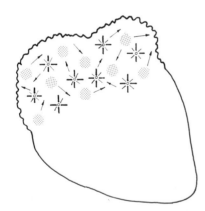

FIG. 3-16

In atrial fibrillation there is chaotic discharge of impulses simultaneously from numerous atrial foci. Most impulses collide with each other in transit through the atria. Only few reach AV junction. Conduction through to the ventricles depends on refractoriness of AV junction and is totally irregular.

Nursing management

Refer to Atrial tachycardia.

ATRIAL FIBRILLATION (Figs. 3-14, 3-15, and 3-16)
Definition

This rhythm is characterized by the chaotic discharge of impulses from numerous atrial foci at a rate of greater than 350 per minute. Electrical activity of the atria is recorded on the ECG as irregular undulations of varying shape and amplitude known as "f" waves. The absence of P waves and a totally irregular ventricular response are the hallmarks of this dysrhythmia.

Atrial fibrillation has been observed to be initiated by a single premature atrial complex or to develop from the progression of atrial flutter.[12] It is thought that the two mechanisms involved in the production of atrial flutter, enhanced automaticity and reentry, are also involved in atrial fibrillation. Maintenance of the fibrillation, however, seems to be favored when there is an enlarged mass of atrial tissue, usually as a result of increased left atrial pressure.[15] The stretch of atrial tissue alters conduction and/or refractory times and contributes to the propagation of the fibrillation.[5]

Fibrillation waves are erratically conducted through the AV junction to the ventricles. Some atrial impulses collide with each other in transit through the atria and are cancelled before they reach the AV junction (see Fig. 3-16). Other impulses arrive at the junction during its refractory period and are blocked. Only those impulses that arrive at the junction when it is completely repolarized are conducted through to the ventricles. Conduction of fibrillatory waves through the AV junction, therefore, is highly variable and accounts for the totally irregular ventricular rhythm.[20] The irregular rhythm also affects ventricular filling and stroke volume.[14]

Etiology

Short paroxysms of atrial fibrillation may occur in the absence of heart disease. Chronic fibrillation, however, is almost always seen in the presence of diseases such as:
1. Coronary artery disease
2. Hypertensive heart disease
3. Rheumatic heart disease (particularly mitral stenosis with left atrial enlargement)
4. Congenital heart disease (atrial septal defect)
5. Pericarditis
6. Cardiomyopathy
7. Pulmonary hypertension
8. Chronic obstructive pulmonary disease

Following cardiac surgery, atrial fibrillation as well as other atrial or ventricular dysrhythmias may occur as a result of transient hypokalemia and hypoxia. Thyrotoxicosis should always be considered as a possible cause of atrial fibrillation in a young person without heart disease.

Characteristics of rhythm

1. Rate: The atrial rate exceeds 350 per minute but is impossible to calculate; the ventricular rate depends entirely upon the degree of AV conduction; in patients with normal AV conduction, the ventricular rate with untreated atrial fibrillation is most commonly 100 to 160 per minute[20]; when the refractory period of the AV node is increased with pharmacological agents, AV conduction is decreased and the ventricular rate slows
2. Rhythm: The hallmark of atrial fibrillation is the totally irregular (irregularly irregular) ventricular rhythm; the rhythm may appear regular when the ventricular response is either very rapid or very slow
3. P waves: The absence of P waves is the key to the diagnosis of atrial fibrillation; in their place, atrial fibrillatory waves ("f" waves) are inscribed on the ECG as irregular undulations of varying shape and amplitude often best seen in leads II and V_1[14]; coarse fibrillation may resemble flutter waves; fine fibrillation may not be seen and appear only to be an isolectric line (often both are seen in the same tracing and the terms "flutter/fibrillation," "impure flutter," or "flutteration" have been used)
4. PR interval: Nonexistent
5. Ratio of P/QRS: Nonexistent; the ratio of "f" waves/QRS cannot be determined
6. QRS interval: Within normal limits
7. QT interval: Cannot be determined

Clinical features

Clinical symptoms depend on the ventricular rate. In rapid fibrillation, a 40% reduction in coronary artery blood flow has been demonstrated,[1] which, if sustained, can result in angina, congestive heart failure, and myocardial infarction. In addition, loss of atrial contraction results in a 20% to 30% decrease in ventricular end-diastolic volume.[5] Subsequent decreased cardiac output is manifested by hypotension, dyspnea, diaphoresis, and cerebral ischemic symptoms such as confusion, dizziness, blurred vision, and syncope. Renal blood flow has also been documented to decrease approximately 20% with resulting ischemia or renal damage if the tachydysrhythmia continues for a prolonged period of time.[9]

When the ventricular response rate is adequately controlled (less than 100) with pharmacological agents, the individual is usually symptom-free, unaware of the dysrhythmia, and capable of carrying on with activities of daily living.

The most common and feared clinical problem associated with chronic atrial fibrillation is pulmonary or systemic arterial embolization. The lack of synchronous atrial contraction promotes stasis of blood and thrombus formation. Friable clots unpredictably dislodge and travel in the circulation, most commonly producing stroke. The highest incidence of stroke (40%) has been found in individuals with atrial fibrillation secondary to rheumatic and ischemic heart disease.[7]

Treatment measures

Like the treatment for atrial flutter, the goal of therapy is to 1) control the ventricular response and 2) restore normal sinus rhythm if possible. Attempts should be made to identify and treat the underlying cause. If the precipitating factor cannot be appropriately or adequately treated (i.e., atrial enlargement), it is unlikely that the fibrillation can be converted to a sinus rhythm.

The patient's clinical status generally dictates the proper approach to treatment.
1. If the onset of atrial fibrillation is sudden and the

patient experiences hypotension or congestive heart failure as a result of the rapid ventricular rate, DC cardioversion should be the initial treatment to terminate the dysrhythmia abruptly. Rapid atrial pacing is ineffective in terminating atrial fibrillation.[20]

2. If the patient's clinical status has not deteriorated, treatment measures outlined under "Treatment of atrial flutter" (3 and 4) are used.

3. DC cardioversion may be attempted once the patient has received therapeutic dosages of quinidine. Adequate serum levels of quinidine reduce the amount of electrical energy required to restore normal sinus rhythm and assist in maintaining it following cardioversion. Digitalis is withheld for 24 to 48 hours before DC cardioversion to decrease the danger of precipitating serious ventricular dysrhythmias. Some physicians choose to anticoagulate patients at high risk for emboli for 2 weeks before and after cardioversion.[20]

4. It is possible that atrial fibrillation will not convert to sinus rhythm with either DC cardioversion or drug therapy, particularly if the underlying cause is left atrial enlargement. In those cases, the goal of drug therapy is to maintain the ventricular response at a resting rate of 60 to 80 per minute and not greater than 100 with exercise.[20] This is usually achieved with daily maintenance doses of digoxin. Quinidine, because it is ineffective except for use before attempted DC cardioversion, is not used.

5. Long-term anticoagulation therapy to reduce the incidence of emboli is controversial. Some physicians recommend it in patients at predictably high risk, such as those who have had previous emboli, atrial enlargement, and those who have a prosthetic mitral valve.

Nursing management

Refer to "Nursing management of atrial tachycardia" for interventions pertaining to patients with rapid atrial fibrillation.

1. Always count the apical rate for 1 full minute in patients with atrial fibrillation. As the ventricular rate increases, the pulse amplitude decreases and the peripheral pulse count becomes inaccurate.

2. Nonprofessional personnel should not be relied on to count rates of patients with atrial fibrillation. Irregular rhythms are tricky to count and require a professional ear to ensure accuracy.

3. The nurse must continuously be alert to complaints or signs and symptoms relating to pulmonary and/or systemic emboli in patients with atrial fibrillation.

Special considerations

1. Patients with prosthetic heart valves tolerate rapid irregular rhythms poorly. Atrial fibrillation in such individuals should be terminated as quickly as possible.

2. The longer atrial fibrillation is allowed to continue, the greater the chance of thrombi developing in the atria, which may then be released as pulmonic or systemic emboli upon conversion to normal sinus rhythm. For this reason individuals with long-standing atrial fibrillation or those with fibrillation of undetermined onset are *not* candidates for DC cardioversion.

WANDERING ATRIAL PACEMAKER (ATRIAL ESCAPE COMPLEX/RHYTHM) (Fig. 3-17)
Definition

Wandering atrial pacemaker refers to a rhythm characterized by a shifting or wandering of the pacemaker impulse from the SA node to other foci within the atrial

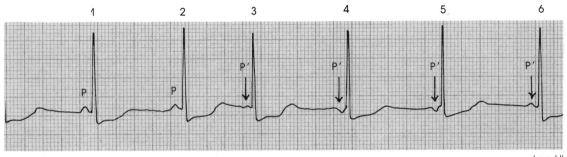

FIG. 3-17

Wandering atrial pacemaker (atrial escape complex). Sinus P waves are seen in first two complexes. Note change in morphology of P' waves as pacemaker impulse wanders to atria (3, 6) and AV junction (4, 5).

Lead II

tissue or AV node. Normally the SA node is the dominant pacemaker because it has the highest inherent rate. However, if the sinus rate slows (bradycardia) or if the transmission of the sinus impulse is blocked, impulses from slower potential pacemakers, specifically the atria and AV node, have the opportunity to discharge spontaneously. This discharge of a lower pacemaker is termed *escape complex* because it has "escaped" from the influence of the faster pacemaker, the SA node.[15] For the length of time the sinus impulses are depressed or blocked, the pacemaker impulse may wander to different foci within the atria and AV node, in which case it is termed an *atrial escape complex/rhythm*. Because this rhythm is a consequence of SA node failure, it is never a primary diagnosis.[15]

Etiology

Wandering atrial pacemaker (atrial escape complex/ rhythm) can be seen as a normal phenomenon in the very young or aged as the result of increased vagal stimulation or the effects of digitalis on the SA node. It is particularly common in athletes who maintain slow heart rates. Underlying heart disease should be suspected, however, if the pacemaker remains in the AV junction for long periods of time.[3]

Characteristics of rhythm

1. Rate: Overall the atrial rate is slow because it is an escape rhythm that occurs only when the sinus rate has slowed or failed; in general, as the pacemaker focus wanders away from the SA node toward the AV junction, the rate slows; conversely, as the focus wanders back toward the SA node, the rate increases; atrial and ventricular rates are equal; the change in rate between complexes may be minute and calculable only on a rhythm strip
2. Rhythm: The rhythm is irregular because of the change in pacemaker focus; the escape complex occurs *late* in relation to the normal PP cycle; the rhythm remains irregular as long as the pacemaker focus wanders; this irregularity is usually detected only on the rhythm strip and not in the peripheral pulse
3. P waves: As the pacemaker wanders to various foci, the morphology of the P′ wave varies (see Fig. 3-8):
   a. If the ectopic focus is close to the SA node, the impulse will be transmitted through the atria in relatively normal fashion and the P′ wave will closely resemble the morphology of the sinus P wave; at times it may be especially difficult to distinguish between P and P′ waves
   b. The farther away from the sinus node the ectopic focus is located, the greater the distortion of the P′

c. When the ectopic focus is located near the AV junction, the atrial impulse is conducted in retrograde fashion and an inverted P′ wave is seen in leads II, III, and aV_F
   d. Therefore, in wandering atrial pacemaker, P′ waves can be upright, bisphasic, or inverted
4. PR interval: Varies, shortening to 0.12 second or less as the pacemaker focus shifts closer to the AV junction
5. Ratio of P/QRS: 1:1
6. QRS interval: Within normal limits
7. QT interval: Within normal limits

Clinical features

The patient is unaware of the variation in heart rate and is asymptomatic. Alternate acceleration and slowing of the heart rate is usually not detected by apical auscultation or radial palpation.

Treatment measures

Because this dysrhythmia is a consequence of SA node dysfunction, it is usually not treated. Atropine may be used to treat the bradycardia. If the bradycardia persists and the patient becomes symptomatic, an artificial pacemaker may be required.

Nursing management

Observe the patient for signs and symptoms related to the bradycardia, such as fatigue, dyspnea on exertion, or dizziness. Report accordingly and plan nursing care activities as tolerated.

REFERENCES

1. Corday, E., et al.: Effect of the cardiac arrhythmias on coronary circulation, Ann. Intern. Med. **50**:535, 1959.
2. Gilman, A.G., et al.: The pharmacological basis of therapeutics, ed. 6, New York, 1980, Macmillan Publishing Co.
3. Goldman, M.: Principles of clinical electrocardiography, ed. 11, Los Altos, California, 1982, Lange Medical Publications.
4. Guyton, A.: Textbook of medical physiology, ed. 6, Philadelphia, 1981, W.B. Saunders Co.
5. Guzzetta, C., and Dossey, B.: Cardiovascular nursing: bodymind tapestry, St. Louis, 1984, The C.V. Mosby Co.
6. Han, J.: The mechanism of paroxysmal atrial tachycardia, Am. J. Cardiol. **26**:329, 1970.
7. Hinton, R.C., et al.: Influence of etiology of atrial fibrillation on incidence of systemic embolism, Am. J. Cardiol. **40**:509, 1977.
8. Hurst, J.W. and Myerburg, R.J.: Introduction to electrocardiography, ed. 2, New York, 1973, McGraw-Hill Inc.
9. Irving, D.W., and Corday, E.: Effect of cardiac arrhythmias on the renal and mesenteric circulation, Am. J. Cardiol. **8**:32, 1961.

10. Josephson, M.E., and Kastor, J.A.: Supraventricular tachycardia: mechanisms and management, Ann. Intern. Med. **87**:346, 1977.

11. Karlsberg, R.P.: Calcium channel blockers for cardiovascular disorders, Arch. Intern. Med. **142**:452, 1982.

12. Killip, T., and Gault, J.H.: Mode of onset of atrial fibrillation in man, Am. Heart J. **70**:172, 1965.

13. Marriott, H.J.L.: Practical electrocardiography, ed. 7, Baltimore, 1983, Williams & Wilkins.

14. McLachlan, E.M.: Fundamentals of electrocardiography, New York, 1981, Oxford University Press.

15. Schamroth, L.: An introduction to electrocardiography, ed. 6, Boston, 1980, Blackwell Scientific Publications.

16. Schamroth, L.: The clinical use of intravenous verapamil, Am. Heart J. **100**:1070, 1980.

17. Schwartz, D.J., et al.: Therapeutic uses of calcium-blocking agents: verapamil, nifedipine, and diltiazem, Compr. Ther. **7**:25, 1981.

18. Singh, B., et al.: New perspectives in the pharmacologic therapy of cardiac arrhythmias, Prog. Cardiovasc. Dis. **22**:243, 1980.

19. Watson, R.M., and Josephson, M.E.: Atrial flutter, I. Electrophysiologic substrates and modes of initiation and termination, Am. J. Cardiol. **45**:732, 1980.

20. Zipes, D.: Specific arrhythmias. In Braunwald, E., editor: Heart disease: a textbook of cardiovascular medicine, ed. 2, Philadelphia, 1984, W.B. Saunders Co.

SUGGESTED LEARNING ACTIVITIES AND EXPERIENCES

A. Locate patients in any of the intensive care units who demonstrate rhythm disturbances related to the atria:
   1. You may ask any ICU nurse for assistance in identifying such patients
   2. Once a rhythm disturbance has been identified, review the patient's record including:
      a. History
      b. Physical examination findings
      c. Diagnosis
      d. Medications received (both scheduled and p.r.n.)
      e. Vital signs
   3. Attempt to identify a possible etiology of the rhythm disturbance
   4. Identify treatment measures and nursing observations and/or management that relate to the specific rhythm disturbance
   5. Write patient care objectives on the nursing care plan in relation to nursing management of the dysrhythmia
B. Practice interpreting atrial dysrhythmias by obtaining as many rhythm strips as possible; analyze each strip according to the format listed on the practice strips in the Supplements section of this module
C. Observe a DC cardioversion; obtain information regarding vital signs, neurovital signs, medications (specifically, cardiac medications and anticoagulants), and blood chemistry (particularly potassium levels); determine the rationale for the cardioversion at this time; observe the patient's response following cardioversion—was it successful?
D. If one has access to an electrophysiology laboratory, it is an excellent resource for new knowledge pertaining to the generation and transmission of all cardiac dysrhythmias

POSTTEST (Answers on p. 82)

Directions: Circle one answer to each question unless otherwise indicated.

A. The dysrhythmia in Fig. 3-18 can be interpreted as:
   1. Sinus tachycardia
   2. Atrial flutter
   3. Atrial tachycardia
   4. Atrial fibrillation
B. The Fig. 3-18 dysrhythmia may be associated with (circle all that apply):

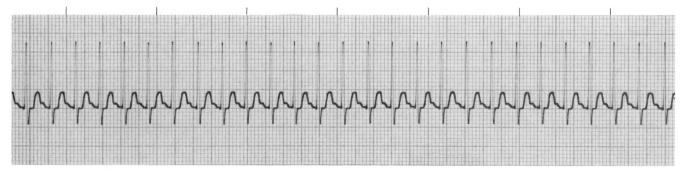

FIG. 3-18

Lead II

1. Chronic pulmonary disease
2. Atrial hypertrophy
3. Hypoxia
4. Increased catecholamines

C. Treatment for the dysrhythmia in Fig. 3-18 might include (circle all that apply):
   1. Carotid sinus massage
   2. Drugs such as verapamil, propranolal, and digitalis
   3. Defibrillation
   4. Overdrive pacing

D. Nursing measures that should be considered for the dysrhythmia in Fig. 3-18 include (circle all that apply):
   1. Documenting the rhythm
   2. Maintaining bedrest in high Fowler's position
   3. Assessing for signs of congestive heart failure and coronary insufficiency
   4. Establishing venous access

E. The dysrhythmia in Fig. 3-19 can be interpreted as:
   1. Atrial fibrillation
   2. Atrial flutter
   3. Premature atrial complexes
   4. Wandering atrial pacemaker

F. The ventricular rhythm in Fig. 3-19 is irregular because:
   1. Conduction of "f" waves is totally irregular

2. Conduction ratio of "F" waves to QRS varies
3. Premature atrial complexes occur in trigeminy
4. The atrial rate varies as the pacemaker impulse wanders throughout the atria

G. Treatment measures for the dysrhythmia in Fig. 3-19 may include (circle all that apply):
   1. Cardioversion
   2. Rapid atrial pacing
   3. Verapamil
   4. Long-term prophylaxis with digitalis and quinidine

H. The rhythm in Fig. 3-20 can be interpreted as:
   1. Wandering atrial pacemaker
   2. Premature atrial complexes in trigeminy
   3. Atrial fibrillation
   4. Atrial flutter

I. The hallmark(s) of the dysrhythmia in Fig. 3-20 is (are) (circle all that apply):
   1. "F" waves replacing P waves
   2. Irregularly irregular ventricular rhythm
   3. Changing P wave morphology
   4. "f" waves replacing P waves

J. The atrial dysrhythmia that most often occurs in the absence of heart disease is:
   1. Paroxysmal atrial tachycardia
   2. Atrial fibrillation

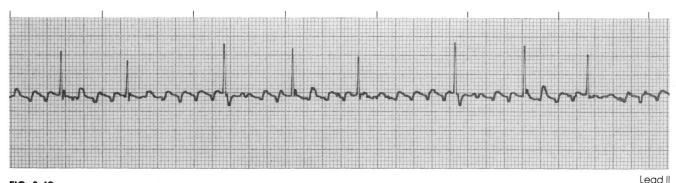

FIG. 3-19   Lead II

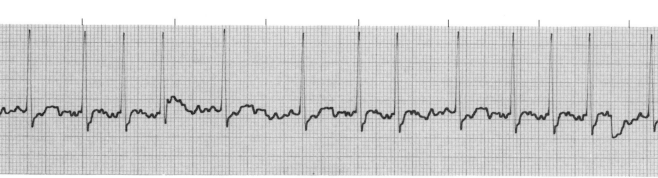

FIG. 3-20   Lead II

3. Wandering atrial pacemaker
4. Atrial flutter

K. The goal of treatment measures in chronic fibrillation is to:
1. Terminate the dysrhythmia immediately
2. Maintain the ventricular rate at less than 100
3. Eradicate atrial irritability with long-term quinidine therapy
4. Correct the underlying cause

L. The action of digitalis in treating atrial dysrhythmias can best be described as:
1. Direct action on atrial tissue to abolish an irritable focus
2. Slowing of the ventricular rate by prolonging the refractory period of the AV node
3. Slowing the atrial rate so that the sinus node can take over as pacemaker
4. Increasing the strength of ventricular contraction

M. When a tachydysrhythmia terminates, the patient should be observed for signs of (circle all that apply):
1. Congestive heart failure
2. Neurological defecits
3. Myocardial infarction
4. Systemic emboli

N. Symptoms patients experience during a tachydysrhythmia are primarily related to:
1. Decreased AV conduction
2. Increased atrial irritability
3. Decreased ventricular filling time and stroke volume
4. Vasoconstriction as a result of hypotension

O. Prophylaxis for paroxysmal atrial tachycardia includes all of the following *except:*
1. Eliminating stimulants such as caffeine
2. Employing vagal maneuvers
3. Anticoagulant therapy
4. Decreasing stress

P. Matching: Match the term in column A with the definition in column B.

| Column A | Column B |
Term	Definition
___ 1. Ectopic	a. Refers to ectopic impulses originating in different foci
___ 2. "f" waves	b. Impulse conduction in a backward direction
___ 3. Multifocal	c. A period during which fibers are unresponsive to a stimulus
___ 4. Escape rhythm	d. Initiated by a lower pacemaker when the sinus node slows or fails
___ 5. Retrograde	e. Originates outside the sinus node
___ 6. Compensatory pause	f. Application of synchronized direct electrical current to terminate a tachycardia
___ 7. Extrasystole	g. Flutter waves
___ 8. "F" waves	h. A delay occurring after a premature beat which resets the sinus cadence
___ 9. Refractory	i. Premature complex arising from an ectopic focus
___10. Cardioversion	j. Fibrillation waves

SUPPLEMENTS

This is a work section. A work space is provided beneath each strip to the left. The answers are to the right. It is suggested that you cover the answer section with a card or paper while you work the strips. Check your answers on the right.

A.

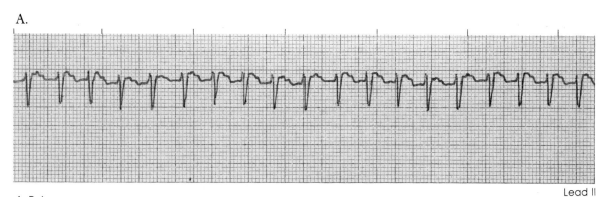

FIG. 3-21

Lead II

1. Rate:	
Atrial:	180
Ventricular:	180
2. P waves:	Present; upright on downslope of T waves
3. PR interval:	0.20 second
4. Ratio of P/QRS:	1:1
5. QRS interval:	0.08 second
6. QT interval:	0.18 second
7. Interpretation:	Atrial tachycardia

B.

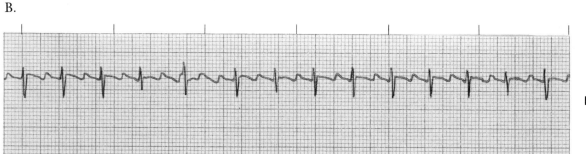

FIG. 3-22

Lead II

1. Rate:	
Atrial:	Approximately 300
Ventricular:	140
2. Rhythm:	
Atrial:	Regular ("F" waves)
Ventricular:	Basically regular; note change between the fifth and sixth complexes
3. P waves:	None; "F" waves seen
4. PR interval:	Nonexistent
5. Ratio of P/QRS:	Nonexistent; "F"/QRS 2:1, 3:1
6. QRS interval:	0.06 second
7. QT interval:	Unable to determine
8. Interpretation:	Atrial flutter with varying conduction

C.

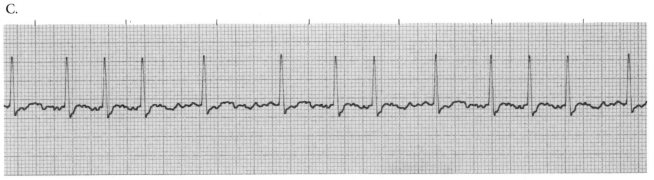

FIG. 3-2

Lead II

1. Rate:
   Atrial: Unable to determine
   Ventricular: 110
2. Rhythm:
   Atrial: Irregular ("f" waves)
   Ventricular: Totally irregular
3. P waves: None; "f" waves
4. PR interval: Nonexistent
5. Ratio of P/QRS: Nonexistent; "f"/QRS varying
6. QRS interval: 0.06 second
7. QT interval: Unable to determine
8. Interpretation: Atrial fibrillation

D.

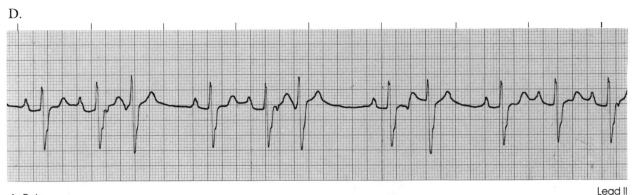

FIG. 3-24

Lead II

1. Rate:
   Atrial: Approximately 80
   Ventricular: Approximately 80
2. Rhythm:
   Atrial: Irregular
   Ventricular: Irregular
3. P waves: Present; buried in T waves preceding each
                                              premature complex
4. PR interval: Sinus complexes, 0.22 second; premature
                                              complexes, unable to determine
5. Ratio of P/QRS: 1:1
6. QRS interval: 0.12 second
7. QT interval: Sinus complexes, 0.40 second
8. Interpretation: Premature atrial complexes; distorted T
                                              wave preceding each premature complex
                                              is clue that P' is buried in T

E.

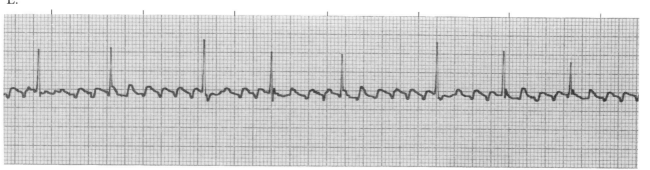

FIG. 3-25

Lead II

1. Rate:	
Atrial:	Approximately 300
Ventricular:	Approximately 70
2. Rhythm:	
Atrial:	Appears regular ("F" waves)
Ventricular:	Irregular
3. P waves:	None; "F" waves
4. PR interval:	Nonexistent
5. Ratio of P/QRS:	Nonexistent; "F"/QRS 4:1, 6:1
6. QRS interval:	0.04 second
7. QT interval:	Unable to determine
8. Interpretation:	Atrial flutter with varying ventricular response

F.

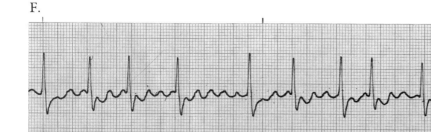

FIG. 3-26

Lead II

1. Rate:	
Atrial:	Approximately 300
Ventricular:	Approximately 80
2. Rhythm:	
Atrial:	Basically regular ("F" waves)
Ventricular:	Irregular
3. P waves:	None; "F" waves
4. PR interval:	Nonexistent
5. Ratio of P/QRS:	Nonexistent; "F"/QRS varies 2:1 to 6:1
6. QRS interval:	Approximately 0.12 second
7. QT interval:	Unable to determine
8. Interpretation:	Atrial flutter with varying ventricular response

G.

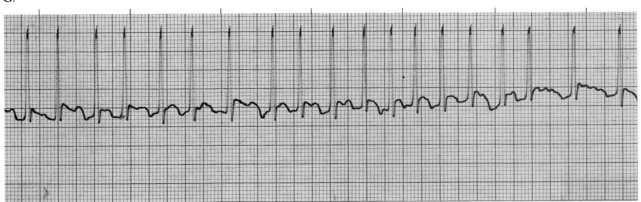

FIG. 3-2?

Lead II

1. Rate:
   Atrial: Unable to determine
   Ventricular: Approximately 170
2. Rhythm:
   Atrial: Irregular
   Ventricular: Irregular
3. P waves: None; few "f" waves seen between last two
                                    complexes
4. PR interval: Nonexistent
5. Ratio of P/QRS: Nonexistent; "f"/QRS varying
6. QRS interval: 0.06 second
7. QT interval: Unable to determine
8. Interpretation: Atrial fibrillation with rapid ventricular re-
                                    sponse; fibrillatory waves are visible only
                                    between last two complexes; totally irreg-
                                    ular ventricular response is the clue

H.

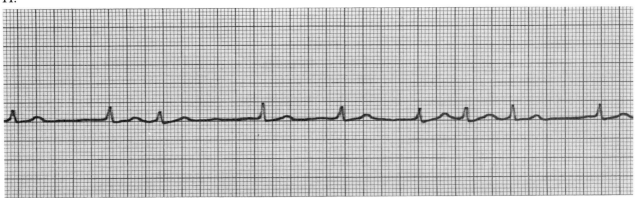

FIG. 3-28

Lead III

1. Rate:
   Atrial: Unable to determine
   Ventricular: Approximately 80
2. Rhythm:
   Atrial: Isoelectric line; unable to determine
   Ventricular: Irregular
3. P waves: None
4. PR interval: Nonexistent
5. Ratio of P/QRS: Nonexistent
6. QRS interval: 0.06-0.08 second
7. QT interval: 0.36-0.40 second
8. Interpretation: Atrial fibrillation; fibrillatory waves not visible
                                    in this lead; totally irregular ventricular re-
                                    sponse is the clue; T waves are visible be-
                                    cause fibrillatory waves are absent and
                                    rate is slow

I.

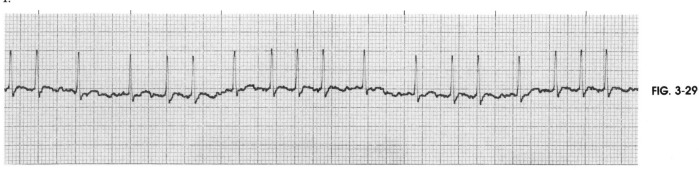

FIG. 3-29

Lead II

1. Rate:
   Atrial:
   Ventricular:
2. Rhythm:
   Atrial:
   Ventricular:
3. P waves:
4. PR interval:
5. Ratio of P/QRS:
6. QRS interval:
7. QT interval:
8. Interpretation:

Unable to determine
Approximately 160

Irregular ("f" waves)
Irregular
None; "f" waves
Nonexistent
Nonexistent; "f"/QRS varying
0.06 second
Unable to determine
Atrial fibrillation with rapid ventricular
response

J.

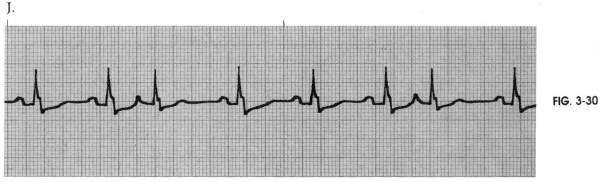

FIG. 3-30

Lead II

1. Rate:
   Atrial:
   Ventricular:
2. Rhythm:
   Atrial:
   Ventricular:
3. P waves:

4. PR interval:
5. Ratio of P/QRS:
6. QRS interval:
7. QT interval:

8. Interpretation:

Approximately 80
Approximately 80

Irregular
Irregular
Present before each complex but shape of
P' differs from P
PR—0.20 seconds; P'R—0.18 second
1:1
0.08 second
Approximately 0.44 second (end of T wave
not clear)
Premature atrial complexes; there is a non-
compensatory pause after both PACs

K.

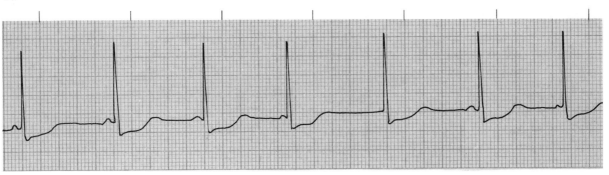

FIG. 3-31

Lead II

1. Rate:
     Atrial: Approximately 70
     Ventricular: Approximately 70
2. Rhythm:
     Atrial: Irregular
     Ventricular: Irregular
3. P waves: Present; morphology differs in each
                                                          complex
4. PR interval: Varies 0.04-0.14 second
5. Ratio of P/QRS: 1:1
6. QRS interval: 0.04 second
7. QT interval: Approximately 0.52 second (end of T wave
                                                          not clear)
8. Interpretation: Wandering atrial pacemaker; P' wave mor-
                                                          phology and P'R interval vary as impulse
                                                          wanders

ANSWERS TO PRETEST AND POSTTEST
Pretest

A. 1, 2, 3, 4	L. 3
B. 2	M. 2
C. 2	N. 3
D. 4	O. 1
E. 3	P. 1
F. 1, 2, 3, 4	Q. Matching:
G. 3	1. b.
H. 2	2. d.
I. 3	3. c.
J. 2	4. a.
K. 4	

Posttest

A. 3	M. 1, 2, 3, 4
B. 1, 2, 3, 4	N. 3
C. 1, 2, or 4	O. 3
D. 1, 3, 4	P. Matching:
E. 2	1. e
F. 2	2. j
G. 1, 3	3. a
H. 3	4. d
I. 2, 4	5. b
J. 1	6. h
K. 2	7. i
L. 2	8. g
	9. c
	10. f

4 Junctional dysrhythmias

PRETEST (Answers on p. 99)

Directions: Circle one answer to each question unless otherwise indicated.

A. The dysrhythmia in Fig. 4-1 can be interpreted as:
1. Sinus bradycardia
2. Junctional escape rhythm
3. Accelerated junctional rhythm
4. Junctional tachycardia

B. Proper therapy of the dysrhythmia in Fig. 4-1 might include which of the following? (Circle all that apply.)
1. Discontinuation of digoxin
2. Administration of atropine intravenously
3. Insertion of a temporary pacemaker
4. Administration of lidocaine intravenously

C. The dysrhythmia in Fig. 4-2 can be interpreted as:
1. Sinus rhythm with a premature atrial complex (PAC)
2. Sinus rhythm with premature ventricular complex (PVC)
3. Sinus rhythm with a junctional escape complex
4. Sinus rhythm with a premature junctional complex (PJC)

D. The dysrhythmia in Fig. 4-2 may be associated with which of the following? (Circle all that apply.)
1. Following open heart surgery
2. Digoxin toxicity
3. Diabetes mellitus
4. Coronary artery disease

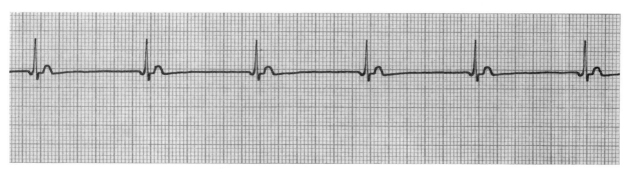

FIG. 4-1　　　　　　　　　　　　　　　　　　　　　　Lead II

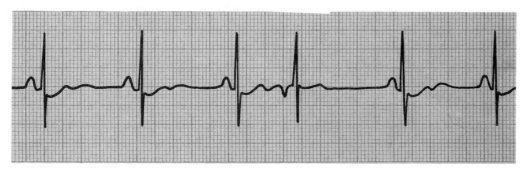

FIG. 4-2　　　　　　　　　　　　　　　　　　　　　　Lead II

E. Treatment/management of the dysrhythmia in Fig. 4-2 would probably include (circle all that apply):
   1. Mild sedation
   2. Administration of quinidine
   3. Administration of propranolol
   4. Administration of atropine
F. The dysrhythmia in Fig. 4-3 can be interpreted as:
   1. Junctional tachycardia
   2. Accelerated junctional rhythm (nonparoxysmal junctional tachycardia)
   3. Atrial fibrillation
   4. Ventricular tachycardia

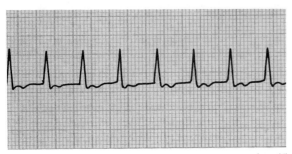

FIG. 4-3   Lead II

G. The dysrhythmia in Fig. 4-3 is most commonly associated with which of the following? (Circle all that apply.)
   1. Acute myocardial infarction
   2. Digoxin toxicity
   3. Chronic obstructive pulmonary disease
   4. Acute rheumatic myocarditis
H. The dysrhythmia in Fig. 4-4 can be interpreted as:
   1. Accelerated junctional rhythm (nonparoxysmal junctional tachycardia)
   2. Sinus tachycardia
   3. Junctional tachycardia
   4. Ventricular tachycardia
I. Which of the following statements is true concerning the dysrhythmia in Fig. 4-4? (Circle all that apply.)

1. This dysrhythmia rarely occurs in patients with heart disease and is considered to be benign
2. If the ventricular rate is rapid enough, the patient may experience chest pain, dyspnea, and dizziness
3. DC cardioversion may be used as a form of treatment
4. Patients with acute myocardial infarction (especially inferior wall MI) may develop this dysrhythmia
J. The dysrhythmia in Fig. 4-5 can be interpreted as:
   1. Sinus rhythm with atrial escape beat
   2. Sinus rhythm with junctional escape beat
   3. Junctional tachycardia
   4. Sinus rhythm with PJC
K. Which of the following statements is true concerning the dysrhythmia in Fig. 4-5? (Circle all that apply.)
   1. It is often the result of SA node depression
   2. Frequently it is seen after pauses that are produced by sinus bradycardia, nonconducted (blocked) PACs, and a Mobitz type I heart block
   3. It is a serious life-threatening dysrhythmia and should be treated aggressively by the use of a lidocaine drip
   4. It is considered to be a passive or default dysrhythmia rather than an active or usurpation dysrhythmia

PURPOSE

The purpose of this module is to provide the learner with basic information and a structural framework to develop skills in identifying and understanding the etiology, clinical significance, and treatment of junctional dysrhythmias.

BEHAVIORAL OBJECTIVES

At the end of this module, the learner should be able to:
A. List possible etiological factors of, define and identify criteria for, recognize on rhythm strips, state clinical

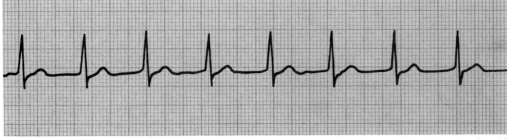

FIG. 4-4   Lead II

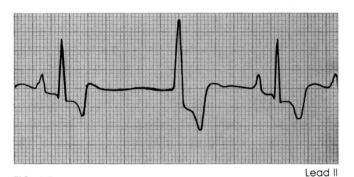

FIG. 4-5

Lead II

features of, and discuss modes of treatment and nursing management for the following dysrhythmias:
1. Premature junctional complex (PJC)
2. Accelerated junctional rhythm (nonparoxysmal junctional tachycardia)
3. Junctional tachycardia
4. AV nodal reentry tachycardia
5. Junctional escape beat
6. Junctional rhythm

VOCABULARY

Aberrant conduction Because of a prolongation of the refractory period in the bundle branches, an impulse(s) is(are) abnormally conducted through the ventricles producing a change in the QRS morphology.

Active rhythm A rhythm initiated by a premature complex (one that is early in the regular cycle) that continues at a rate faster than the normal pacemaker and usurps control of the heart rhythm.

AN region The uppermost part of the AV node (atrionodal), thought to contain potential pacemaker fibers.

Antegrade conduction Impulse conduction that proceeds in a normal (forward) direction.

Atrioventricular junction An area of specialized conduction tissue that includes the AV node and the bundle of His area.

Automaticity Electrical property of cells that permits spontaneous initiation of the cardiac impulse.

Cardiac output The volume of blood pumped by the heart per minute. The normal amount is 4 to 8 liters per minute.

Cardioversion A direct electrical current that is synchronized to be delivered on the R wave of the ECG via paddles applied to the chest in order to terminate a tachycardia.

Compensatory pause A type of pause that occurs after a premature complex. If the interval measured between the R wave of the beat *preceding* the premature beat and the R wave of the beat *following* it is *equal to twice* that of the RR interval between two normal beats, the pause is fully compensatory. This occurs when the premature beat does not interrupt the sinus node cycle.

Ectopic An impulse that originates outside the SA node.

Electrophysiology study A procedure performed with intracardiac catheters to measure impulse formation and the speed of conduction at various sites in the conduction system.

Escape complex/rhythm A complex/rhythm that is initiated by a lower pacemaker when the sinus node fails or slows. Usually

preceded by a pause, it is also termed a passive rhythm or a rhythm by default.

NH region Lowermost part of the AV node (AV node–His bundle area), thought to contain potential pacemaker fibers.

Noncompensatory pause A delay in ventricular systole, following a premature complex, which resets the sinus node cadence. If the interval measured between the R wave of the beat *preceding* the premature beat and the R wave of the beat *following* it is *less than twice* the RR interval between two normal beats, the pause is noncompensatory. This occurs when the premature beat interrupts the sinus node cycle.

N region A midnodal region whose main function is to slow the transmission of the impulse from the atria to the ventricles. It is thought to be void of pacemaking capabilities.

Overdrive pacing The use of a pacemaker for the purpose of artifically stimulating the heart at a faster rate than the patient's intrinsic rate. The purpose of this increased heart rate is to suppress an abnormal tachydysrhythmia.

P′ wave A P wave that differs in shape from the sinus P wave because the impulse originates outside the sinus node.

Refractory The period during which fibers are unresponsive to a stimulus.

Retrograde conduction Impulse conduction in a backward direction from normal.

CONTENT
Suggested review

Before beginning this module on junctional dysrhythmias, it is recommended that the learner review Module 1 on the anatomy and physiology of the AV node.

Junctional dysrhythmias—an overview

The AV node may be divided into three areas: (1) the AN region (atrionodal) or uppermost part of the AV node, (2) the N region or midnodal region, and (3) the NH region (node-His) or lowermost part of the node. The AV junction is the area of specialized conduction that contains the above three regions and ends where the bundle of His bifurcates into the right and the left bundle branches (Fig. 4-6, p. 86).

As previously discussed in the Anatomy and Physiology Module, the main function of the AV node is to slow the transmission of the impulse from the atria to the ventricles. The slowing (delay) of the impulse is important since this allows for complete atrial emptying, including atrial contraction, to occur before ventricular depolarization begins. This delay is thought to occur in the N region. The AN and NH regions contain potential pacemaker fibers, while these fibers are probably not present in the N region.[8,9] These potential pacemaker fibers have an inherent rate of 40 to 60 per minute and have the capacity to act as the pacemaker of the heart if the usual pacemaker, the SA node, fails. The term "junctional rhythm" is preferred over "nodal rhythm" since the rhythm may originate from the AN, NH, or the bundle of His area.

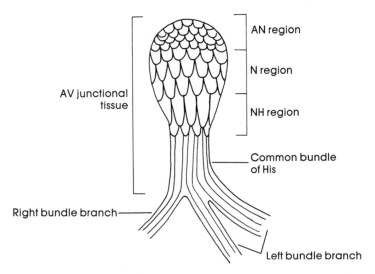

FIG. 4-6

Diagramatic representation of three divisions of AV node. AN region (atrionodal) is area composed of uppermost part of node, N region is midportion of node, and NH is lowermost part of node, which is in close communication with the bundle of His.

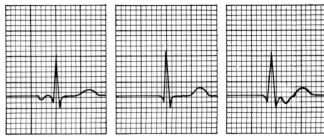

FIG. 4-7

Diagramatic representation of three ways P' wave may appear in junctional rhythm: inverted and preceding QRS, inverted and following QRS, and absent or lost within QRS complex.

FIG. 4-8

Atrial activation occurs in retrograde fashion in junctional rhythm. Leads that have their positive pole on left leg (II, III, and aV$_F$) will inscribe inverted P' waves, while aV$_R$ with its positive pole on right arm will inscribe an upright P' wave.

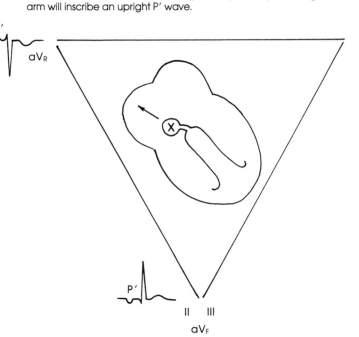

The older classifications of AV junctional rhythms included upper, middle, and lower nodal rhythm. This classification was based on the direction of the P wave in the standard as well as augmented limb leads and also on the timing of the P wave with respect to the QRS complex. Electrophysiological studies have now proven this classification to be of questionable value and the precise site of impulse formation in the AV junction cannot be determined from rhythm strips or the conventional 12-lead ECG.

The normal pacemaker of the heart is the SA node since it has the fastest inherent rate (60 to 100 beats per minute). Activation of the atria occurs normally in an antegrade fashion from the SA node to the AV node. When the AV junction is the pacemaker of the heart, the activation of the atria is retrograde or opposite to that of a sinus impulse, thus affecting the P wave. The P' wave on the ECG may appear in one of the following ways (Fig. 4-7): (1) the P' wave may be inverted and precede the QRS complex with a P'R interval measuring 0.11 seconds or less (in leads that normally should have an upright P wave), (2) the P' wave may not be visible and may be hidden in the QRS complex, or (3) it may be inverted but still following the QRS complex. The P' wave will be inverted in leads II, III, and aV$_F$ (leads that normally have an upright P wave) and upright in lead aV$_R$ (which normally has an inverted P wave) (Fig. 4-8).

Rhythm disturbances
PREMATURE JUNCTIONAL COMPLEX (PJC) (Fig. 4-9)
Definition

A complex that comes early (before the next expected sinus complex in the cycle) has an abnormal P wave (P') and P'R interval with a normal QRS complex. The PJC is usually followed by a pause that may be compensatory or noncompensatory. PJCs as well as both accelerated junc-

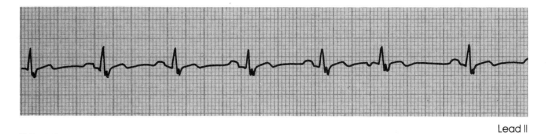

Lead II

FIG. 4-9
Sixth beat is a premature junctional complex (PJC). Note inverted P' wave before QRS complex. PJC produced a compensatory pause.

tional rhythm and junctional tachycardia are the result of active impulse formation by the AV junction. The AV junction usurps or actively gains control of the heart as the dominant pacemaker.

Etiology

1. Digoxin toxicity is commonly a cause
2. PJC may be seen following open heart surgery (as a result of trauma or swelling of the AV junctional area)
3. Acute rheumatic myocarditis is a rare cause
4. Heart disease (especially in patients with inferior or posterior wall myocardial infarction) also causes PJC

Characteristics of rhythm

1. Rate: Usually within limits of sinus rhythm (60-100 per minute)
2. Rhythm: Basically regular except for the premature complex
3. P' waves: Of the PJC may be inverted before or after the QRS complex or may be absent (lost within the QRS complex)
4. P'R interval: 0.11 second or less if the inverted P' wave precedes the QRS or may not be measurable if the P' wave is absent
5. QRS interval: Within normal limits since conduction through the ventricles is not altered (Fig. 4-9)

Clinical features

1. No symptoms may be produced
2. The patient may become anxious and complain of palpitations
3. If the PJCs become frequent enough to alter the patient's cardiac output, symptoms such as dizziness may occur
4. Physical signs include an irregular pulse
5. A drop in blood pressure may occur if the cardiac output is altered because of frequent PJCs
6. Clinical significance is similar to that of premature atrial complexes (PACs) (see Atrial Dysrhythmias Module)

7. Isolated PJCs may lead to accelerated junctional rhythm or junctional tachycardia
8. PJCs are a relatively uncommon occurrence in comparison with PACs and PVCs

Treatment measures

1. If digoxin toxicity is the cause, the drug should be discontinued promptly; potassium may then be administered cautiously since heart block may result because of the additive effect of the two drugs
2. Careful monitoring of the patient may be the only treatment necessary

Nursing management

1. Assess the patient and monitor vital signs
2. Record the dysrhythmia with a rhythm strip or 12-lead ECG for documentation purposes
3. Give reassurance to the patient

ACCELERATED JUNCTIONAL RHYTHM (Fig. 4-10, p. 88)
Definition

Accelerated junctional rhythm is a regular rhythm originating in the AV junction with a ventricular rate of 70 to 130 complexes per minute.[5] The onset and termination of the dysrhythmia is not sudden as is the case with paroxysmal supraventricular tachycardia (PSVT). Accelerated junctional rhythm like PJC is the result of enhanced automaticity of the AV junction. The term "nonparoxysmal junctional tachycardia" is used by some. This rhythm starts and stops more slowly than PSVT does and may not always be regular.

Etiology

1. The same as those for PJCs
2. Hypokalemia is also a cause

Characteristics of rhythm

1. Rate: 70-130 per minute
2. Rhythm: Usually regular but may be slightly irregular

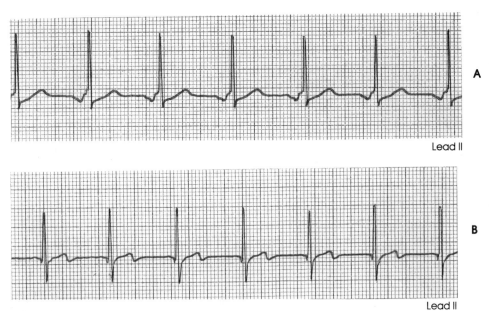

FIG. 4-10

A, Accelerated junctional rhythm recorded at rate of 75 per minute. Note inverted P waves that are inverted before QRS complexes. **B,** This rhythm strip of accelerated junctional rhythm illustrates lack of visible P waves. Junction is firing at rate of 85 per minute.

3. P Waves: See P′ wave appearance for PJCs
4. PR interval: See PR interval for junctional rhythm
5. QRS interval: Within normal limits since interaventricular conduction is undisturbed and continues in a normal antegrade direction (see Fig. 4-10)

Clinical features

1. The patient may experience no symptoms
2. If the rate is rapid the patient may experience symptoms of a decreased cardiac output (dizziness, mental confusion and/or syncope because of decreased cerebral blood flow, chest pain, and/or shortness of breath)
3. The apical/radial pulse will be equal and regular with a rate of 70 to 130 per minute

Treatment measures

1. If digoxin tocicity is the cause, the drug should be discontinued promptly; potassium may then be administered cautiously since heart block may result because of the additive effect of the two drugs
2. If the patient is not taking digoxin and the ventricular rate is rapid enough to produce a decrease in cardiac output, then administration of digoxin is warranted
3. Electrical DC cardioversion may be used if digitalization is not successful and the dysrhythmia is clearly *not* the result of digoxin
4. Phenytoin, propranolol, or lidocaine may be tried

5. Careful observation may be all that is necessary if the patient is tolerating the dysrhythmia well; usually this dysrhythmia will convert spontaneously

Nursing management

1. Assess the patient and monitor all vital signs
2. Withhold further doses of digoxin if applicable
3. Record the patient's dysrhythmia with a rhythm strip or 12-lead ECG for documentation purposes
4. Check the level of the patient's serum potassium
5. Prepare to administer appropriate drugs
6. Observe monitor closely for additional dysrhythmias (especially PVCs and ventricular tachycardia) if digoxin toxicity is thought to be the likely etiology

JUNCTIONAL TACHYCARDIA (FIG. 4-11)
Definition

Junctional tachycardia is a regular rhythm originating in the AV junction with a ventricular rate greater than 100 per minute. The onset and termination of this dysrhythmia is usually sudden; however, it may be a permanent dysrhythmia in children.

Etiology

1. Junctional tachycardia is usually seen in children with uncorrected congenital heart disease
2. It may be the result of hypokalemia
3. Digoxin toxicity may cause this dysrhythmia; however

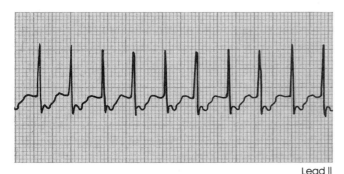

FIG. 4-11

Junctional tachycardia is evident by presence of inverted P' waves following QRS complexes, rate of 195 per minute, and narrow QRS complexes.

accelerated junctional rhythm (nonparoxysmal junctional tachycardia) more commonly results

4. It may be seen following cardiac surgery
5. It may be associated with inferior and posterior wall myocardial infarctions

Characteristics of rhythm

1. Rate: Greater than 100 per minute (in children the rate may exceed 400 per minute)
2. Rhythm: Regular
3. P waves: See P' wave appearance for PJCs
4. PR interval: See PR interval for PJCs
5. QRS interval: Within normal limits (see Fig. 4-11)

Clinical features

1. Individuals may have symptoms of palpitations and may also have anxiety
2. If the ventricular rate is rapid enough to drop the patient's cardiac output, a drop in blood pressure may occur; a decrease in cerebral blood flow may produce symptoms of dizziness, mental confusion or syncope; a decrease in coronary blood flow may produce chest pain and/or shortness of breath

Treatment measures

1. The permanent form of the dysrhythmia, which is more commonly seen in children, is usually resistant to drug therapy and may require surgical intervention
2. If the dysrhythmia is caused by digoxin toxicity, the drug should be promptly discontinued
3. When the dysrhythmia is associated with an inferior or posterior infarction, it lasts for only a few days and is not considered to be associated with a poor prognosis
4. When the dysrhythmia is associated with cardiac surgery, it is also not associated with a poor prognosis and usually will last only a few days

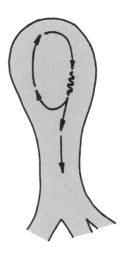

FIG. 4-12

Diagramatic representation of dual pathways present within AV node. One pathway is slow and the other is fast, which sets up ability for a single beat to reenter and produce circus movement tachycardia.

Nursing management

1. Assess the patient and monitor all vital signs
2. Reassure the patient to lessen anxiety
3. Record the patient's dysrhythmia with a rhythm strip or 12-lead ECG for documentation purposes
4. If applicable, withhold further doses of digoxin
5. Be prepared to administer appropriate drugs

AV NODAL REENTRY TACHYCARDIA (Fig. 4-12)
Definition

Paroxysmal supraventricular tachycardia (PSVT) is a dysrhythmia characterized by regularly occurring ventricular complexes that exceed 100 per minute, P waves that may or may not be present, and a narrow QRS. The PSVT may be the result of a reentry mechanism that occurs when an impulse returns to activate a pathway in a particular region of the conduction system. When this impulse repeatedly returns, a circus movement results and produces a tachycardia. The reentry mechanism may be located in the SA node, the atria, the AV node, or the AV node plus an accessory pathway. AV nodal reentry is the most common type of PSVT.

Reentry within the AV node is possible because two separate pathways exist within the AV node.[4,14] These two pathways have different refractory periods and conduction times and are labeled the *slow pathway* and the *fast pathway*. The slow pathway has a shorter refractory period than the fast pathway. If an early beat arrives, such as a PAC, it may be conducted down the slow pathway to the ventricles, which allows time for the fast pathway to recover and the impulse to return via the fast pathway back to the atria. This impulse is then conducted back down the slow pathway to reactivate the ventricles in a circus fashion via the AV node. This circus movement may be initiated by a PAC, PJC, or PVC, each of which produces a PSVT via the nodal reentry mechanism.[11]

Etiology

Two factors must be present: (1) dual pathways must exist within the the AV node and (2) there must be a premature beat (PAC, PJC, or PVC) that precipitates a tachycardia. It is the most common type of PSVT present in children who have undergone cardiac surgery.[6] Tachycardias that are the result of a reentry mechanism can be

distinguished from tachycardias produced by automaticity because the former can be initiated and terminated by cardiac pacing[6]; clinically, the reentry tachycardia is frequently precipitated by a premature beat.[7]

Characteristics of rhythm

1. Rate: Exceeds 100 per minute and usually is from 160-250 per minute[3]
2. Rhythm: Usually begins abruptly and maintains the same rate until it is abruptly terminated
3. P' waves: Commonly the P' is lost within the QRS complex; however, the P' may follow the QRS complex but rarely precedes it[16]
4. QRS interval: Usually narrow since ventricular activation occurs in a normal antegrade fashion (Fig. 4-13)

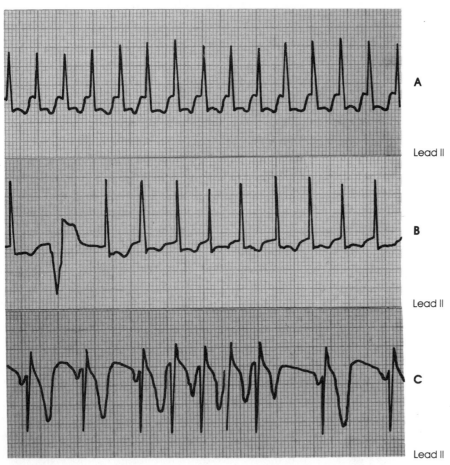

A

Lead II

B

Lead II

C

Lead II

FIG. 4-13

Three rhythm strips illustrating paroxysmal supraventricular tachycardia (PSVT) of the AV nodal reentry variety. **A,** Tachycardia has no visible P waves and has rate of 210 per minute. **B,** PSVT is initiated by a PVC, and **C,** single premature beat initiates four-beat run of PSVT at a rate of 210 per minute.

Clinical features

1. No symptoms may be produced
2. The patient may become anxious and complain of palpitations
3. If the rate is rapid enough, a decrease in cardiac output may result and produce symptoms discussed under "Junctional tachycardia"
4. Symptoms will depend on the rate of the tachycardia, the duration of the tachycardia, and the presence or absence of heart disease[1]

Treatment measures

1. Vagal maneuvers may abruptly terminate the tachycardia by increasing the refractory period of the AV node[10]
2. Verapamil, propranolol, and digoxin depress conduction in slow pathway[12,13]; verapamil is usually the drug of choice in adults if vagal maneuvers fail to terminate the tachycardia[2]
3. Procainamide and quinidine slow conduction through the fast pathway[17]
4. Atrial overdrive pacing may interrupt the circus movement tachycardia[7]
5. Rarely will DC cardioversion be required

Nursing management

1. Assess the patient and monitor vital signs
2. Record the dysrhythmia with a rhythm strip or 12-lead ECG for documentation purposes
3. Give reassurance to the patient
4. Be prepared to administer appropriate drugs

JUNCTIONAL ESCAPE BEATS (FIG. 4-14)
Definition

Junctional escape beat is a complex that occurs late in the cycle (after the interval at which the next expected sinus complex should have occurred) with its origin in the AV junction. These complexes are generated by pas-sive impulse formation to protect the patient from asystole.

Etiology

Junctional escape beats develop when the automaticity of the SA node falls below that of the AV junction or when the impulse from the SA node fails to reach the AV junction as in sinus arrest, sinoatrial block, or second- and third-degree AV block.

Junctional escape complexes are considered passive or default complexes since they usually occur as a result of disturbances in function of the SA node. These disturbances include: (1) vagal stimulation (caused by endotracheal suctioning, a slowing during the exhalation phase of respiration, carotid sinus pressure, or the Valsalva maneuver); (2) injury to the SA node by toxic or infectious processes (myocarditis); (3) digoxin toxicity; (4) effect of certain drugs and electrolytes (quinidine, hyperkalemia); (5) atropine during the initial state of its effect, especially if given in low doses or too slowly; and (6) episodes of sinus bradycardia accompanying acute myocardial infarction.

These escape beats commonly follow the postectopic pause of either a PAC, PJC, or PVC.

Characteristics of rhythm

1. Rate: Will be determined by the underlying rhythm
2. Rhythm: Will become irregular because of the delay in the regularly occurring pacemaker
3. P' waves: See P' wave appearance for PJCs
4. P'R interval: May be the same as that for PJCs
5. QRS interval: Usually normal since ventricular depolarization is unchanged (see Fig. 4-14)

Clinical features

1. No symptoms may result
2. If the escape beat is associated with an extremely slow ventricular rate, the patient's cardiac output may be

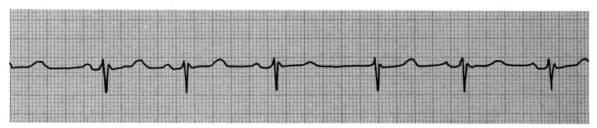

FIG. 4-14

Lead MCL₁

Junctional escape beat is present in fourth complex. This beat occurs because of a pause produced when SA node failed to fire at expected time. P wave is absent and QRS appears like other QRS complexes.

compromised producing symptoms of decreased cerebral blood flow (dizziness, syncope, confusion) and decreased coronary blood flow (chest pain or shortness of breath from congestive heart failure)

Treatment measures

1. Treatment measures are directed at the underlying rhythm producing the pause and not at the escape complexes themselves
2. Escape complexes are not to be treated by trying to abolish them since they are protecting the patient from asystole
3. If pauses are frequent and/or of long duration causing a decrease in cardiac output, a pacemaker may be inserted
4. Atropine or isoproterenol may be administered if the underlying rate is so slow that cardiac output is decreased

Nursing management

1. Assess the patient and monitor vital signs
2. Record the dysrhythmia with a rhythm strip or 12-lead ECG for documentation purposes
3. Prepare for possible pacemaker insertion
4. Endotracheal suctioning should be done with less vigor if overzealous suctioning is the cause

JUNCTIONAL ESCAPE RHYTHM (Fig. 4-15)
Definition

Junctional escape rhythm is a dysrhythmia characterized by regular normal-appearing QRS complexes at a rate from 40 to 60 per minute, abnormal or absent P' waves, with the site of origin of the dysrhythmia located in the AV junction.

Etiology

See "Junctional escape beats."

Characteristics of rhythm

1. Rate: 40-60 per minute
2. Rhythm: Regular
3. P waves: Abnormal appearance because of retrograde activation of the atria; they will be inverted in leads II, III, and aV_F and upright in lead aV_R and may precede or follow the QRS complex; the P' waves may be hidden in the QRS complex thus making them impossible to see
4. PR interval: Abnormally short—usually 0.11 seconds or less when the P' wave is visible
5. QRS interval: Within normal limits since interventricular conduction is undisturbed (see Fig. 4-15)

Clinical features

See "Junctional escape beats."

Treatment measures

1. See "Junctional escape beats"
2. Discontinuation of digoxin, quinidine, or potassium if applicable

Nursing management

1. Assess patient and monitor vital signs
2. Record the dysrhythmia with a rhythm strip or 12-lead ECG for documentation purposes
3. Endotracheal suctioning should be done with less vigor if overzealous suctioning is the cause
4. Withhold further administration of digoxin, quinidine, and potassium if applicable
5. Prepare for possible pacemaker insertion

REFERENCES

1. Bauernfiend, R., et al.: Paroxysmal supraventricular tachycardia. In Mandel, W., editor: Cardiac arrhythmias: their mechanism, diagnosis and management, Philadelphia, 1980, J.B. Lippincott Co.

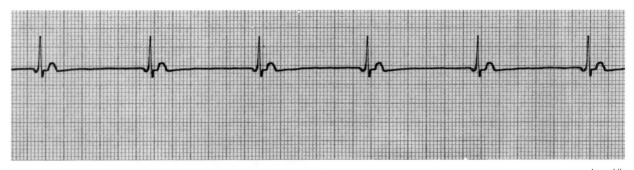

Lead II

FIG. 4-15
Junctional escape rhythm at rate of 50 per minute. Inverted P' waves are visible before QRS complexes.

2. Brugada, P., and Wellens, H.: Electrophysiology, mechanisms, diagnosis, and treatment of paroxysmal recurrent atrioventricular nodal reentrant tachycardia. In Surawicz, B., et al., editors: Tachycardias, Boston, 1984, Martinus Nijhoff Publishing.

3. Conover, M.B.: Understanding electrocardiography: arrhythmias and 12-lead ECG, ed. 4, St. Louis, 1984, The C.V. Mosby Co.

4. Denes, P., et al.: Demonstration of dual A-V nodal pathways in patients with paroxysmal supraventricular tachycardia, Circulation **48**:549, 1973.

5. Fisch, C.: Digitalis-induced tachycardias. In Surawicz, B., et al., editors: Tachycardias, Boston, 1984, Martinus Nijhoff Publishing.

6. Garson, A., Jr.: Supraventricular tachycardia. In Gillette, P., and Garson, A., editors: Pediatric cardiac dysrhythmias, New York, 1981, Grune and Stratton.

7. Goldreyer, B., et al.: The electrophysiologic demonstration of atrial ectopic tachycardia in man, Am. Heart J. **85**:205, 1973.

8. Hoffman, B., and Cranefield, P.: The physiological basis of cardiac arrhythmias, Am. J. Med. 37:670, 1964.

9. Hoffman, B., et al.: Transmembrane potentials of single fibers of the atrioventricular node, Nature **181**:66, 1958.

10. Josephson, M., and Kastar, J.: Supraventricular tachycardia: mechanisms and management, Ann. Intern. Med. **87**:346, 1977.

11. Marriott, H.J.L., and Conover, M.B.: Advanced concepts in arrhythmias, St. Louis, 1983, the C.V. Mosby Co.

12. Wellens, H., et al.: Effect of digitalis in patients with paroxysmal atrioventricular nodal tachycardia, Circulation **52**:779, 1975.

13. Wellens, H., et al.: Effect of verapamil studied by programmed electrical stimulation of the heart in patients with paroxysmal re-entrant supraventricular tachycardia, Br. Heart J. **39**:1058, 1977.

14. Wu, D.: Dual atrioventricular nodal pathways: a reappraisal, PACE **5**:72, 1982.

15. Wu, D., et al.: The effects of propranolol on induction of AV nodal re-entrant tachycardia, Circulation **50**:665, 1974.

16. Wu, D., et al.: Clinical electrocardiographic and electrophysiologic observations in patients with paroxysmal supraventricular tachycardia, Am. J. Cardiol. **41**:1045, 1978.

17. Wu, D., et al.: Effects of procainamide on atrioventricular nodal re-entrant paroxysmal tachycardia, Circulation **57**:1171, 1978.

SUGGESTED LEARNING ACTIVITIES AND EXPERIENCES

A. Visit an intensive care unit and observe patients with junctional dysrhythmias:
1. Review their clinical backgrounds
2. Identify their dysrhythmia
3. Review their treatment plans

B. Visit an electrophysiology laboratory and observe patients undergoing testing:
1. Observe the dysrhythmia induction and termination
2. Review the treatment plan(s)

POSTTEST (Answers on p. 99)

Directions: Circle one answer to each question unless otherwise indicated.

A. The correct interpretation of the rhythm strip in Fig. 4-16 is:
1. Junctional rhythm
2. PSVT (AV nodal reentry tachycardia)
3. Atrial fibrillation
4. Sinus tachycardia

B. The dysrhythmia in Fig. 4-16 may be treated with which of the following therapy measures? (Circle all that apply.)
1. Verapamil
2. Overdrive pacing
3. Atropine
4. Isoproterenol

C. The dysrhythmia in Fig. 4-17 on p. 94 can be interpreted as which one of the following?
1. Sinus bradycardia

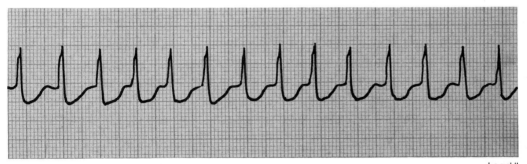

FIG. 4-16

Lead II

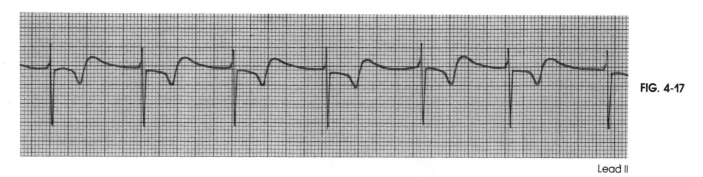

FIG. 4-17

Lead II

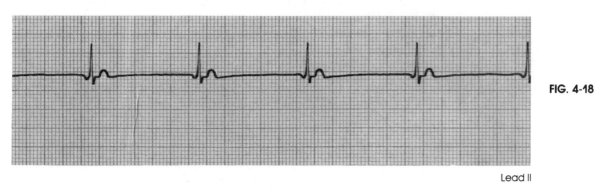

FIG. 4-18

Lead II

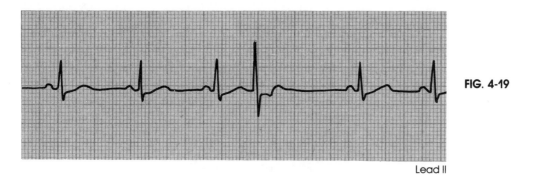

FIG. 4-19

Lead II

2. Accelerated junctional rhythm
3. Junctional rhythm
4. Atrial flutter

D. Which of the following statements are true with regard to the dysrhythmia in Fig. 4-17? (Circle all that apply.)
1. It is often the result of SA node depression and is seen in patients with SA block, sinus arrest, and sinus bradycardia
2. It is a serious life-threatening dysrhythmia and should be aggressively treated by the use of a lidocaine drip
3. It is commonly seen in patients with acute myocardial infarction and is considered to be associated with a poor prognosis
4. It is considered to be a passive rather than an active dysrhythmia

E. The dysrhythmia in Fig. 4-18 can be interpreted as:
1. Junctional rhythm
2. Nonparoxysmal junctional tachycardia (accelerated junctional rhythm)
3. Sinus bradycardia
4. Sinus rhythm

F. Proper therapy of the dysrhythmia in Fig. 4-18 might include (circle all that apply):
1. Administration of lidocaine I.V. push
2. Insertion of a temporary pacemaker
3. Administration of atropine intravenously
4. Discontinuation of digoxin

G. The dysrhythmia in Fig. 4-19 can be interpreted as:
1. Sinus rhythm with a PVC
2. Sinus rhythm with a junctional escape beat
3. Sinus rhythm with a PAC
4. Sinus rhythm with a PJC

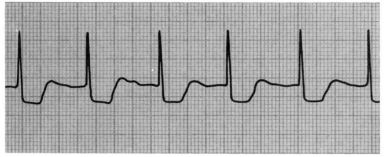

FIG. 4-20

Lead II

H. Proper therapy of the dysrhythmia in Fig. 4-19 might include the following (circle all that apply):
1. If these beats occur infrequently, the dysrhythmia is considered to be benign and requires no therapy
2. These beats are frequently the precursor of ventricular dysrhythmias (ventricular tachycardia and fibrillation) and therefore should be treated with a lidocaine drip
3. The patient may be treated with rest and sedation
4. If the patient experiences bothersome palpitations, propranolol may be given

I. The dysrhythmia in Fig. 4-20 can be interpreted as:
1. Atrial fibrillation
2. Sinus tachycardia
3. Junctional tachycardia (paroxysmal)
4. Nonparoxysmal junctional tachycardia (accelerated junctional rhythm)

J. Which of the following statements are true with regard to the dysrhythmia in Fig. 4-20? (Circle all that apply.)
1. Patients with acute inferior wall myocardial infarction may develop this dysrhythmia
2. DC cardioversion may be used if the patient's condition deteriorates
3. If the ventricular rate is rapid enough, the patient may experience chest pain, dyspnea, and lightheadedness
4. This dysrhythmia rarely occurs in patients with heart disease and is considered benign because of the relatively slow ventricular rate

SUPPLEMENTS

This is a work section. A work space is provided beneath each strip to the left. The answers are to the right. It is suggested you cover the answer section with a card or paper while you work the strips. Check your answers on the right.

A.

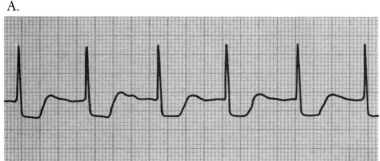

FIG. 4-21

Lead II

1. Rate:
   Atrial: Not measurable
   Ventricular: 80 per minute
2. Rhythm: Regular
3. P waves: Not present
4. PR interval: Not measurable
5. QRS interval: 0.04 second
6. Ratio of P/QRS: No P waves visible
7. QT interval: 0.44 second (difficult to measure since T
                                              waves are not easily discernible).
8. Interpretation: Accelerated junctional rhythm

B.

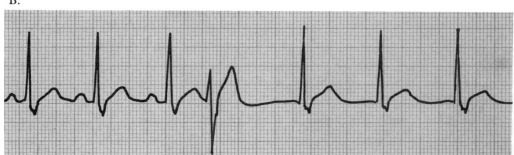

FIG. 4-22

Lead II

1. Rate:
   Atrial and
   ventricular: At the beginning of rhythm strip, the atrial
                                              and ventricular rates are both 75 per
                                              minute; after the premature complex, the
                                              atrial rate is not measurable and the ven-
                                              tricular rate is 72 per minute
2. Rhythm: The rhythm is regular until the premature
                                              complex occurs and then once again be-
                                              comes regular
3. P waves: Upright for first three complexes and then
                                              the P waves are absent
4. PR interval: 0.20 second for first three complexes
5. QRS interval: 0.06 second for all complexes except the
                                              fourth complex, which is 0.12 second
6. Ratio of P/QRS: 1:1 for first three complexes, then P waves
                                              are absent
7. Interpretation: Sinus rhythm with a PVC (fourth complex),
                                              followed by a pause that is interrupted by
                                              an accelerated junctional rhythm

C.

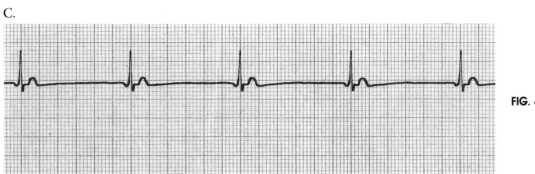

Lead II

FIG. 4-23

1. Rate:
   Atrial and
   ventricular: 50
2. Rhythm: Regular
3. P waves: Inverted before the QRS complexes
4. PR interval: 0.08 second
5. QRS interval: 0.06 second
6. Ratio of P/QRS: 1:1
7. Interpretation: Junctional rhythm

D.

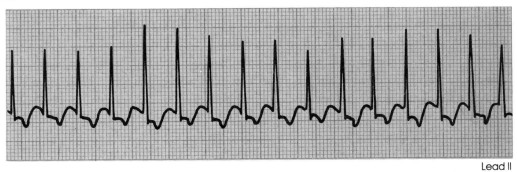

Lead II

FIG. 4-24

1. Rate:
   Atrial: No P waves visible to measure atrial rate
   Ventricular: Ventricular rate is 195 per minute
2. Rhythm: Regular
3. P waves: Not visible
4. PR interval: Not measurable
5. QRS interval: 0.06 second
6. Ratio of P/QRS: P waves not visible
7. Interpretation: Junctional tachycardia (this could be PSVT caused by nodal reentry); the distinction between the two cannot be made by evaluation of this rhythm strip alone and instead would require clinical information about the patient

E.

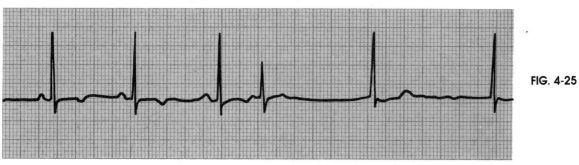

FIG. 4-25

Lead II

1. Rate:
   Atrial:

   Ventricular:

2. Rhythm:

3. P waves:

4. PR interval:
5. QRS interval:
6. Ratio of P/QRS:

7. Interpretation:

Atrial rate of 66 per minute for the first four complexes and then P waves are not visible
Ventricular rate is 66 per minute also for the first four complexes and then 42 per minute for the last two complexes
Regular for the first four complexes and then becomes irregular
Visible for the first four complexes and then are not visible
0.14 second for the first four complexes
0.08 second for all complexes
1:1 for the first four complexes and then P waves are not visible
Sinus rhythm with a PJC for the fifth complex, followed by two junctional escape complexes

F.

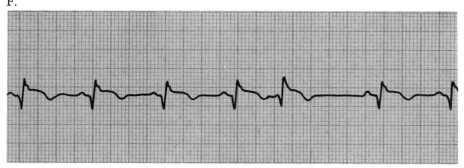

FIG. 4-26

Lead II

1. Rate:
   Atrial and
   ventricular:
2. Rhythm:
3. P waves:

4. PR interval:
5. QRS interval:
6. Ratio of P/QRS:
7. Interpretation:

77
Regular except for the premature complex
P waves are visible and upright except for the premature complex, which does not have a clearly visible P wave
0.14 second
0.04 second
1:1 except for the premature complex
Sinus rhythm with a PJC (fifth complex)

G.

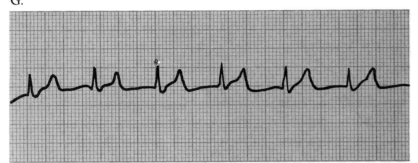

FIG. 4-27

Lead II

1. Rate:
     Atrial:
     Ventricular:
2. Rhythm:
3. P waves:
4. PR interval:
5. QRS interval:
6. Ratio of P/QRS:
7. Interpretation:

No P waves visible to measure an atrial rate
The ventricular rate is 90 per minute
Regular
Not visible
Not measurable
0.10 second
No P waves present
Accelerated junctional rhythm

ANSWERS TO PRETEST AND POSTTEST

Pretest	Posttest
A. 2	A. 2
B. 1, 2, 3	B. 1, 2
C. 4	C. 3
D. 1, 2, 4	D. 1, 4
E. 1, 2, 3	E. 1
F. 1	F. 2, 3, 4
G. 1, 2, 4	G. 4
H. 1	H. 1, 3, 4
I. 2, 3, 4	I. 4
J. 2	J. 1, 3
K. 1, 2, 4	

Atrioventricular blocks

PRETEST (Answers on pp. 115-116)

Directions: Circle one answer to each question unless otherwise indicated.

A. The dysrhythmia in Fig. 5-1 most likely represents:
   1. First-degree AV block
   2. Second-degree AV block, type I
   3. Second-degree AV block, type II
   4. Third-degree (complete) AV block

B. Which of the following might be considered as appropriate treatment for the dysrhythmia in Fig. 5-1? (Circle all that apply.)

   1. I.V. procainamide
   2. Isoproterenol
   3. Discontinue lidocaine drip
   4. Transvenous pacemaker

C. The dysrhythmia in Fig. 5-2 most likely represents:
   1. First-degree AV block
   2. Second-degree AV block, type I
   3. Second-degree AV block, type II
   4. Third-degree (complete) AV block

D. Which of the following are commonly associated with the dysrhythmia in Fig. 5-2? (Circle all the apply.)

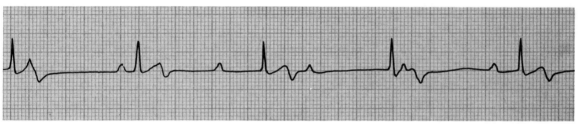

FIG. 5-1   Lead II

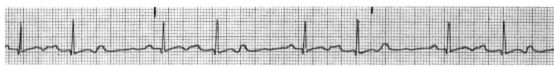

FIG. 5-2   Lead II

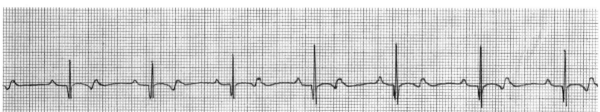

FIG. 5-3   Lead II

1. Digoxin, propranolol, quinidine, and other antidysrhythmic drugs
2. Necrosis in the area of block
3. Anterior wall myocardial infarction
4. Inferior wall myocardial infarction

E. Treatment/management of the dysrhythmia in Fig. 5-2 would probably include:
   1. Close monitoring to observe for progression to greater degrees of AV block
   2. Withholding of digoxin until physician is notified
   3. Assessment of the patient's clinical status
   4. Insertion of a transvenous pacemaker

F. The dysrhythmia in Fig. 5-3 would most probably be diagnosed as:
   1. First-degree AV block
   2. Second-degree AV block, type I
   3. Second-degree AV block, type II
   4. Third-degree (complete) AV block

G. Which of the following statements supports your answer to the preceding question?
   1. Because the PR interval is greater than 0.20 second, it favors first-degree AV block
   2. Without the patient's clinical history, this rhythm strip is difficult to diagnose, but because of the narrow QRS complex and the atrial rate, it favors second-degree AV block, type I
   3. Because there is no gradual prolongation of the PR intervals and the PR intervals of the conducted complexes are constant, the rhythm favors second-degree AV block, type II
   4. Because the atrial rate is regular and is faster than the ventricular rate, the rhythm favors third-degree AV block

H. The dysrhythmia in Fig. 5-4 most likely represents:
   1. First-degree AV block
   2. Second-degree AV block, type I
   3. Second-degree AV block, type II
   4. Third-degree (complete) AV block

I. Which one of the following statements concerning the dysrhythmia illustrated in Fig. 5-4 are true? (Circle all that apply.)
   1. It is commonly caused by digoxin, quinidine, procainamide, myocardial ischemia, or acute infections
   2. The treatment of choice is pacemaker insertion
   3. Generally, no therapy is required unless the rate slows to such an extent that the patient becomes symptomatic
   4. The nurse should carefully monitor the PR interval and report any increase in duration

J. Interpret the rhythm strip in Fig. 5-5.
   1. Rate:
      Atrial:
      Ventricular:
   2. Rhythm:
      Atrial:
      Ventricular:
   3. P waves:
   4. PR interval:
   5. Ratio of P/QRS:
   6. QRS interval:
   7. QT interval:
   8. Interpretation:

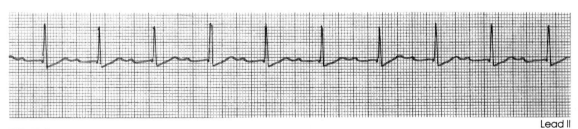

Lead II

FIG. 5-4

Lead II

FIG. 5-5

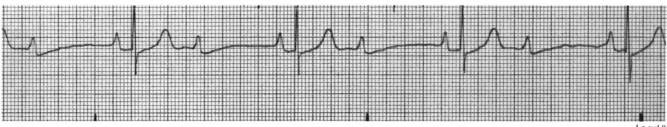

FIG. 5-6   Lead II

K. Interpret the rhythm strip in Fig. 5-6.
   1. Rate:
      Atrial:
      Ventricular:
   2. Rhythm:
      Atrial:
      Ventricular:
   3. P waves:
   4. PR interval:
   5. Ratio of P/QRS:
   6. QRS interval:
   7. QT interval:
   8. Interpretation:
L. T F   Blocks occurring below the bundle of His
          bifurcation are generally not nearly as severe as
          those occurring above the bifurcation.
M. Third-degree AV block (complete) generally occurs at
   the level of:
   1. AV node
   2. Bundle of His
   3. Left bundle branch
   4. Both bundle branches
N. The ventricular rate in third-degree heart block is:
   1. Faster than the atrial rate
   2. Usually between 45 to 60 per minute
   3. Is usually less than 45 per minute
   4. Not important
O. The atrial rhythm in third-degree heart block can be
   (circle all that apply):
   1. Normal sinus
   2. Sinus tachycardia
   3. Atrial tachycardia
   4. Atrial fibrillation

PURPOSE

The purpose of this module is to provide the learner
with basic information and a structural framework within
which to develop skills in identifying and understanding
the etiology, characteristics, clinical significance, and
management of atrioventricular (AV) blocks.

BEHAVIORAL OBJECTIVES

Upon completion of this module, the learner should
be able to:

A. List possible etiological factors of, define and identify
   criteria for, recognize on rhythm strips, state clinical
   features of, and discuss modes of treatment and
   nursing management for the following dysrhythmias:
   1. First-degree AV block
   2. Second-degree AV block
      a. Type I
      b. Type II
   3. Third-degree (complete) AV block

VOCABULARY

Idiojunctional rhythm (escape rhythm—passive rhythm) A rhythm
arising from the branching area of the bundle of His at its own
inherent rate (40 to 50 per minute) and producing a normal QRS
complex.
Idioventricular rhythm (escape rhythm—passive rhythm) A rhythm
arising in and controlling only the ventricles at their slow inherent
rate.
Stokes-Adams syndrome Episodes characterized by sudden syncope or seizures resulting from intermittent severe bradycardia,
third-degree AV block, or ventricular tachycardia, fibrillation, or
standstill.
Ventricular escape rhythm See Idioventricular rhythm.

CONTENT
Suggested review

Before beginning this module on atrioventricular
blocks, it is recommended that the learner review the
following in Module 1 on the anatomy and physiology of
the AV node.

1. Anatomy of the normal conducting pathways of the
   heart
2. Anatomy of the AV junctional area of the heart
3. Normal and potential pacemaking sites of the heart
4. Normal PR and QRS intervals
5. Calculation of heart rate by use of calipers and use of
   ECG paper time increments
6. Escape complex (junctional and ventricular)

Atrioventricular blocks—an overview

AV block occurs when there is an interference with conduction of impulses between the atria and ventricles. These blocks are caused by ischemia, edema, and/or damage to the tissues of the AV node, bundle of His, and/or the bundle branches. The treatment and prognosis of the patient are generally related to the specific area affected. Blocks occurring in the AV node are usually transient and/or benign, whereas blocks occurring infranodally tend to be more serious and permanent. Past experience and the patient's clinical status often help to identify the area of involvement from the surface ECG.[2]

For the purposes of simplicity, heart blocks are usually categorized as first-, second- or third-degree AV blocks.

In first-degree AV block, *all* impulses from the sinus node are conducted through the AV junction but are abnormally delayed, usually at the AV node itself. The PR interval is greater than 0.20 second and is the same for each impulse.

In second-degree AV block, *some,* but not all, of the atrial impulses are conducted to the ventricles. There are two basic types of second-degree block, each with its own degree of severity and area of involvement. As more information has become available over the years, terminology used for types of second-degree block has changed. Wenckebach[7] (1899) described AV conduction disturbances using jugular pulse tracings, which developed into a classification of blocks, including the term "Wenckebach block." Mobitz[5] (1924), using electrocardiography as a basis, classified second-degree AV block as "type I" and "type II," with the terms "Mobitz I" and "Mobitz II" resulting. Today, we more commonly hear the terms "type I" and "type II" AV block, which will be used in this text.

In third-degree (complete) AV block, *none* of the impulses from the atria are conducted to the ventricles; hence, the term "complete heart block" is used. In this situation the atria and ventricles function independently of each other, with the ventricular rate being much slower than the atrial rate.

Fig. 5-7 illustrates locations where the various types of heart blocks occur.

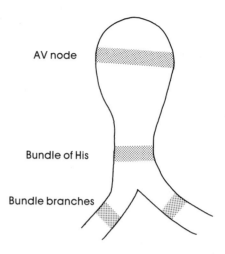

FIG. 5-7

AV junctional pathways illustrating various locations where blocks can occur: *AV node*—first degree; second degree, type I; and third degree. *Bundle of His*—third degree. *Bundle branches*—second degree, type II, and third degree.

Rhythm disturbances
FIRST-DEGREE AV BLOCK (FIG. 5-8)
Definition

1. First-degree AV block is manifested on the ECG by prolongation of the PR interval; this prolongation generally represents delayed conduction of the cardiac impulse through the AV node
2. Each atrial impulse is conducted to the ventricles, resulting in a regularly occurring ventricular rhythm

Etiology

1. First-degree AV block is commonly associated with:
   a. Digoxin, propranolol, quinidine, procainamide, and/or other antidysrhythmic drugs
   b. Ischemia of the AV node caused by coronary artery disease
2. It has been reported to occur in 7% to 13% of patients with acute myocardial infarction[2]

PR interval = 0.32 sec

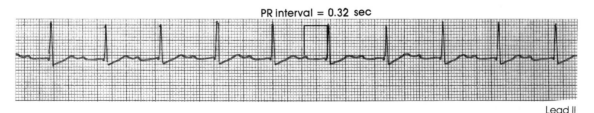

Lead II

FIG. 5-8

Normal sinus rhythm with first-degree AV block.

3. It may be caused by:
   a. A variety of acute infectious diseases such as pericarditis
   b. Acute rheumatic fever
4. It may occur in the absence of heart disease

Characteristics of rhythm

1. Rate:
   Atrial: Usually within normal limits of 60-100 per minute; however, first-degree AV block can be present with sinus bradycardia (rate less than 60 per minute)
   Ventricular: Same as atrial
2. Rhythm:
   Atrial: Regular, although first-degree AV block can also occur with sinus arrhythmia, in which case the rhythm would be irregular
   Ventricular: Same as atrial
3. P waves: Normal, originating in the SA node
4. PR interval: Prolonged beyond 0.20 second; however, all the PR intervals are the same
5. QRS interval: Usually within normal limits, although first-degree block can also be seen in association with bundle branch blocks (wide and/or notched QRSs)
6. Ratio of P/QRS: 1:1
7. QT interval: Less than 0.43 second or less than one half of the preceding RR interval

Clinical features

1. No physical signs or symptoms are related to this dysrhythmia
2. The diagnosis is made only from ECG where the PR interval can be measured

Treatment measures

1. No treatment is necessary if the delay in conduction is only slight (0.21 to 0.25 second) and the patient is asymptomatic

2. If the PR interval increases in duration and is greater than 0.26 second, the physician may decide to hold any drugs that the patient may be receiving that are known to slow AV conduction

Nursing management

1. Assess the patient and monitor vital signs, neurovital signs, level of consciousness, etc.
2. Carefully measure and record the PR interval every 2 to 4 hours, depending on the amount of PR prolongation
3. If the PR interval becomes progressively longer or is greater than 0.26 second, notify the physician
4. Carefully observe the cardiac monitor for the appearance of a second- or third-degree AV block; if either of these advanced forms of heart block occur, notify the physician immediately
5. The patient's need for digoxin or antidysrhythmic drugs should be assessed by the physician

Special considerations

When first-degree block occurs in individuals with no history of heart disease, there is usually no further progression of the block. However, when first-degree heart block is associated with a myocardial infarction, it is not uncommon for the block to progress to second-degree AV block, type I, and on to third-degree AV block with an adequate junctional pacemaker rate.

SECOND-DEGREE AV BLOCK

Second-degree heart block is characterized by the presence of P waves with associated QRS complexes and other P waves that are not followed by QRS complexes. This occurs because some atrial impulses are blocked in the AV junction or below the bundle of His and do not reach the ventricles. In this type of conduction disturbance, impulses may be blocked at regular or irregular

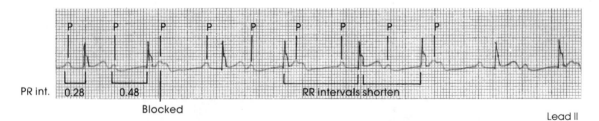

FIG. 5-9

Second-degree AV block, type I with 3:2 conduction. Strip shows progressive prolongation of PR interval (0.28 second and 0.48 second) and blocked or nonconducted QRS complex. PR interval following "dropped" or nonconducted complex is shortest in series of cycles. As PR intervals lengthen, RR intervals shorten before "dropped" complexes.

intervals. There are basically two types of second-degree AV block:

Second-degree AV block, type I
(Mobitz type I or Wenckebach block) (Figs. 5-9 and 5-10)
Definition

1. In a cyclical fashion an atrial impulse is blocked at the AV node and a ventricular complex is "dropped" or nonconducted
2. The shortest PR interval of the cycle occurs with the first complex following the dropped QRS complex
3. Then, because of lengthening AV conduction time, the PR interval becomes progressively longer with each succeeding complex until the AV junction is refractory and does not conduct an atrial impulse; hence, no ventricular stimulation occurs (a QRS complex fails to appear, or is "dropped")
4. The duration of the pause following the nonconducted P wave is less than two times the shortest cycle
5. The ratio of atrial impulses to ventricular responses is frequently 5:4, 4:3, 3:2 or 2:1
6. The increment of the PR lengthening is greatest with the second complex of the cycle
7. As the PR intervals lengthen, the RR intervals shorten before the nonconducted complexes

Etiology

1. Second-degree AV block, type I is commonly associated with:
   a. Inferior wall myocardial infarction that tends to cause temporary inflammation and edema only to the area of the AV node—sparing the bundle of His and the bundle branches, which usually have an adequate inherent rate
   b. Postoperative phase of open heart surgery
   c. Digoxin toxicity[2]
   d. Propranolol

2. It may be caused by:
   a. Almost any acute infectious disease
   b. Rheumatic fever
   c. Myocarditis
   d. Many illnesses, including myxedema, scleroderma,[1] etc.
3. It may occur in the absence of organic heart disease

Characteristics of rhythm

1. Rate:
   Atrial: May be normal or slow
   Ventricular: Depends on atrial rate and number of dropped complexes
2. Rhythm:
   Atrial: Usually regular
   Ventricular: Irregular because of dropped complexes (unless the ratio of atrial impulses to ventricular impulses is 2:1) and progressive prolongation of the PR intervals
3. P waves: Normal in appearance; the number of P waves is always greater than the number of QRS complexes
4. PR interval: Lengthens progressively until an atrial impulse is completely blocked at the AV node, resulting in the loss of a QRS complex (a "dropped" complex)
5. QRS interval: Usually normal
6. Ratio of P/QRS: Variable, but always more P waves than QRS complexes
7. QT interval: Usually normal (less than 0.43 second)

Clinical features

1. Depends on ventricular rate; the patient is unaware of this conduction disturbance unless the rate is exceptionally slow
2. The diagnosis can be established by ECG findings

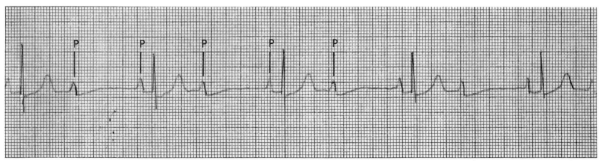

FIG. 5-10
Second-degree AV block, type I, with 2:1 conduction. See text for rationale for designating type I vs. type II block.

Lead II

Treatment

1. Many physicians do not treat this rhythm disturbance since progression to a more serious dysrhythmia usually does not occur; typically, this type of block is transient
2. In patients who are symptomatic and who have very slow ventricular rates, atropine, in 0.5 mg increments I.V., or isoproterenol, 1 to 2 μg/min, may be used to increase conduction through the AV node
3. Although uncommon, pacemaker therapy may be used if the block persists after drug therapy[1]
4. Although drugs seldom cause this dysrhythmia, digoxin or certain antidysrhythmic drugs should be withheld if the block persists

Nursing management

1. Assess the patient, monitor vital signs, neurovital signs, level of consciousness, etc.
2. Identify and document this conduction disorder on a rhythm strip
3. Determine variability and progressive lengthening of the PR interval
4. Prepare for possible administration of atropine and/or isoproterenol
5. Withhold digoxin and other antidysrythmic drugs, if applicable
6. Observe monitor closely for progression to a greater degree of AV block

Special considerations

1. If the conduction ratio of atrial impulses to ventricular impulses is 2:1, one may misdiagnose this rhythm as second-degree AV block, type II, which carries a more significant prognosis and treatment regime than does type I AV block; type I AV block usually occurs at the AV node level, whereas type II AV block generally occurs below the bifurcation of the bundle of His
2. Although one cannot be absolutely sure from the surface ECG which of the two types it is, experience has shown that the width of the QRS is a good predictor of the location of the block; with a QRS of normal duration, the block usually is above the bifurcation of the bundle of His at the AV node; with a QRS greater than 0.12 second, the block is usually below the bifurcation of the bundle of His[7]
3. A clinical measurement that should be used in the differential diagnosis of 2:1 block as type I or type II is the type of myocardial infarction that is present, if applicable; an inferior wall myocardial infarction usually only temporarily affects the AV node, whereas an anterior wall myocardial infarction often causes permanent damage (necrosis) to the area below the bundle of His

Second-degree AV block, type II (Mobitz type II)
(Fig. 5-11)
Definition

1. This type of block almost always occurs in the bundle branches; one bundle branch is usually completely blocked causing a wide QRS complex and the other is intermittently blocked causing nonconducted QRS complexes[2]
2. Some atrial impulses are blocked in the AV junction and do not reach the ventricles, but the PR intervals of the impulses that *do* conduct to the ventricles are all identical to each other; hence there is no progressive lengthening of the PR interval as there is in type I AV block
3. The PR intervals of the conducted impulses may be prolonged greater than 0.20 second (an associated first-degree block), or they may be normal
4. The PP interval is generally constant and the atrial rhythm is regular
5. The ventricular rate can be normal or dangerously slow and the rhythm can be regular or irregular

Etiology

1. Second-degree AV block, type II is most commonly associated with an anterior wall myocardial infarction that can cause extensive necrosis to the uppermost portion of the interventricular septum; often the AV node and bundle of His are spared, but severe damage is done to the bundle branches and complete AV block may develop
2. Second-degree block can be associated with open heart surgery

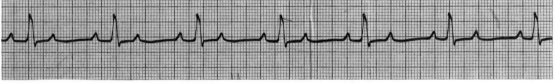

FIG. 5-11   Lead II

Widened QRS complex in second-degree AV block, type II, with 2:1 conduction.

3. It can be caused by numerous degenerative processes, including[1]:
   a. Fibrosclerosis of the cardiac skeleton
   b. Fibrosis of the conduction system
   c. Coronary artery disease
   d. Myodarditis
   e. Cardiomyopathies
4. It is occasionally associated with various diseases, such as:
   a. Scleroderma
   b. Myxedema
   c. Chagas' disease
   d. Lenegre's disease
   e. Lev's disease[1]

Characteristics of rhythm

1. Rate:
   Atrial: Variable, depending on whether sinus bradycardia, sinus tachycardia, or another dyshythmia is the atrial mechanism; typically, however, the atrial rhythm is regular and the rate is normal, 60-100 per minute
   Ventricular: If the block is periodic and occurs only occasionally, the rate may be near normal; however, if the block is a constant 2:1 to 3:1, etc., the ventricular rate will be slow
2. Rhythm:
   Atrial: Usually regular
   Ventricular: Regular or irregular, depending on whether atrial impulses are blocked at irregular or constant intervals; if only periodic atrial impulses are blocked, the ventricular rhythm will be irregular; if the block is 2:1, 3:1, 4:1, etc. and constant, the ventricular rhythm will be regular
3. P waves: Usually normal
4. PR interval: In the conducted complexes the PR interval is constant; may be normal or may be prolonged more than 0.20 second
5. QRS interval: May be within normal limits (0.06-0.12 second) but is usually prolonged beyond 0.12 second; if the block is in the AV junction, the QRS is normal; if the block is below the junction (bundle branches), which is the most common occurrence, the QRS is prolonged
6. Ratio of P/QRS: Can be variable if the block is periodic or can be 2:1, 3:1, 4:1, etc., if the block is constant
7. QT interval: Usually normal (less than 0.43 second)

Clinical features

1. Symptoms are related to the ventricular rate and cardiac output; the patient is unaware that this conduction disorder is present if the ventricular rate is near normal; if the ventricular rate is slow, the patient may experience angina, heart failure, dyspnea, and/or syncope
2. The diagnosis is made from ECG findings

Treatment measures

1. If the patient has had an acute myocardial infarction (MI), a temporary transvenous pacemaker should be inserted as soon as this type of block is identified; this is a precautionary measure since there is the imminent danger of a complete heart block or ventricular standstill occurring
2. When the QRS complexes are widened, drug therapy cannot be relied on, but if the QRS complexes are within normal limits, isoproterenol may be administered while awaiting insertion of a temporary pacemaker; atropine is not a drug of choice because it tends to increase the atrial rate without decreasing the block and may cause more atrial impulses to block and decrease the ventricular rate even more[1]
3. All antidysrhythmic drugs and/or digoxin should be withheld if the patient receiving them develops a second-degree AV block

Nursing management

1. Assess patient and monitor vital signs, neurovital signs, level of consciousness, etc.
2. Identify this dysrhythmia and document it on a rhythm strip
3. Measure the PR intervals throughout the rhythm strip to determine if they are constant
4. Measure the QRS intervals; if they are greater than 0.12 second, be alerted to the possibility of a complete heart block or ventricular standstill developing
5. Prepare to administer isoproterenol I.V.
6. Prepare for insertion of a transvenous pacemaker
7. If applicable, withhold further doses of antidysrhythmic agents and digoxin
8. Observe monitor closely for progression of rhythm to a complete heart block or ventricular standstill

Special considerations

Type II AV block has a very serious prognosis if one of the following is present: anterior wall MI and evidence that block is below the AV junction

THIRD-DEGREE AV BLOCK (COMPLETE)
(Figs. 5-12 and 5-13, p. 108)
Definition

1. With this conduction disturbance, the atria and ventricles depolarize entirely independently of one another because all atrial impulses are blocked; the ventricular rhythm is an "escape" or "passive" rhythm

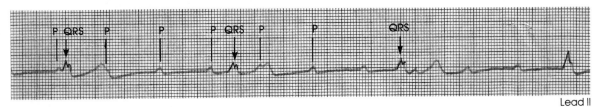

Lead II

FIG. 5-12

Third-degree (complete) AV block. Note that atrial rate is faster than ventricular rate and that atrial and ventricular complexes are totally dissociated from each other. Also note very slow ventricular rate and widened QRS complex, indicating that ventricular escape focus is low within ventricles.

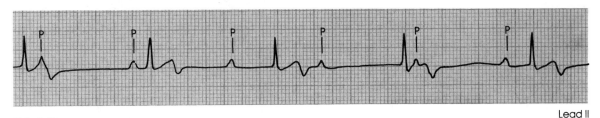

Lead II

FIG. 5-13

Third-degree (complete) AV block. Note total dissociation between atrial and ventricular complexes.

2. The atrial pacemaker is usually the sinus node and therefore produces a normal sinus rhythm; however, ectopic foci may produce atrial tachycardia or fibrillation

3. The ventricular pacemaker may be above or below the bundle of His, depending on the location of the block

4. If it is above the bundle of His, it is supraventricular and the QRS may be narrow with a rate of 40 to 50 per minute or faster; this is called an "idiojunctional" rhythm

5. If the ventricular pacemaker is below the bundle of His, the QRS is wide and the rate will be 40 or below, depending on the location of the site; this is called a "idioventricular" rhythm

Etiology

1. Third-degree AV block is most commonly associated with an anterior wall MI that can cause extensive necrosis to the uppermost portion of the interventricular septum; often the AV node and bundle of His are spared, but severe damage is done to the bundle branches; complete AV block may develop

2. Third-degree block can be associated with open heart surgery

3. It can be caused by numerous degenerative processes, including[1]:
   a. Fibrosclerosis of the cardiac skeleton
   b. Fibrosis of the conduction system
   c. Coronary artery disease
   d. Myocarditis
   e. Cardiomyopathies

4. It is frequently associated with various diseases, including[1]:
   a. Scleroderma
   b. Myxedema
   c. Chagas' disease
   d. Lenegre's disease
   e. Lev's disease

Characteristics of rhythm

1. Rate:
   Atrial: Generally from 60-120 per minute; always faster than the ventricular
   Ventricular: Less than 50 per minute

2. Rhythm: Both atrial and ventricular rhythms are generally regular, but are not related to each other

3. P waves: The number of P waves *always* exceeds the number of QRS complexes; the P waves have a normal

appearance if the pacemaker is the sinus node; if an ectopic focus is the pacemaker, atrial activity will take on respective characteristics

4. PR interval: PR interval is never constant because the atria and ventricles have independent pacemakers; P waves, in this case, have no relation to QRS complexes, and PR intervals should not be measured
5. QRS interval: The width and configuration of the complex depends on the location of the ectopic pacemaker; if the pacemaker is in the AV junctional site, the QRS complexes will appear normal; if the pacemaker is below the bundle of His, the QRS complexes will be widened and bizarre
6. Ratio of P/QRS: Variable; there are more P waves than QRS complexes
7. QT interval: Generally less than 0.43 second

Clinical features

1. If the ventricular rate is slow enough to lower cardiac output, signs of decompensation occur:
   a. The blood pressure commonly drops
   b. Episodes of dizziness and syncope are common and convulsions may occur as a result of cerebral ischemia
2. The patient may be symptomatic with any physical activity if the onset of the block is acute
3. Angina may occur in the patients with preexisting coronary artery disease
4. Individuals with long-standing third-degree AV block may be totally asymptomatic and tolerate the rhythm well

Treatment measures

1. Transvenous cardiac pacing is the immediate treatment of choice for a block that is not long-standing
2. If the patient is in danger, isoproterenol may be given by I.V. infusion while preparing for insertion of the pacemaker
3. If the complete heart block persists because of irreversible damage to the conduction system, a permanent pacemaker should be inserted

Nursing management

1. Assess patient and monitor vital signs, neurovital signs, etc.
2. Identify and document this conduction disturbance with a rhythm strip
3. Notify the physician immediately
4. Limit the patient's activity and administer oxygen if indicated
5. Prepare an infusion of isoproterenol
6. Prepare for insertion of temporary transvenous pacemaker

7. Have a defibrillator at the bedside because of the possibility of ventricular fibrillation in the presence of an extremely slow ventricular rate (idioventricular rhythm)
8. Keep a 100-mg syringe of lidocaine at the bedside
9. Assess the patient for signs or symptoms of left ventricular failure
10. Carefully watch the monitor for premature ventricular contractions that forewarn of ventricular tachycardia or fibrillation
11. If ventricular standstill occurs, immediately initiate CPR

Special considerations

1. The Stokes-Adams syndrome related to complete AV block has a serious prognosis; death can occur from ventricular fibrillation or ventricular standstill
2. Anterior infarction carries a more serious prognosis than inferior or posterior infarction for third-degree AV blocks

REFERENCES

1. Andreoli, K.G., et al.: Comprehensive cardiac care, ed. 5, St. Louis, 1983, The C.V. Mosby Co.
2. Conover, M.B.: Understanding electrocardiography: arrhythmias and the 12-lead ECG, ed. 4, St. Louis, 1984, The C.V. Mosby Co.
3. Goldman, M.J.: Principles of clinical electrocardiography, ed. 10, Los Altos, Calif., 1979, Lange Medical Publications.
4. Marriott, H.J.L., and Conover, M.B.: Advanced concepts in arrhythmias, St. Louis, 1983, The C.V. Mosby Co.
5. Mobitz, W.: Über die Unvoldstandige storung der erregungsuberleitung zwischen vorhof und kammer des menschlichen, Herzens, Z. Gesamte, Exp. Med. **41**:180, 1984.
6. Watanabe, Y., and Driefus, L.S.: Atrioventricular block: basic concepts. In Mandel, W., editor: Cardiac arrhythmias, Philadelphia, 1980, J.B. Lippincott Company.
7. Wenckebach, K.F.: Zur Analyse des unregelmgssigen pulses, Z. Klin. Med. **37**:475, 1899.

SUGGESTED LEARNING ACTIVITIES AND EXPERIENCES

A. Find patients in any of the critical care areas who demonstrate AV blocks
B. Once a conduction disturbance is identified, review the patient's record, including:
   1. History
   2. Physical examination
   3. Diagnosis
   4. Medications (both scheduled and p.r.n.)
   5. Vital signs
   6. Laboratory data

7. Any other treatment modality, such as pacemaker, etc.

C. Attempt to identify a possible etiology of the conduction disturbance

D. Identify treatment measures and nursing observations and/or management that relates to the particular conduction disturbance

E. Write patient care objectives on the nursing process record in relation to the disturbance

F. Study the available and suggested references on AV blocks

POSTTEST (Answers on p. 116)

Directions: Circle one answer to each question unless otherwise indicated.

A. In 80% to 90% of the population, the AV node receives its blood supply from the:
1. Right coronary artery
2. Left anterior descending coronary artery
3. Left circumflex
4. Diagonal branch

B. Stimulation of the sympathetic nerve causes which of the following:
1. Decreased speed of conduction through the AV node
2. Increased speed of conduction through the AV node
3. No influence on the AV node
4. Decreased heart rate

C. Which one of the following are true concerning first-degree AV block? (Circle all that apply.)
1. There is a 1:1 ratio of P/QRS
2. Conduction through the junction is prolonged more than 0.20 second
3. The most common cause is anterior wall myocardial infarction
4. The rhythm is irregular

D. As the PR intervals lengthen, the RR intervals shorten before "dropped complexes." This statement best describes:
1. Type II AV block with variable block
2. Third-degree AV block
3. First-degree AV block
4. Type I AV block

E. Some atrial impulses are blocked in the AV junction and do not reach the ventricles, but the PR intervals of those that *do* conduct are all identical to each other. The QRS complex is 0.14 second. These statements best describe:
1. Type II AV block

2. Third-degree AV block
3. First-degree AV block
4. Type I AV block

F. If the patient has had an acute anterior MI, a temporary transvenous pacemaker may be inserted as soon as this type of heart block is identified. This is a precautionary measure since there is danger of complete AV block or ventricular standstill occurring. These statements most probably refer to:
1. Type II AV block with a slow ventricular response
2. First-degree AV block
3. Type I AV block
4. Type I AV block

G. Type II AV block has a very serious prognosis if the following are present (circle all that apply):
1. Anterior wall MI
2. Inferior wall MI
3. Evidence that heart block is below the AV junction
4. Evidence that heart block is in the AV node

H. In this conduction disturbance, the ventricular rate is slow with wide bizarre complexes, and the atrial rate may be normal or abnormal, as in atrial tachycardia or fibrillation:
1. Type II AV block
2. Third-degree AV block
3. First-degree AV block
4. Type I AV block

I. Which of the following concerning third-degree AV block are true? (Circle all that apply.)
1. All patients with third-degree heart block are symptomatic and require a pacemaker
2. Angina can occur because of decreased cardiac output in patients with preexisting coronary artery disease
3. Individuals may be totally asymptomatic and tolerate the conduction disturbance well
4. Episodes of dizziness, syncope, and/or convulsions may occur

J. List at least five causes of third-degree AV block:
1. _____
2. _____
3. _____
4. _____
5. _____

K. Interpret the rhythm in Fig. 5-14.
1. Rate:
   Atrial:
   Ventricular:
2. Rhythm:
   Atrial:
   Ventricular:

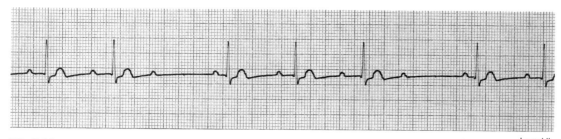

FIG. 5-14   Lead II

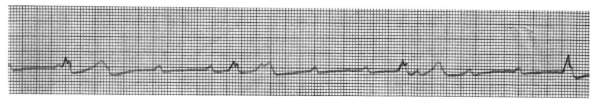

FIG. 5-15   Lead II

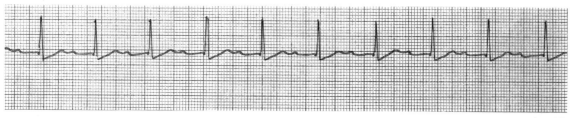

FIG. 5-16   Lead II

3. P wave morphology (all the same or different?):
4. PR interval:
5. Ratio of P/QRS:
6. QRS interval:
7. QT interval:
8. Interpretation (identify basic rhythm *and* rhythm disturbance):
9. Common cause(s):
10. Management (treatment and nursing management):

L. Interpret the rhythm in Fig. 5-15.
  1. Rate:
    Atrial:
    Ventricular:
  2. Rhythm:
    Atrial:
    Ventricular:
  3. P wave morphology (all same or different?):
  4. PR interval:
  5. Ratio of P/QRS:

6. QRS interval:
7. QT interval:
8. Interpretation: (identify basic rhythm *and* rhythm disturbance):
9. Common cause(s):
10. Management (treatment and nursing management):

M. Interpret the rhythm in Fig. 5-16.
  1. Rate:
    Atrial:
    Ventricular:
  2. Rhythm:
    Atrial:
    Ventricular:
  3. P wave morphology (all same or different?):
  4. PR interval:
  5. Ratio of P/QRS:
  6. QRS interval:
  7. QT interval:

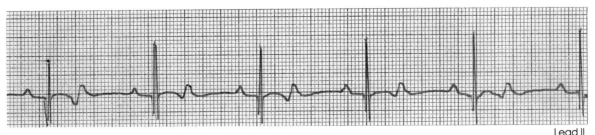

FIG. 5-17   Lead II

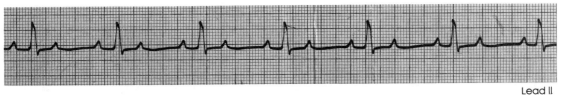

FIG. 5-18   Lead II

8. Interpretation: (identify basic rhythm *and* rhythm disturbance):
9. Common cause(s):
10. Management (treatment and nursing management):

N. Interpret the rhythm in Fig. 5-17.
   1. Rate:
      Atrial:
      Ventricular:
   2. Rhythm:
      Atrial:
      Ventricular:
   3. P wave morphology (all same or different?):
   4. PR interval:
   5. Ratio of P/QRS:
   6. QRS interval:
   7. QT interval:
   8. Interpretation: (identify basic rhythm *and* rhythm disturbance):
   9. Common cause(s):
  10. Management (treatment and nursing management):

O. Interpret the rhythm in Fig. 5-18.
   1. Rate:
      Atrial:
      Ventricular:
   2. Rhythm:
      Atrial:
      Ventricular:
   3. P wave morphology (all same or different?):
   4. PR interval:

5. Ratio of P/QRS:
6. QRS interval:
7. QT interval:
8. Interpretation: (identify basic rhythm *and* rhythm disturbance):
9. Common cause(s):
10. Management (treatment and nursing management):

P. Matching: Match the term in Column A with the definition in Column B.

Column A Term	Column B Definition
___ 1. Idiojunctional rhythm ___ 2. Type I AV block ___ 3. Stokes-Adams syndrome ___ 4. Third-degree AV block ___ 5. Idioventricular rhythm	a. Episodes characterized by sudden syncope or seizures resulting from intermittent severe bradycardia, third-degree AV block, or ventricular tachycardia, fibrillation, or standstill b. A rhythm arising in the branching area of the bundle of His at its own inherent rate and producing a normal QRS complex c. A rhythm arising in and controlling the ventricles at their inherent rate d. A rhythm in which the atrial rate is faster than the ventricular rate and the two rhythms are independent of each other e. A rhythm characterized by gradual prolongation of PR intervals with "dropped" complexes

SUPPLEMENTS

This is a work section. A work space is provided beneath each strip to the left. The answers are to the right. It is suggested that you cover the answer section with a card or paper while you work the strips. Check your answers on the right.

A.

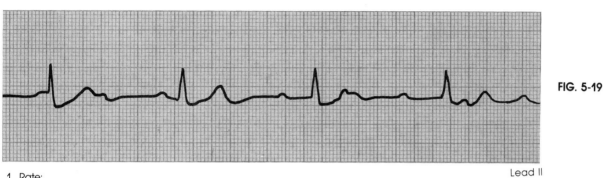

FIG. 5-19

Lead II

1. Rate:	
Atrial:	95
Ventricular:	Approximately 42
2. Rhythm:	
Atrial:	Regular
Ventricular:	Regular
3. P waves:	Upright
4. PR interval:	Not relevant
5. Ratio of P/QRS:	Not relevant
6. QRS interval:	0.10 second
7. QT interval:	Approximately 0.56 to 0.60 second
8. Interpretation:	Third-degree AV block

B.

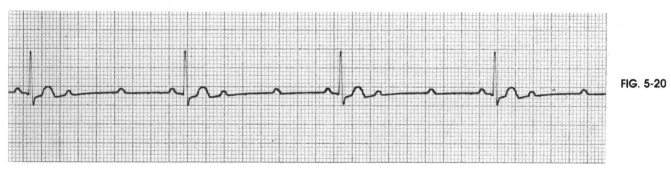

FIG. 5-20

1. Rate:	
Atrial:	102
Ventricular:	36
2. Rhythm:	
Atrial:	Regular
Ventricular:	Regular
3. P waves:	Upright
4. PR interval:	0.16 second
5. Ratio of P/QRS:	3:1
6. QRS interval:	0.08 second
7. QT interval:	0.32 second
8. Interpretation:	Second-degree heart block with 3:1 conduction

C.

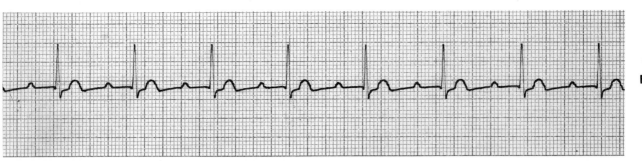

FIG. 5-21

Lead II

1. Rate:
    Atrial: 70
    Ventricular: 70
2. Rhythm:
    Atrial: Regular
    Ventricular: Regular
3. P waves: Upright
4. PR interval: 0.30 second
5. Ratio of P/QRS: 1:1
6. QRS interval: 0.08 second
7. QT interval: 0.32 second
8. Interpretation: Normal sinus rhythm with first-degree AV
                                     block

D.

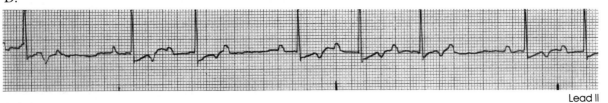

FIG. 5-22

Lead II

1. Rate:
    Atrial: 75
    Ventricular: 54
2. Rhythm:
    Atrial: Regular
    Ventricular: Regular
3. P waves: Upright
4. PR interval: Variable—0.28-0.40 second
5. Ratio of P/QRS: 3:2
6. QRS interval: 0.07-0.08 second
7. QT interval: 0.36 second
8. Interpretation: Type I AV block with 3:2 conduction

E.

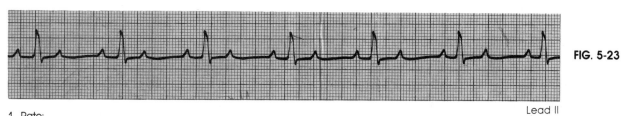

FIG. 5-23

Lead II

1. Rate:	
Atrial:	100
Ventricular:	50
2. Rhythm:	
Atrial:	Regular
Ventricular:	Regular
3. P waves:	Upright
4. PR interval:	0.28 second
5. Ratio of P/QRS:	2:1
6. QRS interval:	0.14 second
7. QT interval:	Not able to measure
8. Interpretation:	Most likely type II AV block with 2:1 conduction; rationale for type II vs. type I— wide QRS complex

F.

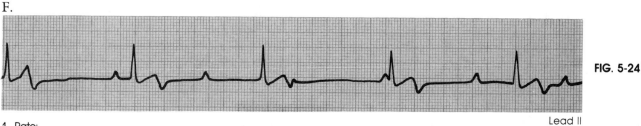

FIG. 5-24

Lead II

1. Rate:	
Atrial:	48
Ventricular:	34
2. Rhythm:	
Atrial:	Regular
Ventricular:	Regular
3. P waves:	Upright
4. PR interval:	Variable—not relevant
5. Ratio of P/QRS:	Not relevant
6. QRS interval:	0.08-0.10 second
7. QT interval:	0.52 second
8. Interpretation:	Third-degree AV block

ANSWERS TO PRETEST AND POSTTEST
Pretest

A. 4

B. 2, 3, 4

C. 2

D. 1, 4

E. 1, 2, 3

F. 2

G. 2

H. 1

I. 1, 3, 4

J. Fig. 5-5.
  1. Rate:
    Atrial: 78
    Ventricular: 78

2. Rhythm:
  Atrial: Regular
  Ventricular: Regular
3. P waves: Upright, peaked and notched
4. PR interval: 0.28 second
5. Ratio of P/QRS: 1:1
6. QRS interval: 0.08-0.09 second
7. QT interval: 0.32 second
8. Interpretation: Normal sinus rhythm with first-degree AV block

K. Fig. 5-6.
  1. Rate:

Atrial: 66
Ventricular: 33
2. Rhythm:
   Atrial: Regular
   Ventricular: Regular
3. P waves: Upright
4. PR interval: 0.22 second
5. Ratio of P/QRS: 2:1
6. QRS interval: 0.08 second
7. QT interval: 0.48 second
8. Interpretation: Most likely type I AV block with 2:1 conduction; rationale for type I vs. type II—narrow QRS complex

L. F
M. 4
N. 3
O. 1, 2, 3, 4

Posttest

A. 1   F. 1
B. 3   G. 1, 3
C. 1, 2   H. 2
D. 4   I. 2, 3, 4
E. 1

J. Anterior wall MI, open heart surgery, degenerative fibrosis of cardiac skeleton, fibrosis of conduction system, coronary artery disease myocarditis, cardiomyopathies, and systemic disease (scleroderma, myxedema, Chagas' disease, Lenegre's disease, Lev's disease)

K. Fig. 5-14.
   1. Rate:
      Atrial: 69
      Ventricular: Approximately 50
   2. Rhythm:
      Atrial: Regular
      Ventricular: Regular
   3. P waves: Upright
   4. PR interval: Variable; 0.18-0.32 second
   5. P/QRS ratio: 3:2
   6. QRS interval: 0.08 second
   7. QT interval: 0.32 second
   8. Interpretation: Type I second-degree AV block with 3:2 conduction

L. Fig. 5-15.
   1. Rate:
      Atrial: 83
      Ventricular: Approximately 25
   2. Rhythm:
      Atrial: Regular
      Ventricular: Regular
   3. P waves: Upright
   4. PR interval: Variable—not relevant
   5. Ratio of P/QRS: Not relevant
   6. QRS interval: 0.14 second
   7. QT interval: Approximately 0.66 second
   8. Interpretation: Third-degree AV block

M. Fig. 5-16.
   1. Rate:
      Atrial: 79
      Ventricular: 79
   2. Rhythm:
      Atrial: Regular
      Ventricular: Regular
   3. P waves: Upright
   4. PR interval: 0.32 second
   5. Ratio of P/QRS: 1:1
   6. QRS interval: 0.08 second
   7. QT interval: 0.38 second
   8. Interpretation: Normal sinus rhythm with first-degree AV block

N. Fig. 5-17.
   1. Rate:
      Atrial: 104
      Ventricular: Approximately 52
   2. Rhythm:
      Atrial: Regular
      Ventricular: Regular
   3. P waves: Upright
   4. PR interval: 0.28 second
   5. Ratio of P/QRS: 2:1
   6. QRS interval: 0.08 second
   7. QT interval: Not able to measure
   8. Interpretation: Most likely type I AV block with 2:1; rationale for type I vs. type II—narrow QRS complex

O. Fig. 5-18.
   1. Rate:
      Atrial: 100
      Ventricular: 50
   2. Rhythm:
      Atrial: Regular
      Ventricular: Regular
   3. P waves: Upright
   4. PR interval: 0.28 second
   5. Ratio of P/QRS: 2:1
   6. QRS interval: 0.14 second
   7. QT interval: Not able to measure
   8. Interpretation: Most likely type II AV block with 2:1; rationale for type II vs. type I—wide QRS complex

P. Matching:
   1. b   3. a   5. c
   2. e   4. d

6 Ventricular dysrhythmias

PRETEST (Answers on p. 148)

Directions: Circle one answer to each question unless otherwise indicated.

A. A continuous rhythm strip showing each normal complex followed by a premature ventricular complex (PVC) would be *best* interpreted as:
1. Ventricular trigeminy
2. Irregular rhythm
3. Ventricular bigeminy
4. Frequent PVCs

B. A single ventricular ectopic focus may fire once or may fire in a series of rapid successive impulses to produce:
1. Ventricular escape rhythm
2. Ventricular fusion complexes
3. Ventricular fibrillation
4. Ventricular tachycardia

C. Ventricular tachycardia (circle all that apply):
1. Is usually a serious finding and indicates the presence of underlying heart disease
2. Can be caused by smoking or alcohol
3. Usually ends spontaneously and requires no treatment
4. Is often propagated by the electrophysiological mechanism of reentry

D. The most likely treatment to be used in correcting the rhythm in Fig. 6-1 would be:
1. A pacemaker
2. Quinidine p.o.
3. DC countershock
4. External chest compression (CPR)

E. The rhythm is Fig. 6-2 would most likely be treated with (circle all that apply):

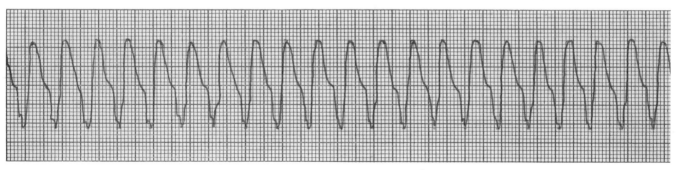

FIG. 6-1 Lead II

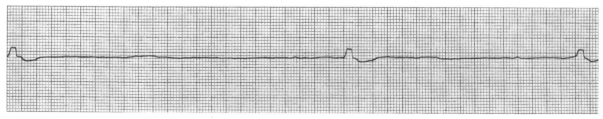

FIG. 6-2 Lead II

117

1. Atropine and/or isoproterenol and a pacemaker
2. Lidocaine
3. DC countershock
4. External chest compression (CPR)

F. The ectopic complexes in Fig. 6-3 would most likely be classified as:
1. R-on-T PVCs
2. Interpolated PVCs
3. Aberrantly conducted complexes
4. End-diastolic PVCs

G. The fast rhythm on the last part of the strip in Fig. 6-4 was probably initiated by:
1. Fusion complex
2. Angina
3. Myocardial infarction (MI)
4. R-on-T PVC

H. Interpret the rhythm in Fig. 6-5.
1. Rate:
   Atrial:

Ventricular:
2. Rhythm:
   Atrial:
   Ventricular:
3. PR interval:
4. QRS interval:
5. Interpretation:
6. Common cause:
7. Initial treatment:

I. Interpret the rhythm in Fig 6-6.
1. Rate:
   Atrial:
   Ventricular:
2. Rhythm:
   Atrial:
   Ventricular:
3. PR interval:
4. QRS interval:
5. Interpretation:

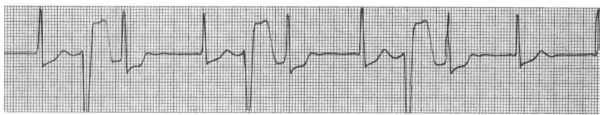

Lead II

FIG. 6-3

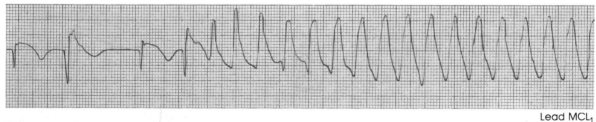

Lead MCL₁

FIG. 6-4

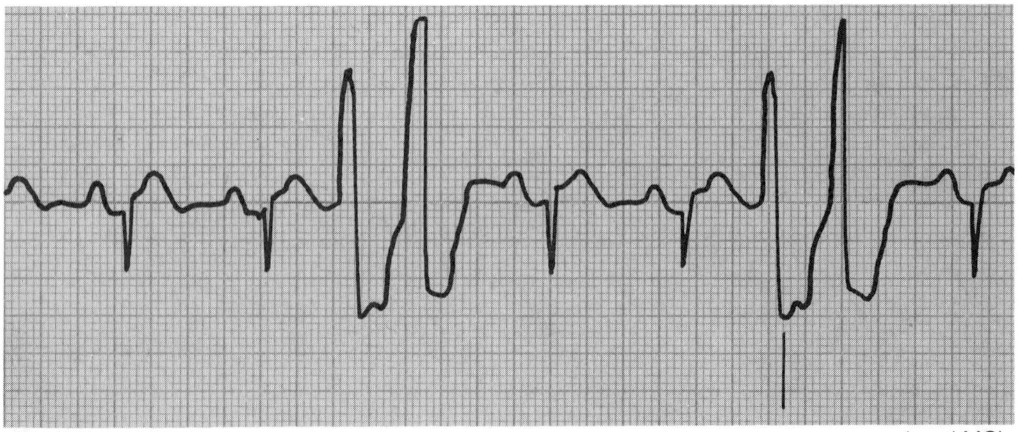

Lead MCL₁

FIG. 6-5

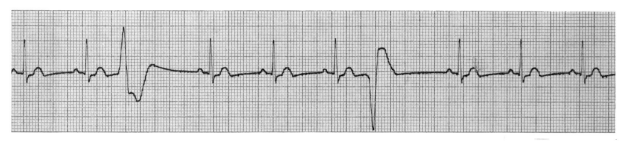

FIG. 6-6

Lead II

6. Common cause:

7. Initial treatment:

J. An essentially regular rhythm with a rate of 40 per minute or less, no preceding P wave, and a QRS complex greater than 0.12 second most probably describes:

1. Bradycardia

2. Second-degree AV block

3. Ventricular escape rhythm

4. Accelerated idioventricular rhythm

K. A wide and bizarre complex that occurs slightly prematurely and is preceded by a sinus P wave that is on time most probably describes:

1. R-on-T PVC

2. PAC with aberrant conduction

3. Junctional escape complex

4. End-diastolic PVC

L. Active impulse formation from a ventricular focus may produce the following (circle all that apply):

1. PVC

2. Idioventricular rhythm

3. Ventricular tachycardia

4. Ventricular escape complex

M. Passive impulse formation from a ventricular focus occurs:

1. When higher and faster pacemaker sites fail

2. When a ventricular focus is unstable and fires prematurely

N. ECG characteristics of PVCs generally include (circle all that apply):

1. P waves related to QRS complex

2. QRS usually wider than 0.12 second

3. Noncompensatory pause

4. Large T wave in opposite direction of QRS

O. Treatment for PVCs that are frequent, multiform, and associated with heart disease might include the following

1. Doing nothing

2. Atropine or isoproterenol if underlying rhythm is fast

3. Lidocaine I.V. bolus, followed by drip

4. Pacemaker

PURPOSE

The purpose of this module is to provide the learner with basic information and a structured framework within which to develop skills in identifying and understanding the etiology, characteristics, clinical significance, and management of ventricular dysrhythmias.

BEHAVIORAL OBJECTIVES

At the end of this module, the learner should be able to:

A. List possible etiological factors of, define and identify criteria for, recognize on rhythm strips, state clinical features of, and discuss modes of treatment and nursing management for:

1. Premature ventricular complexes (PVCs)

2. Unifocal PVCs

3. Ventricular bigeminy

4. Ventricular trigeminy

5. Multifocal PVCs

6. R-on-T PVCs

7. End-diastolic PVCs

8. Interpolated PVCs

9. Sequential PVCs

10. Ventricular tachycardia

11. Ventricular fibrillation

12. Escape (idioventricular) rhythm

13. Accelerated ventricular rhythm

14. Ventricular standstill

VOCABULARY

Aberrant conduction Because of a prolongation of the refractory period in the bundle branches, an impulse(s) is/are abnormally conducted through the ventricles producing a change in the QRS morphology.

Active rhythm A rhythm initiated by a premature complex (one early in the regular cycle) that continues at a rate faster than the normal pacemaker and usurps control of the heart rhythm.

Cardioversion A direct electrical current synchronized to be delivered on the R wave of the ECG via paddles applied to the chest in order to terminate a tachycardia.

Compensatory pause (complete) A type of pause that occurs after a premature complex. If the interval measured between the R wave of the complex preceding the premature complex and the R wave of the complex following it is equal to twice that of the RR interval between two normal complexes, the pause is fully compensatory. This occurs when the premature complex does not interrupt the sinus node cycle.

Defibrillation A direct unsynchronized electrical current delivered via paddles applied to the chest in order to terminate ventricular fibrillation.

Escape complex/rhythm (passive complex/rhythm) A complex/rhythm that is initiated by a lower pacemaker when the sinus node slows or fails. It is usually preceded by a pause. It is also termed a passive rhythm or rhythm by default.

Overdrive pacing The use of a pacemaker for the purpose of artificially stimulating the heart at a faster rate than the heart's intrinsic rate. The purpose of this increased heart rate is to suppress an abnormal dysrhythmia.

Passive complex rhythm See escape complex/rhythm.

Retrograde conduction Impulse conducted in a backward direction from normal.

Sine wave A smooth biphasic wave representing end-stage hyperkalemia and ventricular tachycardia. A disparity in the depolarization process in the myocardium widens the QRS complex, which merges with the T wave, producing the sine wave.

CONTENT
Suggested review

Before beginning this module on ventricular dysrhythmias it is recommended that the learner review the following:

1. Module 1
   a. Anatomy of the conduction system of the ventricles
   b. Normal conduction through the ventricles
   c. Normal P-QRS-T complex
2. Module 8
   Drugs used for ventricular dysrhythmias.

Ventricular dysrhythmias—an overview

Just as the sinus node, atria, and junction may function as pacemakers for the heart, the conduction system and muscle fibers of the ventricles may also send out electrical impulses that bring about cardiac depolarization and contraction.

Ventricular dysrhythmias may be generated by either "active" or "passive" impulse formation. Active impulse formation from a ventricular focus may produce a premature ventricular complex (PVC), ventricular tachycardia, and/or fibrillation. These rhythm disturbances occur *regardless* of underlying cardiac rhythm.

In contrast to active impulse formation, passive impulse formation of the ventricle occurs when higher and faster pacemaking sites fail to produce an impulse or when atrial impulses are blocked at the AV junction. The ventricle then produces impulses at its own very slow rate and the rhythm is termed "ventricular escape rhythm" or "idioventricular rhythm."

Dysrhythmias, regardless of the fundamental mechanism, may originate from any location in the ventricle.

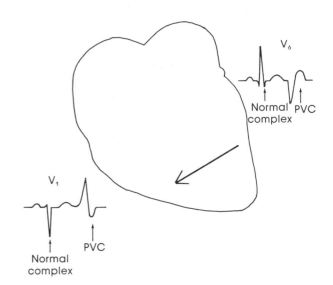

FIG. 6-7

Ventricles being depolarized toward V_1. Impulse originating from focus in left ventricles travels away from its point of origin to right side of heart, thus producing a positive deflection in V_1 and a negative deflection in V_6.

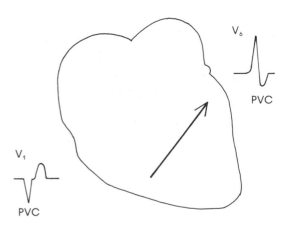

FIG. 6-8

Ventricles being depolarized toward V_6. Impulse originating from focus in right ventricle travels away from its point of origin to left side of heart, thus producing a negative deflection in V_1 and a positive deflection in V_6.

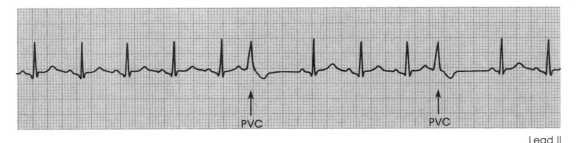

FIG. 6-9
Two PVCs in otherwise normal sinus rhythm.

Lead II

The configuration of the QRS complex is greatly influenced by the location of the ectopic focus (Figs. 6-7 and 6-8).

The impulse begins at the site of the focus and travels toward the rest of the ventricular muscle mass. Because the impulse cannot travel through its usual accelerated path via the bundle of His and bundle branches, conduction is delayed, causing a characteristically abnormal complex.

Rhythm disturbances
PREMATURE VENTRICULAR COMPLEXES (PVCS) (FIG. 6-9)
Definition

PVC is an early or premature complex initiated by an ectopic site in either the right or left ventricle below the branching portion of the bundle of His. PVCs are the most common of ventricular dysrhythmias and may be observed in practically every individual at some time during his or her lifetime. Although PVCs are commonly found in healthy adults—especially following excessive ingestion of coffee or tea, heavy smoking, or emotional excitement—the frequent occurrence of this dysrhythmia, especially when multiform, usually indicates organic heart disease and/or digoxin intoxication.

PVCs may originate from a single focus or from multiple foci anywhere in the ventricles. They may occur rarely, occasionally or frequently, and regularly or irregularly. There may be two or more consecutive PVCs, which may lead to ventricular tachycardia or fibrillation.

There are several mechanisms that are responsible for the development of PVCs, one being the reentry phenomenon. Fig. 6-10 illustrates conduction passing through the His-Purkinje fibers. It travels normally through healthy tissue but is blocked at depressed tissue, which is still refractory. Conduction continues to travel through the normal tissue, and, when it reaches the opposite end of the depressed tissue, it may find such tissue now re-polarized so it can slowly travel through this area in the opposite direction. When the impulse again reaches the healthy tissue, one of two things can occur: (1) it may be blocked because the healthy tissue has not repolarized; therefore no PVC is produced; or (2) it may find the healthy tissue nonrefractory and will "reenter" the same tissue and go on to produce a PVC. If the relationship between the healthy and depressed tissue remains the same, the phenomenon could continue to produce a continuous rhythm—ventricular tachycardia[8] (see Fig. 6-10).

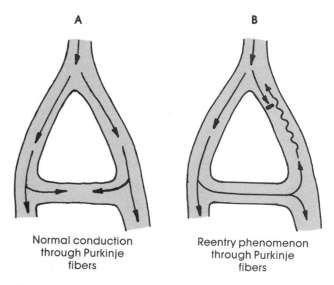

Normal conduction through Purkinje fibers

Reentry phenomenon through Purkinje fibers

FIG. 6-10
Conduction travels normally through healthy tissue (A) but is blocked in depressed tissue (B), which is still refractory from previous impulses. Conduction continues through normal tissue and when it reaches the opposite end of depressed tissue may find it now repolarized and will slowly travel through this area in the opposite direction (as indicated by wavy line). When the impulse reaches healthy tissue it may be blocked because such tissue has not yet repolarized, or it may "reenter" and activate such tissue for a second time.

More in-depth discussion of reentry and the other types of mechanisms responsible for ventricular dysrhythmias is reserved for the advanced learner and will not be discussed here.

Etiology

1. PVCs can occur in normal hearts, especially in association with excessive ingestion of coffee, tea, or alcohol, heavy smoking, emotional excitement, or exercise; incidence tends to increase with age, paralleling coronary artery disease[6]
2. They also occur with:
   a. Myocardial ischemia or infarction
   b. Congestive heart failure
   c. Organic heart disease such as myocarditis, pericarditis, or infiltrative diseases
   d. Prolapsed mitral valve
   e. Hypotension
   f. Hypoglycemia
   g. Anemia
   h. Electrolyte imbalance
   i. Anoxia
   j. Acid-base imbalance
   k. Digoxin or other drug intoxication such as amphetamines, quinidine, etc.

Characteristics of rhythm

1. Premature occurrence of QRS complex is initiated in ventricle
2. Contour is different from normal supraventricular complex
3. Wide bizarre complex, usually greater than 0.12 second because impulse cannot travel on its usual accelerated path via the bundle branches
4. Large T wave generally in opposite direction of the major deflection of the QRS complex

5. P wave, if present, is unrelated to QRS complex; if P wave is present it occurs at its expected time because the premature focus does not usually affect the atrium; there will be no ventricular response to the P wave proximate to the PVC because the ventricle will be refactory and thus unable to respond; there will, however, be a response to the following P wave and this sequence causes what is called a full compensatory pause (Fig. 6-11)

Clinical features

1. Patient may be asymptomatic
2. There may be symptoms of palpitations or discomfort in chest or neck because of greater than normal contractile force of the beat following the PVC
3. Patient may have feeling that the heart has stopped because of long pause following the PVC
4. Frequent PVCs in patients who have heart disease may produce angina or hypotension
5. PVCs may progress to ventricular tachycardia or fibrillation especially if they:
   a. Fall close to the preceding T wave
   b. Occur at a rate greater than 5 or 6 per minute
   c. Occur in a bigeminal pattern
   d. Are multiform
   e. Occur in sequence (two or more together)
   f. Are extremely wide[10]

Treatment measures

1. None, if PVCs are infrequent or not associated with heart disease
2. Treat underlying cause, such as:
   a. Congestive heart failure
   b. Hypotension
   c. Hypoglycemia
   d. Anemia

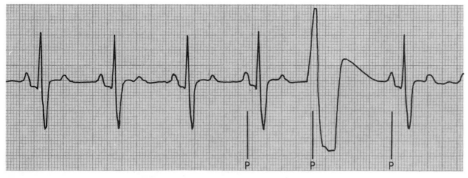

FIG. 6-11
PVCs with apparent full compensatory pause. Although the P wave can not be fully appreciated in repolarization wave of the premature complex, the sinus rhythm does not appear to be disturbed by the premature complex, thus suggesting a PVC with non-penetration to the atria.

e. Electrolyte imbalance

f. Anoxia

g. Acid-base imbalance

3. If associated with very slow heart rates, the PVCs may be abolished by increasing the basic heart rate with atropine or isoproterenol or by pacing at a faster rate with an artificial pacemaker; however, this treatment should be used with extreme caution because faster heart rates increase the oxygen need of the heart and may increase the degree of ischemia

4. For PVCs of immediate concern, lidocaine 1 to 2 mg/kg/min (50 to 100 mg) should be administered I.V. bolus and should be followed by 50-mg doses I.V. bolus 5 minutes apart, up to 225 mg; after the first bolus is administered, a lidocaine I.V. drip should be infused at a rate of 1 to 4 mg/min[2]

5. If lidocaine is unsuccessful in controlling the PVCs or if the patient is allergic to this drug, other drugs may be used, including:

a. Procainamide—I.V. and/or oral

b. Phenytoin—especially if PVCs occur with digoxin toxicity

c. Quinidine

d. Disopyramide

e. Bretylium tosylate

f. Amiodarone

Nursing management

1. Observe patient's ECG pattern closely

2. Treat serious dysrhythmias promptly according to standing orders (do not initiate treatment of dysrhythmia if the patient is stable hemodynamically or if the rhythm is unlikely to worsen)

3. Be thoroughly familiar with drugs that may be administered for dysrhythmias and closely observe patient for adverse effects; if adverse effects *do* occur, discontinue the drug and notify the physician

4. Be familiar with the patient's laboratory data so that values contributing to the dysrhythmia may be corrected

5. Provide emotional and psychological support to patient and family

6. Document strips, treatment, patient response

Special considerations

1. As above

2. Continue to monitor patient as described in "Nursing management" section

TYPES OF PREMATURE VENTRICULAR COMPLEXES (PVCS)
Unifocal PVCs (Fig. 6-12)
Definition

Unifocal PVCs occur from the same focus in the ventricle. All PVCs generally have the same configuration because they all originate from a single focus in the ventricle; however, more recent studies have shown that because of varying refractoriness in tissue surrounding the ectopic focus, pathways may vary, producing "multiform" PVCs from the same focus.[1]

Characteristics of rhythm

1. Rate:
   Atrial: Same as ventricular
   Ventricular: Determined by basic rate and number of PVCs

2. Rhythm:
   Atrial: May be regular or irregular depending on extent of retrograde conduction into AV junction and atria by the PVCs

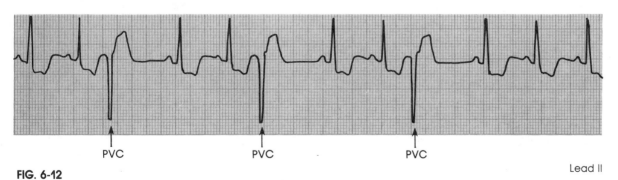

FIG. 6-12

Normal sinus rhythm with unifocal PVCs. Because of uniform size and shape of PVCs, it is assumed that they are arising from one focus and traveling the same pathway through ventricles each time.

Lead II

Ventricular: Irregular because of premature complexes; may be regular irregularity as in bigeminy or trigeminy

3. P waves: Generally normal if present; often lost in QRS or T wave of PVC; may follow PVC and be inverted because of retrograde conduction into atria

4. PR interval: Not relevant

5. QRS of PVC: Wide and bizarre; greater than 0.12 second

6. Ratio of P/QRS: 1:1 with normal complexes; not relevant with PVCs

7. QT interval: Less than 0.43 second in normal complexes; variable with PVCs

Special significance

If associated with heart disease, PVCs may need to be treated if they occur at a rate of more than 5 or 6 per minute.

Ventricular bigeminy (Fig. 6-13)
Definition

Ventricular bigeminy describes two successive complexes, one normal and one ectopic, which occur repetitively as couplets.

Characteristics of rhythm

1. Rate:
   Atrial: Same as ventricular
   Ventricular: Determined by basic rate and number of PVCs

2. Rhythm:
   Atrial: Regular or irregular, depending on extent of retrograde conduction into AV node and atria
   Ventricular: Regularly irregular because of premature complexes

3. P waves: Generally normal but often lost in QRS or T wave of PVCs; can also precede PVC if PVC is end-diastolic or may follow PVC

4. PR interval: Less than 0.20 second with normal complexes; not relevant with PVCs

5. QRS of PVC: Wide and bizarre; greater than 0.12 second; PVC alternates with normal complex

6. Ratio of P/QRS: 1:1, but not relevant with PVCs

7. QT interval: Less than 0.43 second with normal complexes; variable and often times not measurable with PVCs

Special significance

1. PVCs may be the result of digoxin intake

2. PVCs usually occur in a stable rhythm but may precipitate ventricular tachycardia

3. Digoxin may need to be withheld

4. Antidysrhythmic agents may need to be administered

Ventricular trigeminy (Fig. 6-14)
Definition

Ventricular trigeminy describes three successive complexes, normal and ectopic, which occur repetitively as triplets; the rhythm may involve two normal complexes followed by a PVC (see Fig. 6-14) or two PVCs followed by one normal complex (Fig. 6-15).

Characteristics of rhythm

1. Rate:
   Atrial: Same as ventricular
   Ventricular: Determined by basic rate and number of PVCs

2. Rhythm:
   Atrial: Regular or regularly irregular
   Ventricular: Regularly irregular

3. P waves: Generally normal but often lost in QRS or T wave of PVCs; can also precede PVC if PVC is end-diastolic or may follow PVC

4. PR interval: Less than 0.20 second with normal complexes; not relevant with PVCs

5. QRS of PVC: Wide and bizarre; greater than 0.12 second

6. Ratio of P/QRS: 1:1, but not relevant with PVCs

7. QT interval: Less than 0.43 second with normal complexes; variable and often times not measurable with PVCs

Special significance

Same as with ventricular bigeminy; triplets involving two PVCs followed by a normal complex have greater clinical significance than those involving two normal complexes followed by a PVC.

Multifocal or multiform PVCs (Fig. 6-16)
Definition

Formerly called multifocal PVCs because it was thought that if PVCs had varying configurations, they were originating from different foci within the ventricles[1]; but, with a surface ECG, it is difficult to discern whether PVCs with varying contours represent more than one active focus in the ventricles or whether one focus is displaying various activation patterns.

Characteristics of rhythm

1. Rate:
   Atrial: Same as ventricular
   Ventricular: Determined by basic rate and number of PVCs

2. Rhythm:
   Atrial: Regular or irregular, depending on degree of retrograde conduction from PVCs
   Ventricular: Irregular

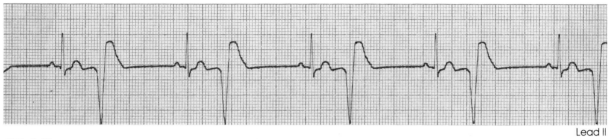

Lead II

FIG. 6-13

Ventricular bigeminy. In this rhythm each normal complex is followed
by a PVC to produce a rhythm of couplets or pairs. One possible
mechanism for this type of rhythm is reentry.

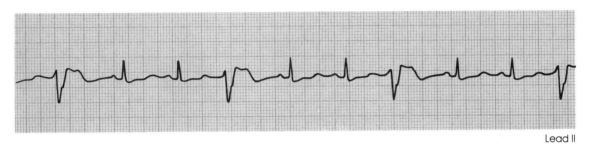

Lead II

FIG. 6-14

Ventricular trigeminy. In this rhythm a series of triplets occur with two
normal complexes being followed by a PVC.

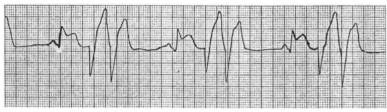

Lead II

FIG. 6-15

Ventricular trigeminy. In this rhythm a series of triplets occur with two
PVCs (couplets) preceded by a normal complex. (From Conover,
M.B.: Understanding electrocardiography: arrhythmias and the
12-lead ECG, ed. 5, St. Louis, 1988, The C.V. Mosby Co.)

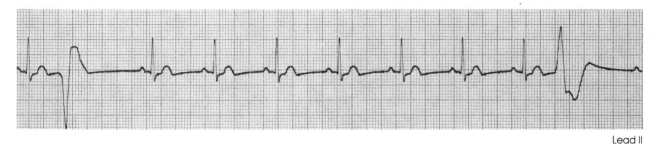

Lead II

FIG. 6-16

Multifocal/multiform PVCs. PVCs with varying configurations, which
indicate that they arise from different foci or that one focus has
varying activation patterns.

3. P waves: Generally normal but often lost in QRS or T wave of PVCs; can also precede PVC if PVC is end-diastolic or may follow PVC
4. PR interval: Less than 0.20 second with normal complexes; not relevant with PVCs
5. QRS of PVC: Wide and bizarre; greater than 0.12 second, with varying contours
6. Ratio of P/QRS: 1:1, but not relevant with PVCs
7. QT interval: Less than 0.43 second with normal complexes; variable and often times not measurable with PVCs

Special significance

In a person with cardiac disease, multifocal PVCs are considered to have serious implications and can precipitate ventricular tachycardia or fibrillation; generally, they should be treated as soon as possible.

R-on-T PVCs (Fig. 6-17)
Definition

R-on-T PVCs are those that occur on the descending limb of a T wave.

Characteristics of rhythm

1. Rate:
   Atrial: Same as ventricular (unless ventricular tachycardia or ventricular fibrillation occurs)
   Ventricular: Determined by basic rate and number of PVCs and possible subsequent rhythm (ventricular tachycardia or fibrillation)
2. Rhythm:
   Atrial: Usually regular
   Ventricular: Irregular due to premature complexes
3. P waves: Generally normal but often lost in QRS or T wave of PVCs

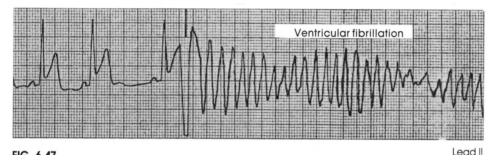

FIG. 6-17

Ventricular fibrillation initiated by an R-on-T PVC. Because the ventricles do not completely repolarize, a stimulus occurring during this phase can cause a chaotic dysrhythmia. (From Conover, M.B.: Understanding electrocardiography: arrhythmias and the 12-lead ECG, ed. 5, St. Louis, 1988, The C.V. Mosby Co.)

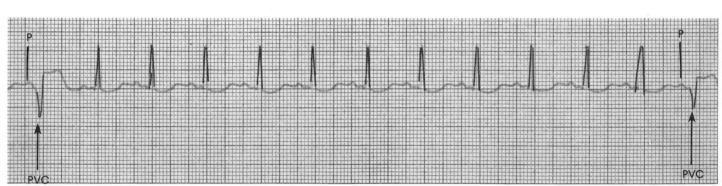

FIG. 6-18   Lead II

Normal sinus rhythm with two end-diastolic PVCs. When the PVCs are just barely premature, a P wave that is on time may be seen in front of the bizarre QRS complex.

4. PR interval: Less than 0.20 second with normal complexes; not relevant with PVCs
5. QRS of PVC: Wide and bizarre; greater than 0.12 second
6. Ratio of P/QRS: 1:1, but not relevant with PVCs
7. QT interval: Less than 0.43 second with normal complexes; variable and often times not measurable with PVCs

Special significance

The term "R-on-T phenomenon" is used to indicate that a PVC has occurred during repolarization of the ventricles (T wave). Because the heart is not yet ready to respond to a stimulus in an organized fashion, a serious ventricular dysrhythmia may result if a stimulus occurs at the time. (NOTE: In a patient with a recent myocardial infarction, this type of PVC should be considered a potential threat and should be treated.)

End-diastolic PVCs (Fig. 6-18)
Definition

When a PVC is just barely premature, a P wave may be seen immediately in front of the bizarre QRS complex since the ectopic site in the ventricles fires just before the sinus impulse had an opportunity to reach the ventricles. This occurrence represents a "late" or "end-diastolic" PVC; the P wave of the entire complex comes on schedule, but the PR interval is shortened and the QRS complex is slightly premature.

Characteristics of rhythm

1. Rate:
   Atrial: Same as ventricular
   Ventricular: Determined by basic rate and number of PVCs
2. Rhythm:
   Atrial: Regular
   Ventricular: Only slightly irregular
3. P waves: Generally normal and occur on time just prior to PVC but not related to PVCs
4. PR interval: Because of slight prematurity of PVC, PR interval of PVC is shorter than PR interval of normal complexes
5. QRS of PVC: Wide and bizarre; greater than 0.12 second
6. Ratio of P/QRS: 1:1, but not relevant with PVCs
7. QT interval: Less than 0.43 second with normal complexes; variable and often times not measurable with PVCs

Special significance

At times, the sinus impulse penetrates and contributes to ventricular activation along with the premature focus.

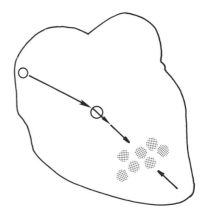

FIG. 6-19
Diagram depicting mechanism of fusion complex. At times, the sinus impulse penetrates and contributes to ventricular activation along with the premature focus.

In this situation the two impulses collide and a "fusion" complex occurs (Figs. 6-19 and 6-20, p. 128); the QRS takes on some characteristics of the normal complex and some of the PVC. (NOTE: El-Sherif and colleagues[4] have shown through recent studies that ventricular vulnerability during acute myocardial infarction may extend throughout most of the cardiac cycle and is not confined to the T wave; therefore, end-diastolic PVCs should be treated as other types of PVCs.)

Interpolated PVCs (Fig. 6-21, p. 128)
Definition

When a sinus-initiated P wave immediately following the PVC conducts to the ventricles with a long PR interval, the PR interval following the PVC is prolonged owing to incomplete recovery of the AV node because of partial penetration by the interpolated PVC; thus the usual compensatory pause is not present. The interpolated PVC does not replace a normally conducted complex but occurs in *addition* to the normally conducted complex.

Characteristics of rhythm

1. Rate:
   Atrial: Same as ventricular
   Ventricular: Determined by basic rate and PVCs
2. Rhythm:
   Atrial: Slightly irregular because of penetration of PVCs into atria
   Ventricular: Irregular because of PVCs
3. P waves: See definition (above)
4. PR interval: See definition (above)
5. QRS of PVC: Wide and bizarre; greater than 0.12 second
6. Ratio of P/QRS: 1:1

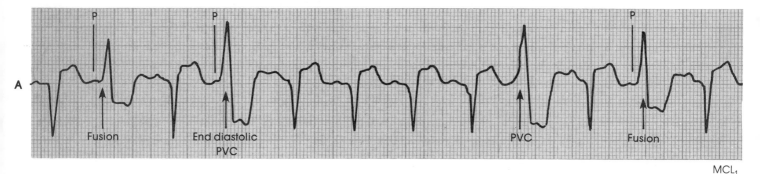

A

P   P   P

Fusion   End diastolic   PVC   Fusion
                     PVC

MCL₁

Normal sinus rhythm   Fusion complexes and PVCs

Initial deflection

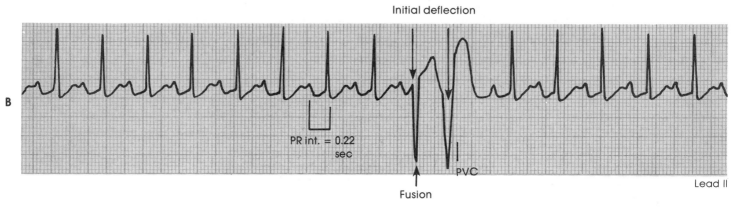

B

PR int. = 0.22
sec

PVC

Fusion

Lead II

FIG. 6-20

A. The above dysrhythmia depicts normal sinus rhythm with two fusion complexes, one end-diastolic PVC, and one PVC. QRS of the fusion complexes are smaller than QRS complexes of the other PVCs. P waves are present before the fusion complexes at the end-diastolic PVC, but the PR interval is slightly longer before the fusion complexes, allowing one of the sinus impulses to penetrate the

ventricles. **B,** Sinus tachycardia with first-degree heart block (PR interval—0.22 second), one end-diastolic fusion complex (QRS has some characteristics of sinus-induced QRS and some characteristics of PVC), and one PVC (which is wider and more bizarre than the fusion complex and has an initial deflection opposite the fusion complex).

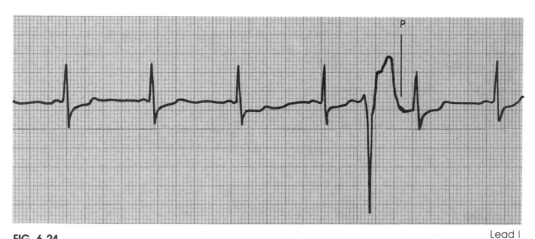

P

FIG. 6-21

Normal sinus rhythm with one interpolated PVC. A sinus-initiated P wave immediately following the PVC conducts to the ventricle with a longer than normal PR interval because of incomplete recovery of AV node, caused by partial penetration of the PVC.

Lead I

7. QT interval: Less than 0.43 second with normal complexes; variable and often times not measurable with PVCs

Sequential PVCs (Figs. 6-22 and 6-23)
Definition

Sequential PVCs involve two or more PVCs occurring consecutively (in sequence).

Characteristics of rhythm

1. Rate:
   Atrial: Same as ventricular
   Ventricular: Determined by basic rate and PVCs
2. Rhythm: Irregular because of PVCs
3. P waves: Generally normal but often lost in QRS or T wave of PVCs; can also precede PVC if PVC is end-diastolic or may follow PVC
4. PR interval: Less than 0.20 second with normal complexes; not relevant with PVCs

5. QRS of PVC: Wide and bizarre; greater than 0.12 second
6. Ratio of P/QRS: 1:1, but not relevant with PVC
7. QT interval: Less than 0.43 second with normal complexes; variable and often times not measurable with PVCs

Special significance

These PVCs are considered to have serious implications since there is a very real danger that the second of the pair will meet with tissue that is repolarizing and consequently produce electrical chaos, such as ventricular tachycardia or fibrillation. They should be treated as soon as possible.

VENTRICULAR TACHYCARDIA (FIG. 6-24, p. 130)
Definition

A series of three or more consecutive PVCs occurring at a rate of 110 to 250 per minute.

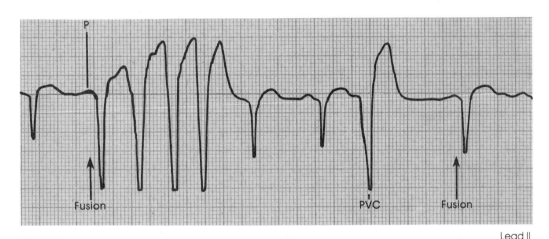

Lead II

FIG. 6-22

Normal sinus rhythm with an end-diastolic fusion complex followed by a run of PVCs (burst of ventricular tachycardia), then a normal complex, followed by a single PVC and another normal complex. Note that the fusion complex is not quite as wide and bizarre as succeeding PVCs.

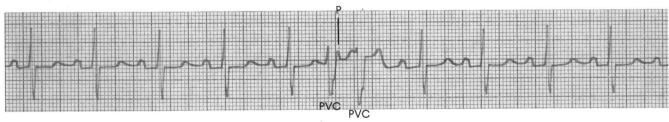

Lead II

FIG. 6-23

Normal sinus rhythm with first-degree AV block (PR interval—0.24 second) and two sequential PVCs. Note P wave in QRS complex of the first PVC, which indicates no penetration of PVC into atria and, therefore, regularity of sinus rhythm.

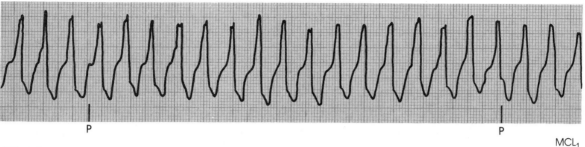

P   P

MCL₁

FIG. 6-24

Ventricular tachycardia. Note wide and bizarre complexes with occasional evidence of P waves occurring totally unrelated to QRS complexes, giving evidence of dissociation between atria and ventricles.

Etiology

1. Ventricular tachycardia is most common in patients with myocardial infarction or coronary artery disease but has also been reported in patients with presumably normal hearts
2. Same as PVCs
3. Ventricular tachycardia is caused by frequent PVCs, especially if they:
   a. Occur more than 5 to 6 times per minute
   b. Occur on the T wave of the preceding complex
   c. Become multifocal/multiform
   d. Occur sequentially

Characteristics of rhythm

1. Rate:
   Atrial: Can be any rate from a slow bradycardia to a tachycardia, but slower than the ventricular rate
   Ventricular: 110 to 250 per minute
2. Rhythm:
   Atrial: May be regular or irregular
   Ventricular: May be very regular or somewhat irregular
3. P waves: May be seen to "march through" the QRS; however, at times they are obscured by the QRS or T wave; this occurs when the ventricular ectopic focus does not ascend the atria, therefore, allowing the sinus node to fire at its own rhythm; there is no relationship between P waves and QRS complexes.
4. PR interval: Not relevant
5. QRS interval: Wide and bizarre, greater than 0.12 second
6. Ratio of P/QRS: Greater number of QRS complexes than P waves; however, not relevant in ventricular tachycardia
7. QT interval: Variable; often times not measurable

8. The distinction between supraventricular and ventricular tachycardia may be difficult to determine at times because the features of both dysrhythmias frequently are the same, and, in fact, sometimes supraventricular tachycardia meets the criteria for ventricular tachycardia; ventricular complexes with wide configurations only indicate that conduction through the ventricles is not traveling through the normal pathways; impulses from the atria can travel through the ventricles through aberrant pathways (bundle branch blocks, etc.), which prolong conduction and widen the QRS complex[1]

Clinical features

1. Symptoms depend on the ventricular rate, the duration of the tachycardia, and the severity of the underlying heart disease
2. Although ventricular tachycardia may be tolerated well hemodynamically by a few individuals, for most persons, because of inadequate filling, this dysrhythmia causes a significant decrease in the amount of blood pumped out of the heart
3. The patient may have a significant drop in blood pressure and may lose consciousness within a matter of minutes

Treatment measures

1. If ventricular tachycardia is not extremely fast and the patient shows no signs of decompensation, this dysrhythmia is best treated medically by administering lidocaine 1 to 2 mg/kg (50 to 100 mg) I.V. bolus, followed by 50 mg doses I.V. bolus 5 minutes apart, up to 225 mg; the total dosage should not exceed 400 to 500 mg per hour and should be reduced in patients who have liver disease, heart failure, or shock; a

lidocaine I.V. drip should then be infused at the rate 1 to 4 mg per minute[2]

2. If the patient does not respond to lidocaine, other drugs that may be tried include:
   a. Procainamide
   b. Bretylium tosylate
   c. Amiodarone
   d. Ethmozine

3. If the dysrhythmia is not responsive to medical therapy, synchronized DC countershock (cardioversion) should be applied at low energy levels (10 to 50 watt/sec)[1]

4. Conditions that may be contributing factors to this dysrhythmia, such as hypokalemia, hypotension, hypoxia, etc., should be corrected

5. In cases where ventricular tachycardia is recurrent, other modes of treatment may include:
   a. "Overdrive" pacing via an electrode inserted into the right ventricle; with this technique, the heart can be artificially stimulated at a rate faster than the tachycardia in order to suppress the dysrhythmia[1]
   b. Synchronized cardioversion performed in the awake patient through a catheter electrode designed to deliver shocks of 0.25 watt/sec[14]
   c. Surgery (performed in conjunction with electrophysiological mapping in order to determine the focus of the dysrhythmia) to ablate the area causing the rhythm disturbance[5]
   d. Combinations of the aforementioned drugs—often determined by performing electrophysiology studies—to see which drug is or drugs are effective

6. When ventricular tachycardia produces the same clinical features as ventricular fibrillation (loss of consciousness, seizures, apnea), nonsynchronized DC countershock (defibrillation) at 200 to 360 watt/sec should be applied immediately[1]; the earlier this stage of ventricular tachycardia is treated, the fewer the metabolic derangements and the more successful the therapy

Nursing management

1. Observe patient's ECG and hemodynamic status closely

2. Treat those dysrhythmias and conditions that may *cause* ventricular tachycardia

3. Be familiar with patient's laboratory data and other conditions that could contribute to ventricular tachycardia and notify the physician and/or treat as appropriate

4. Be familiar with the defibrillator and know when its use is indicated

5. Be thoroughly familiar with drugs that may be administered for dysrhythmias and closely observe the patient for adverse effects

6. Be familiar with pacemakers if they are used for "overdrive suppression"

7. Provide emotional and psychological support to the patient and family

8. Document strips, treatment, patient response

Special considerations

1. There is a subgroup of ventricular tachycardia and/or fibrillation in which the QRS complexes and T waves become fused and produce a sine wave; the rate is between 150 and 300 per minute and is sometimes called "ventricular flutter" (Fig. 6-25)[10]
   The term "ventricular flutter" is a term going out of vogue because it represents a very brief transitory period between classic ventricular tachycardia and fibrillation; the causes, hemodynamic consequences, treatment, and nursing management of this rhythm disturbance are the same as for ventricular fibrillation; the ECG characteristics include the following:
   a. Rapid, uniform regular undulations with a sine wave appearance
   b. A nondistinct QRS that is greater than 0.12 seconds in duration

2. Another type of ventricular tachycardia that is not

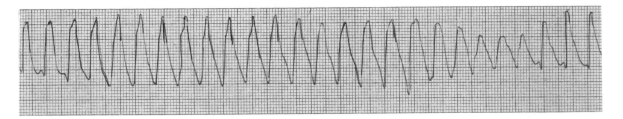

FIG. 6-25

Ventricular flutter. Note that QRS complexes and T waves have become fused to produce a sine wave.

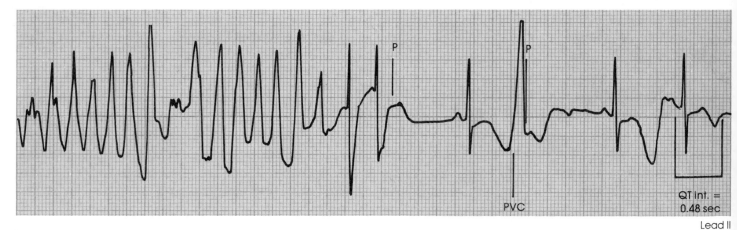

FIG. 6-26

Torsade de pointes presents a rhythm that is not uniform in appearance and which has phasic variation in polarity. After termination of the tachycardia, one PVC occurs in the normal sinus rhythm. Note QT interval of 0.48 second on last complex.

uniform in appearance and that has a phasic variation in polarity is known as *torsade de pointes* (a French term meaning "twisting of the points"); the QRS "twists" around the isoelectric line[12] (Fig. 6-26)

The classification of this rhythm has been significant in the diagnosis and treatment of this disorder, which formerly was called by such names as "transient ventricular fibrillation"[11] "paroxysmal ventricular fibrillation,"[7] and "transient recurrent ventricular fibrillation"[13]

a. Etiology

Torsade de pointes is associated with a prolonged QT interval caused by drugs (quinidine, procainamide, disopyramide, and amiodarone), severe bradycardia, electrolyte imbalances (hyperkalemia and hypomagnesemia), and congenital QT prolongation syndromes[6]; these increase the QT interval (vulnerable period) and set the stage for ectopic foci to occur

b. Characteristics of rhythm

(1) Rate: Between 150-250 per minute

(2) Rhythm: Irregular

(3) P waves: Not identified

(4) QRS complex: various contours and heights; generally wide and bizarre; tends to occur in undulating groups of a few to 20 or more complexes "twisting around the baseline"[11]

(5) Generally initiated by a R-on-T PVC that occurs on a prolonged QT interval

(6) Generally terminates spontaneously

(7) May progress to ventricular fibrillation

c. Clinical features

Generally none unless rhythm is sustained, in which case syncope may occur

d. Treatment measures

Torsade de pointes, if associated with a prolonged QT interval, is not treated with drugs used for other forms of ventricular tachycardia since these tend to prolong the QT interval even further and enhance initiation of the dysrhythmia

Treatment, therefore, includes discontinuing any drugs that may be instrumental in the onset of this particular ventricular tachycardia, using defibrillation as necessary, and, possible overdrive pacing[3]; more in-depth discussion of *torsade de pointes* is reserved for the advanced learner

VENTRICULAR FIBRILLATION (Figs. 6-27, 6-28, and 6-29)
Definition

Ventricular fibrillation is a rapid, chaotic, unsynchronized quivering or twitching of the myocardium in which there is no effective pumping (Fig. 6-27). This represents the most serious dysrhythmia so far discussed and is fatal unless it is corrected within the first 5 minutes of onset.

Etiology

1. Same as for ventricular tachycardia

2. Occurs frequently as terminal event in a variety of diseases

3. Can occur during[1]:

a. Cardiac pacing

b. Cardiac catheterization and other cardiovascular invasive procedures

c. Surgery

d. Anesthesia

4. Can be caused by drug toxicity, such as a reaction to digoxin, quinidine, or procainamide

5. Can occur after electric shock is applied for cardioversion

6. Can be accidental because of improperly grounded electrical equipment

7. Can be caused by electrocution

Characteristics of rhythm

1. Rate:
   Atrial: May be any rate; any type of independent atrial rhythm may exist
   Ventricular: 400-600

2. Rhythm:
   Atrial: Regular or irregular
   Ventricular: Grossly irregular

3. P waves: Generally not identified

4. PR interval: Not relevant

5. QRS interval: Irregular undulations of varying contour and amplitude

6. Ratio of P/QRS: Not relevant

7. QT interval: Not relevant; no distinct QRS complexes, ST segments, or T waves identified

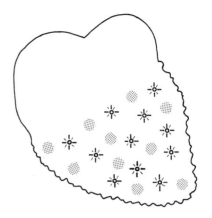

FIG. 6-27
Schematic illustrations showing rapid, chaotic unsynchronized quivering or twitching of myocardium during which no effective pumping can be done.

Clinical features

1. Faintness, followed by loss of consciousness, seizures, and apnea

2. Since no blood is pumped out of the heart during ventricular fibrillation, the dysrhythmia is death producing; no pulse or blood pressure will be detectable

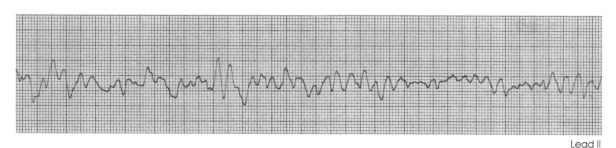

Lead II

FIG. 6-28
"Coarse" ventricular fibrillation. Note rapid, chaotic unsynchronized electrical activity. It is at this stage that defibrillation is most successful.

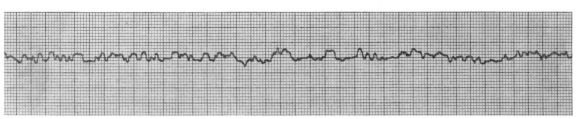

Lead II

FIG. 6-29
Note deterioration in almost all activity. Defibrillation at this stage is highly unsuccessful.

Treatment measures

1. Immediate DC cardioversion using 200 to 360 watt/sec is the only effective treatment
2. Ventricular fibrillation quickly produces severe metabolic acidosis; sodium bicarbonate (1 mEq/kg) should be administered immediately; blood gases should be obtained and sodium bicarbonate should be administered thereafter to correct blood gas abnormalities
3. All contributing factors such as laboratory abnormalities, hypotension, etc. must be identified and treated
4. If ventricular fibrillation is not immediately converted, regular cardiopulmonary resuscitation is employed
5. If fibrillation has deteriorated from "coarse" fibrillation (Fig. 6-28, p. 133) to "fine" fibrillation (Fig. 6-29, p. 133), 0.5 to 1 mg I.V. epinephrine should be administered in an attempt to stimulate the heart back to "coarse" activity

Nursing management

1. Observe patient's ECG and hemodynamic status closely
2. Treat those dysrhythmias and conditions that may predispose to ventricular fibrillation
3. Be familiar with a patient's laboratory data and other conditions that could contribute to ventricular fibrillation, notify physician, and treat as appropriate
4. Be familiar with defibrillator and know when its use is indicated
5. Be thoroughly familiar with advanced life support drugs and closely observe patient for both beneficial and adverse effects
6. Provide emotional and psychological support to patient and family
7. Document strips, treatment, and patient response

Special considerations

1. Termination of ventricular fibrillation within 30 to 45 seconds may prevent major chemical derangements accompanying this dysrhythmia and, hopefully, will eliminate the need for endotracheal intubation and other forms of advanced life support
2. *There must be no delay* in administering DC countershock; if the patient is not monitored and it cannot be determined what rhythm is present, the electric shock should be applied without wasting time attempting to obtain an ECG pattern[1]

ESCAPE (IDIOVENTRICULAR) RHYTHM (FIG. 6-30)
Definition

Also called "passive rhythm" or "rhythm by default," escape rhythm is a rhythm arising in and controlling only the ventricles at their own slow inherent rate (40 or below).

Etiology

An idioventricular escape complex/rhythm occurs when the rate of the supraventricular pacemaker (sinus node and AV junctional) become slower than that of potential ventricular pacemakers, or when supraventricular impulses do not penetrate to the region of the escape focus because of SA or AV block; this dysrhythmia is often associated with myocardial infarction

Characteristics of rhythm

1. Rate:
   Atrial: Usually very slow or nonexistent but independent of ventricles
   Ventricular: 20-40 per minute (inherent rate of ventricles)
2. Rhythm:
   Atrial: No rhythm, or can be regular or irregular depending on independent rhythm

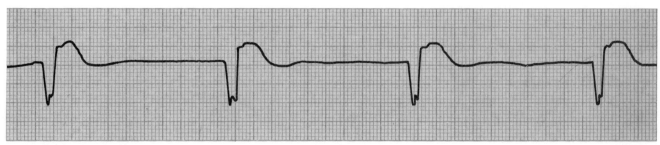

FIG. 6-30
Idioventricular rhythm.

Lead II

Ventricular: Usually regular
3. P waves: Nonexistent, normal, or abnormal, depending on independent atrial rhythm
4. PR interval: Not relevant
5. QRS interval: Wide and bizarre, greater than 0.12 second
6. Ratio of P/QRS: Depends on atrial activity; not relevant
7. QT interval: Variable and often times not measurable

Clinical features

Depending on rate of ventricular rhythm:
1. Rate may be rapid enough to produce adequate cardiac output and prevent immediate symptoms
2. If rate is extremely slow, patient may show, progressive signs of decompensation:
   a. Decreased blood pressure
   b. Deterioration of vital signs
   c. Syncope/unconsciousness
   d. Congestive heart failure
   e. Asystole/death

Treatment measures

Depending on the cause, atropine, isoproterenol, or temporary transvenous pacing generally represent the therapeutic approach

Nursing management

1. Assess patient's clinical status continually, notify the physician and administer atropine I.V. bolus when patient begins to show first signs of decompensation
2. Withhold digoxin or other drugs, if indicated
3. If patient does not respond to atropine, prepare an isoproterenol drip and make preparations for insertion of transvenous pacemaker
4. If no response is shown to above therapy and patient's clinical status so warrants, initiate cardiopulmonary resuscitation
5. Be thoroughly familiar with all drugs that may be administered and closely observe patient for both desired and adverse effects

6. Maintain proficiency in all emergency skills
7. Provide emotional and psychological support to the patient and family
8. Document strips, treatment, and patient response

ACCELERATED IDIOVENTRICULAR RHYTHM (FIG. 6-31)
Definition

A rhythm being initiated in an area of enhanced automaticity within the ventricles at a rate faster than the normal inherent rate of the ventricles (40 per minute) and less than 100 per minute is known as "accelerated idioventricular rhythm"; other terms occasionally used include "slow ventricular tachycardia," "nonparoxysmal ventricular tachycardia," and "idioventricular tachycardia."[6]

Typically, the rate of the ventricular focus and the sinus node are similar and as the sinus node slows and/or the ectopic focus accelerates, the control of the cardiac rhythm alternates between the two foci; usually the change of rate in either focus is gradual and as control of the pacemaker alternates between the two foci, fusion complexes occur (Fig. 6-32, p. 136).

Etiology

An accelerated idioventricular rhythm may be caused by:
1. Acute myocardial infarction
2. Digoxin toxicity
3. Other forms of heart disease
4. Various other drugs

Characteristics of rhythm

1. Rate:
   Atrial: Usually 60-100, but any independent atrial dysrhythmia may exist
   Ventricular: 40-100
2. Rhythm:
   Atrial: Usually regular
   Ventricular: Generally regular although may be irregular

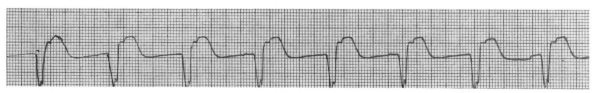

Lead II

FIG. 6-31
Accelerated idioventricular rhythm.

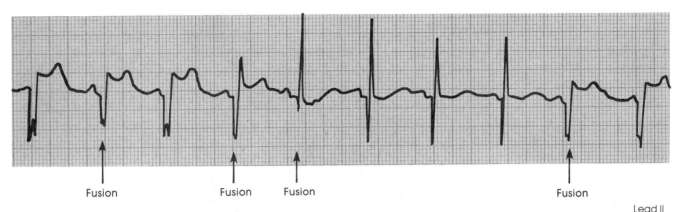

Fusion   Fusion   Fusion   Fusion

Lead II

FIG. 6-32
Accelerated idioventricular rhythm alternating with normal sinus
rhythm. Note that ventricular rhythm takes over when ventricular focus
becomes faster than sinus rhythm, as indicated by fusion complex
on end of strip. When ventricular rhythm slows below rate of sinus
node, as indicated by fusion complexes in beginning of strip,
rhythm then becomes normal sinus.

3. P waves: Often lost in QRS; may be independent or may be inverted because of atrial depolarization by the ectopic focus upward in retrograde fashion
4. PR interval: Not measureable
5. QRS complex: Wide and bizarre, greater than 0.12 second
6. Ratio of P/QRS: Varies according to atrial activity; often there are more QRS complexes than P waves because ventricular focus accelerates to a rate slightly faster than the sinus node rate
7. QT interval: Variable; often times not measurable
8. Special consideration:
   a. Ventricular tachycardia is rarely seen with this dysrhythmia
   b. The rhythm usually ends gradually as the sinus rate increases or as the ectopic ventricular rate decreases
   c. It is generally transient with episodes lasting short periods of time, up to a minute or more

Clinical features

1. Often times, the patient experiences no hemodynamic changes because the rate is adequate to maintain a good pulse and blood pressure
2. If the ventricular rate is too rapid to produce adequate pulses or blood pressure, symptoms associated with ventricular tachycardia occur
3. If the initiating complex of the rhythm is a PVC that produces ventricular fibrillation, clinical manifestations will be those described with fibrillation; (ventricular

fibrillation rarely occurs as a result of accelerated idioventricular rhythm)[1]

Treatment measures

1. The best therapeutic approach is to closely observe the patient's clinical status and ECG pattern and to treat the underlying heart disease
2. If digoxin is the cause of the dysrhythmia, it should be withheld
3. Atropine 0.5 mg may be administered I.V. initially and repeated if necessary to a total dose of 2 mg to speed the sinus rate and override the ectopic ventricular focus
4. Lidocaine may be given to suppress the ectopic ventricular focus[1]

Nursing management

1. Closely observe and document ECG pattern for any excessively slow or fast rhythms
2. Closely observe patient's hemodynamic status and promptly notify the physician of any changes in blood pressure, pulse, level of consciousness, etc.
3. Be knowledgeable about drugs possibly used for treatment and be prepared to administer if necessary
4. Maintain skills with emergency equipment should ventricular tachycardia or fibrillation occur
5. Provide support to the patient and family should the need arise
6. Document rhythm strips, treatment, and patient response

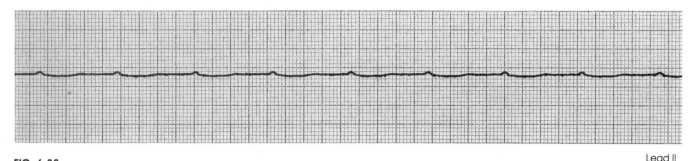

FIG. 6-33   Lead II

Ventricular standstill. Note total lack of ventricular activity; only atrial
depolarization remains.

Special considerations

Care should be taken not to give lidocaine or other antidysrhythmic agents to abolish accelerated idioventricular rhythms unless the patient becomes symptomatic and there is evidence of the presence of higher pacemaker[3]

VENTRICULAR STANDSTILL (CARDIAC ARREST/ASYSTOLE)
(FIG. 6-33)
Definition

Ventricular standstill represents cessation of electrical activity and of contraction in the ventricles or a lack of any ventricular rhythm (QRS complexes); evidence of electrical activity in the atria may be seen as only P waves on the ECG; when *all* electrical activity and contraction has ceased, a cardiac arrest has occurred.

Etiology

Ventricular standstill may be caused by:

1. Acute myocardial infarction
2. Coronary artery disease
3. "Dying heart"
4. Hypoxia from impaired respiratory function
5. Drug overdose
6. Hemorrhage
7. Anaphylactic reaction
8. Severe acidosis
9. Hyperkalemia

Characteristics of rhythm

1. Ventricular standstill:
   a. Absence of QRS complexes
   b. Atrial activity:
      (1) May be regular normal P waves
      (2) May be fibrillatory waves with atrial fibrillation
      (3) May be atrial tachycardia
2. Cardiac arrest/asystole:
   a. Absence of all activity by evidence of a straight line

Clinical features

1. No cardiac output; no pulses or blood pressure present
2. Loss of consciousness
3. Apnea

Treatment measures

1. If ventricular standstill *alone* occurs, a precordial thump may be sufficient to stimulate the ventricular muscle to resume function
2. If the precordial thump is not successful and cardiac standstill is present, immediate cardiopulmonary resuscitation both basic and advanced must be employed
   a. External chest compression
   b. Sodium bicarbonate I.V.
   c. Epinephrine I.V.
   d. Calcium I.V.
   e. Vasopressor I.V.
   f. Transvenous pacemaker
   g. Intraaortic balloon pump[9]

Nursing management

Same as for idioventricular rhythm

Special considerations

If CPR is not successful within the first 3 to 4 minutes, irreversible brain damage will occur.

REFERENCES

1. Andreoli, K.G., et al.: Comprehensive cardiac care, ed. 5, St. Louis, 1983, The C.V. Mosby Co.
2. Briggs, J.T., Jr.: Management of arrhythmias. In Braunwald, E., editor: Heart disease: a textbook of cardiovascular medicine, Philadelphia, 1980, W.B. Saunders Co.
3. Conover, M.B.: Understanding electrocardiography: arrhythmias and the 12-lead ECG, ed. 5, St. Louis, 1988, The C.V. Mosby Co.
4. El-Sherif, N., et al.: Electrocardiographic antecedents of primary ventricular fibrillation: value of the R-on-T phe-

nomenon in myocardial infarction, Br. Heart J. **38**:415, 1976.

5. Horowitz, L.N., et al.: Ventricular resection guided by epicardial and endocardial mapping for treatment of recurrent ventricular tachycardia, N. Engl. J. Med. **302**:589, 1980.

6. Krikler, D.: Ventricular tachycardia and ventricular fibrillation. In Mandel, W.J., editor: Cardiac arrhythmias, Philadelphia, 1980, J.B. Lippincott Co.

7. Loeb, H.S. et al.: Paroxsymal ventricular fibrillation in two patients with hypomagnesemia: treatment by transvenous pacing, Circulation **37**:210, 1968.

8. Marriott, H.J.L., and Conover, M.H.: Advanced concepts in arrhythmias, St. Louis, 1983, The C.V. Mosby Co.

9. McIntyre, K., et al.: Sudden cardiac death. In McIntyre, K., and Lewis, A.J., editors: Textbook of advanced cardiac life support, 1983, The American Heart Association.

10. Scherf, D., and Schott, A.: Extrasystoles in allied arrhythmias, London, 1953, William Heinemann.

11. Schwartz, S.P., et al.: Transient ventricular fibrillation: I. The prefibrillatory period during established auriculoventricular dissociation with a note on the phonocardiograms obtained at such times, Am. Heart J. **37**:21, 1949.

12. Soffer, J., et al.: Polymorphous ventricular tachycardia associated with normal and long QT intervals, Am. J. Cardiol. **49**:2021, 1982.

13. Tamura, K., et al.: Transient recurrent ventricular fibrillation due to hypopotassemia with a special note on the U wave, Jpn. Heart J. **8**:652, 1967.

14. Zipes D.P., et al.: Clinical transvenous cardioversion of recurrent life-threatening ventricular tachyarrhythmias: low energy synchronized cardioversion of ventricular tachycardia and termination of ventricular fibrillation in patients using a catheter electrode (abstract), Am. J. Cardiol. **103**:189, 1982.

SUGGESTED LEARNING ACTIVITIES AND EXPERIENCES

A. Find patients in any critical care area or telemetry-monitored unit who demonstrate ventricular rhythm disturbances

B. Once a rhythm disturbance is identified, review the patient's record, including:
   1. History
   2. Physical examination
   3. Diagnosis
   4. Medications (both scheduled and p.r.n.)
   5. Vital signs
   6. Laboratory data

C. Attempt to identify a possible etiology of rhythm disturbances

D. Identify treatment measures and nursing observations and/or management that relate to the particular rhythm disturbances

E. Write patient care objectives on the nursing process record in relation to the dysrhythmia

F. Study other references available on ventricular dysrhythmias

POSTTEST (Answers on pp. 148-150)

Directions: Circle one answer to each question unless otherwise indicated.

A. A continuous rhythm strip showing each normal complex followed by a PVC is diagnosed as:
   1. Frequent PVCs
   2. Ventricular bigeminy
   3. Irregular rhythm
   4. Ventricular trigeminy

B. At times, the sinus impulse penetrates and contributes to ventricular activation along with a premature focus in the ventricles. The complex produced by this collision is referred to as:
   1. R-on-T PVC
   2. Fusion complex
   3. Sequential PVCs
   4. Ventricular escape complex

C. The best immediate form of therapy for *torsade de pointes* ventricular tachycardia is:
   1. Lidocaine 1 to 2 mg/kg I.V. bolus, followed by 1 to 4 mg per minute I.V. drip and I.V. bolus doses of 50 mg to a total of 225 mg
   2. Discontinuing drugs, such as lidocaine and procainamide, and performing defibrillation as necessary
   3. Insertion of transvenous pacemaker
   4. Cardiopulmonary resuscitation

D. The most likely treatment to be immediately used for the rhythm in Fig. 6-34 is:
   1. Pacemaker
   2. Quinidine p.o.
   3. DC countershock
   4. External chest compression

E. The rhythm in Fig. 6-35 would most likely be treated with (circle all that apply):
   1. Atropine and/or isoproterenol and possibly a pacemaker
   2. Lidocaine
   3. DC countershock
   4. External chest compression

F. The ectopic complex in Fig. 6-36 most likely represents:
   1. R-on-T PVC
   2. Aberrantly conducted complex

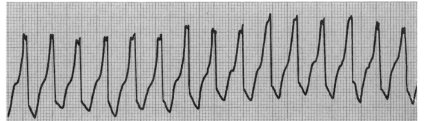

FIG. 6-34

Lead MCL₁

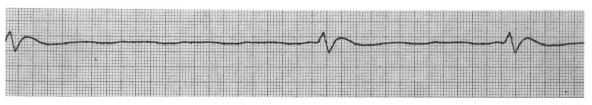

FIG. 6-35

Lead II

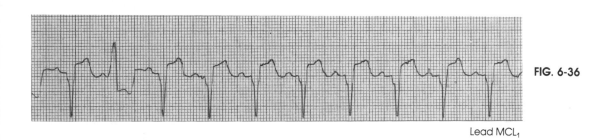

FIG. 6-36

Lead MCL₁

3. Interpolated PVC
4. End-diastolic PVC
G. Dysrhythmias that could progress to ventricular fibrillation and for which the nurse must be continually alert include (circle all that apply):
1. First degree AV block
2. R-on-T PVCs
3. PACs
4. Multifocal/multiform PVCs (more than six per minute)
5. Ventricular tachycardia
H. If "fine" ventricular fibrillation is noted on the ECG monitor, the best immediate action to take is:
1. DC countershock using 200 to 400 watt/sec
2. Lidocaine 1 to 2 mg/kg I.V. bolus, followed by 1 to 4 mg per minute I.V. drip
3. Administration of NAHCO₃, 1 mEq/kg
4. Administration of I.V. epinephrine, 0.5 to 1 mg followed by DC countershock

I. The initial action to be taken for the rhythm shown in Fig. 6-37 on p. 140 is to:
1. Telephone the operator
2. Provide artificial respiration
3. Check blood pressure
4. Provide immediate defibrillation
J. Interpret the rhythm in Fig. 6-38 on p. 140.
  1. Rate:
    Atrial:
    Ventricular:
  2. Rhythm:
    Atrial:
    Ventricular:
  3. P waves:
  4. PR interval:
  5. Ratio of P/QRS:
  6. QRS interval:
  7. QT interval:
  8. Interpretation:

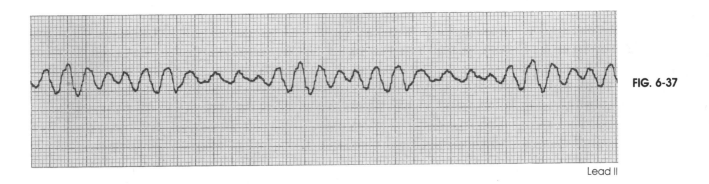

FIG. 6-37

Lead II

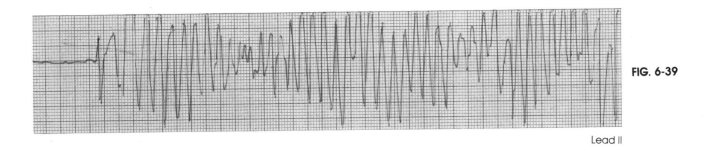

FIG. 6-38

Lead II

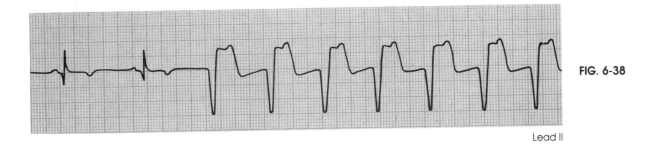

FIG. 6-39

Lead II

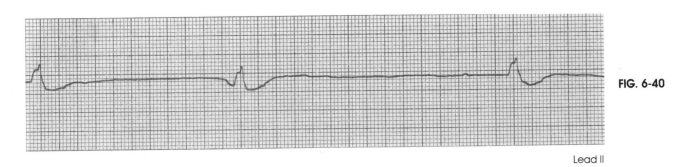

FIG. 6-40

Lead II

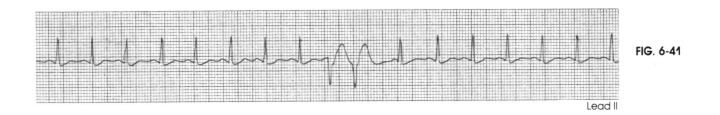

FIG. 6-41

Lead II

9. Common cause(s):

10. Management (treatment and nursing management):

K. Interpret the rhythm in Fig. 6-39.
   1. Rate:
      Atrial:
      Ventricular:
   2. Rhythm:
      Atrial:
      Ventricular:
   3. P waves:
   4. PR interval:
   5. Ratio of P/QRS:
   6. QRS interval:
   7. QT interval:
   8. Interpretation:
   9. Common cause(s):
   10. Management (treatment and nursing management):

L. Interpret the rhythm in Fig. 6-40.
   1. Rate:
      Atrial:
      Ventricular:
   2. Rhythm:
      Atrial:
      Ventricular:
   3. P waves:
   4. PR interval:

5. Ratio of P/QRS:
6. QRS interval:
7. QT interval:
8. Interpretation:
9. Common cause(s):
10. Management (treatment and nursing management):

M. Interpret the rhythm in Fig. 6-41.
   1. Rate:
      Atrial:
      Ventricular:
   2. Rhythm:
      Atrial:
      Ventricular:
   3. P waves:
   4. PR interval:
   5. Ratio of P/QRS:
   6. QRS interval:
   7. QT interval:
   8. Interpretation:
   9. Common cause(s):
   10. Management (treatment and nursing management):

N. Interpret the rhythm in Fig. 6-42.
   1. Rate:
      Atrial:
      Ventricular:

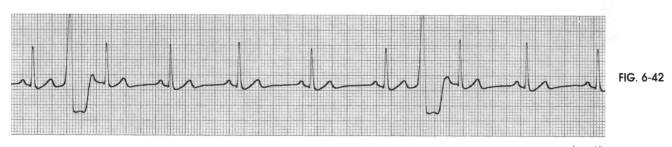

FIG. 6-42

Lead II

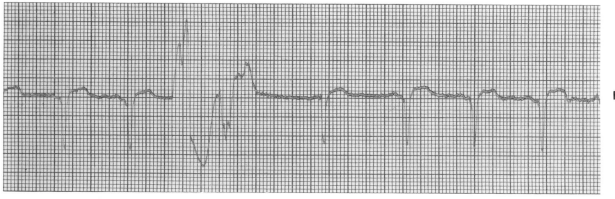

FIG. 6-43

Lead MCL₁

2. Rhythm:
    Atrial:
    Ventricular:
3. P waves:
4. PR interval:
5. Ratio of P/QRS:
6. QRS interval:
7. QT interval:
8. Interpretation:
9. Common cause(s):
10. Management (treatment and nursing management):

O. Interpret the rhythm in Fig. 6-43 on p. 141.
1. Rate:
    Atrial:
    Ventricular:
2. Rhythm:
    Atrial:
    Ventricular:
3. P waves:
4. PR interval:
5. Ratio of P/QRS:
6. QRS interval:
7. QT interval:
8. Interpretation:
9. Common cause(s):
10. Management (treatment and nursing management):

P. Matching: Match the term in column A with the definition in column B.

Column A
Term

___ 1. Active rhythm
___ 2. Cardioversion
___ 3. Defibrillation
___ 4. Fusion complex
___ 5. Idioventricular
___ 6. "Overdrive" pacing
___ 7. Reentry
___ 8. Retrograde conduction
___ 9. *Torsade de pointes*
___ 10. Ventricular tachycardia

Column B
Definition

a. The use of a pacemaker to suppress an abnormal rhythm by artificially stimulating the heart at a faster rate than the heart's intrinsic rate

b. An emergency therapy in which a nonsynchronized direct electrical current is delivered to the myocardium via metal paddles applied to the chest

c. A rhythm initiated by a premature complex (one early in the cycle), that continues at a rate faster than the normal pacemaker usurping control of the heart rhythm

d. A rhythm arising in and controlling only the ventricles at their slow inherent rate

e. Backward conduction from the ventricles or the AV junction into the atria

f. A direct electrical current, syncronized to be delivered on the R wave in order to terminate a tachycardia

g. Reactivation of a tissue more than one time by the same impulse

h. The "collision" of two impulses (often one from the atria and one from the ventricles) in the ventricles, producing a complex with characteristics of both

i. A series of three or more consecutive PVCs, occurring at a rate of 110 to 250 per minute

j. A tachycardia that is not uniform in appearance and which has a phasic variation in polarity

SUPPLEMENTS

This is a work section. A work space is provided beneath each strip to the left. The answers are to the right. It is suggested that you cover the answers while you work the strips. Check your answers on the right.

A.

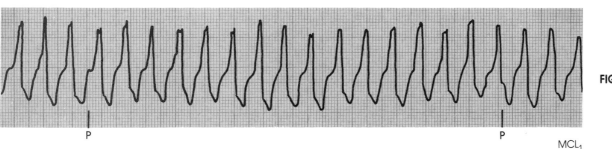

FIG. 6-44

P   P   MCL₁

1. Rate:
   Atrial: Not identifiable
   Ventricular: Approximately 166
2. Rhythm:
   Atrial: Not identifiable
   Ventricular: Essentially regular
3. P waves: P waves not identifiable
4. PR interval: Not applicable
5. Ratio of P/QRS: Not applicable
6. QRS interval: 0.12 second
7. QT interval: Not measurable
8. Interpretation: Ventricular tachycardia

B.   **FIG. 6-45**

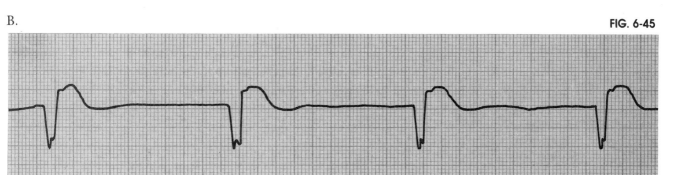

Lead II

1. Rate:
   Atrial: Not present
   Ventricular: Approximately 30
2. Rhythm:
   Atrial: Not applicable
   Ventricular: Essentially regular
3. P waves: Not present
4. PR interval: Not applicable
5. Ratio of P/QRS: Not applicable
6. QRS interval: 0.14 second
7. QT interval: 0.52 second (difficult to ascertain)
8. Interpretation: Ventricular escape rhythm (idioventricular rhythm)

C.

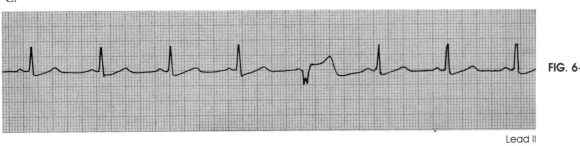

FIG. 6-46

Lead II

1. Rate:
   Atrial: 64
   Ventricular: 64
2. Rhythm:
   Atrial: Regular
   Ventricular: Essentially regular except for one PVC
3. P waves: All the same and upright
4. PR interval: 0.16 second; not relevant with PVC
5. Ratio of P/QRS: 1:1
6. QRS interval: 0.06 second in normal complexes; 0.12 second in PVC
7. QT interval: 0.48 second; 0.48 with PVC
8. Interpretation: Normal rhythm with one end-diastolic PVC

D.

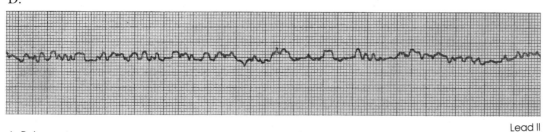

FIG. 6-47

Lead II

1. Rate:
   Atrial: Not identifiable
   Ventricular: Not measurable
2. Rhythm:
   Atrial: Not identifiable
   Ventricular: Grossly irregular
3. P waves: Not identifiable
4. PR interval: Not applicable
5. Ratio of P/QRS: Not applicable
6. QRS interval: Not applicable
7. QT interval: Not applicable
8. Interpretation: Ventricular fibrillation

E.

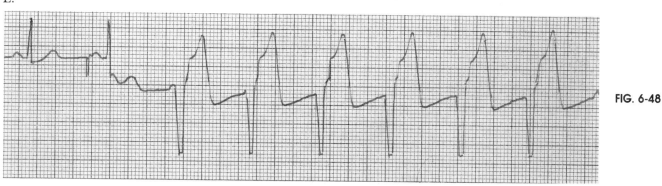

FIG. 6-48

Lead II

1. Rate:
   Atrial: Approximately 72
   Ventricular: Approximately 74
2. Rhythm:
   Atrial: Irregular
   Ventricular: Each rhythm regular unto itself
3. P waves: Identifiable and upright in first part of strip; not identifiable in rhythm with wide, bizarre QRS complexes
4. PR interval: 0.18 second in first part of strip
5. Ratio of P/QRS: 1:1 first part of strip; not applicable to remainder of strip
6. QRS interval: 0.08 second first part of strip; 0.11-0.12 second remainder of strip
7. QT interval: 0.36 second first part of strip; 0.40 remainder of strip
8. Interpretation: Normal sinus rhythm first two complexes with usurpation of sinus node by accelerated idioventricular rhythm

F.

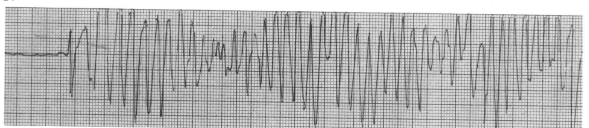

FIG. 6-49

Lead II

1. Rate:
   Atrial: Not identifiable
   Ventricular: Approximately 375
2. Rhythm:
   Atrial: Not identifiable
   Ventricular: Somewhat irregular
3. P waves: Not identifiable
4. PR interval: Not applicable
5. Ratio of P/QRS: Not applicable
6. QRS interval: 0.12 second (difficult to measure)
7. QT interval: Not measurable
8. Interpretation: Ventricular flutter/fibrillation initiated by R-on-T PVC

G.

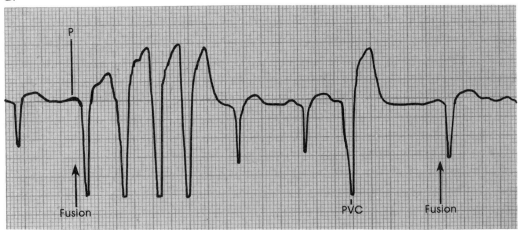

FIG. 6-50

MCL₁

1. Rate:	
Atrial:	Approximately 75
Ventricular:	Approximately 95
2. Rhythm:	
Atrial:	Essentially regular
Ventricular:	Irregular because of PVCs
3. P waves:	Upright and visible in normal part of strip; not visible with PVCs
4. PR interval:	0.20 second
5. Ratio of P/QRS:	1:1 in normal part of strip; not applicable with PVCs
6. QRS interval:	0.09-0.10 in normal part of strip; 0.14-0.16 with PVCs
7. QT interval:	0.38 in normal part of strip; 0.44 with PVCs
8. Interpretation:	Normal sinus rhythm with a sequential run of PVCs, first of which is a fusion complex, and one single PVC

H.

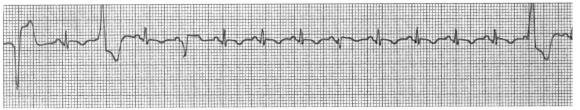

FIG. 6-51

Lead II

1. Rate:	
Atrial:	107
Ventricular:	107
2. Rhythm:	
Atrial:	Regular
Ventricular:	Irregular because of PVCs
3. P waves:	Upright
4. PR interval:	0.12 second in normal part of strip; not applicable with PVCs
5. Ratio of P/QRS:	1:1 in normal part of strip; not relevant with PVCs
6. QRS interval:	0.08 second in normal part of strip; 0.11-0.12 second with PVCs
7. QT interval:	0.32 second in normal part of strip and first PVC; not measurable with remaining PVCs
8. Interpretation:	Sinus tachycardia with three multiform PVCs and one fusion complex; first, second, and fourth are end-diastolic PVCs; the third is a fusion complex

I.

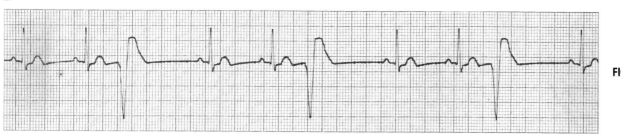

FIG. 6-52

Lead II

1. Rate:
   - Atrial: 69
   - Ventricular: 69
2. Rhythm:
   - Atrial: Regular
   - Ventricular: Irregular because of PVCs
3. P waves: Upright with normal complexes; not visible with PVCs
4. PR interval: 0.16 second with normal complexes; not relevant with PVCs
5. Ratio of P/QRS: 1:1 with normal complexes; not applicable with PVCs
6. QRS interval: 0.08 second with normal complexes; 0.12 second with PVCs
7. QT interval: 0.32 second with normal complexes; 0.38 second with PVCs
8. Interpretation: Ventricular trigeminy

J.

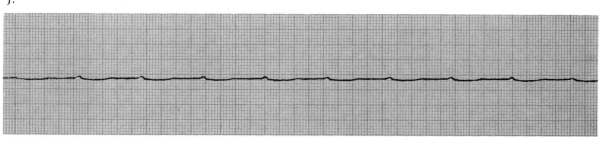

FIG. 6-53

Lead II

1. Rate:
   - Atrial: 69
   - Ventricular: 0
2. Rhythm:
   - Atrial: Regular
   - Ventricular: Not applicable
3. P waves: Upright
4. PR interval: Not applicable
5. Ratio of P/QRS: Not applicable
6. QRS interval: Not applicable
7. QT interval: Not applicable
8. Interpretation: Ventricular standstill

ANSWERS TO PRETEST AND POSTTEST
Pretest

A. 3

B. 4

C. 1, 4

D. 3

E. 1, 4

F. 2

G. 4

H. Fig. 6-5.
1. Rate:
   Atrial: 75
   Ventricular: Approximately 75
2. Rhythm:
   Atrial: Regular
   Ventricular: Basically regular except for abnormal complexes
3. PR interval: 0.22 second
4. QRS duration: 0.06 second normal complex; 0.14 second abnormal complex
5. Interpretation: Normal sinus rhythm with two sets of sequentially occurring PVCs
6. Common cause(s): Myocardial ischemia or infarction, CHF, organic heart disease, prolapsed mitral valve, hypotension, hypoglycemia, anemia, electrolyte imbalance, anoxia, acid-base imbalance, digoxin intoxication, etc.
7. Initial treatment: Lidocaine 1 mg/kg initially, followed by I.V. drip of 1-4 mg/min

I. Fig. 6-6.
1. Rate:
   Atrial: 72
   Ventricular: Approximately 72
2. Rhythm:
   Atrial: Regular
   Ventricular: Essentially regular except for two abnormal complexes
3. PR interval: 0.14 second
4. QRS duration: 0.08 second normal complexes; 0.12 to 0.16 second abnormal complexes
5. Interpretation: Normal sinus rhythm with multiform PVCs
6. Common cause(s): Same as H
7. Initial treatment: Same as H

J. 3

K. 4

L. 1, 3

M. 1

N. 2, 4

O. 3

Posttest

A. 2

B. 2

C. 2

D. 3

E. 1, 4

F. 4

G. 2, 4, 5

H. 4

I. 4

J. Fig. 6-38.
1. Rate:
   Atrial: Undiscernable
   Ventricular: Approximately 75
2. Rhythm:
   Atrial: Undiscernable
   Ventricular: Regular at end of strips
3. P waves: Upright and present before first two complexes; not detectable thereafter
4. PR interval: 0.12 second before first two complexes
5. Ratio of P/QRS: No P waves detected in last part of strip
6. QRS interval: 0.08 second first two complexes; 0.11-0.12 in last part of strip
7. QT interval: 0.46 second first two complexes; 0.42 second remainder of strip
8. Interpretation: Sinus bradycardia (rate 59) with an onset of accelerated idioventricular rhythm at a rate of 83
9. Common cause(s): Acute myocardial infarction, digoxin toxicity, other forms of heart disease, and various other drugs
10. Management: Observe patient's clinical status and ECG pattern and treat underlying heart disease; withhold digoxin if applicable; administer lidocaine if necessary; closely observe and document ECG pattern for excessively slow or fast rhythms; closely observe patient's hemodynamic status and notify physician of any changes in blood pressure, pulse, level of consciousness, etc.; be knowledgeable about drugs that could possibly be used for treatment and be prepared to administer if necessary; maintain skills with emergency equipment should ventricular tachycardia or ventricular fibrillation occur; provide support to the patient and family should the need arise; document strips, treatment, and patient response

K. Fig. 6-39.
   1. Rate:
      Atrial: Not measurable
      Ventricular: Approximately 375
   2. Rhythm:
      Atrial: Not discernable
      Ventricular: Irregular
   3. P wave: Not discernable
   4. PR interval: Not discernable
   5. Ratio of P/QRS: Not applicable
   6. QRS interval: Approximately 0.14-0.16 second
   7. QT interval: Not discernable
   8. Interpretation: Ventricular flutter-fibrillation initiated by an R-on-T PVC
   9. Common cause(s): A PVC occurring in the vulnerable phase of the cardiac cycle (T wave) before the heart is completely repolarized may initiate chaotic activity
   10. Management: Perform immediate DC cardioversion using 200 to 360 watt/sec; administer sodium bicarbonate (1 mEq/kg) immediately since ventricular fibrillation produces metabolic acidosis; obtain blood gases and give sodium bicarbonate to correct blood gas abnormalities; identify and treat all contributing factors such as laboratory abnormalities, hypotension, etc.; employ regular cardiopulmonary resuscitation if ventricular fibrillation is not immediately converted; administer 0.5 to 1 mg I.V. epinephrine if fibrillation has deteriorated from "coarse" to "fine"; observe patient's ECG and hemodynamic status closely; treat dysrhythmias that may predispose to ventricular fibrillation and become familiar with patient's laboratory data; become familiar with defibrillator use and advanced life support drugs; provide emotional and psychological support to patient and family; document strips, treatment, and patient response

L. Fig. 6-40.
   1. Rate:
      Atrial: Not discernable
      Ventricular: Approximately 25
   2. Rhythm:
      Atrial: Not discernable
      Ventricular: Irregular
   3. P waves: Not discernable
   4. PR interval: Not discernable
   5. Ratio of P/QRS: Not applicable
   6. QRS interval: 0.16-0.17 second
   7. QT interval: 0.44 second
   8. Interpretation: Slow idioventricular rhythm

   9. Common cause(s): Most commonly associated with an anterior wall myocardial infarction that can cause extensive necrosis to the uppermost portion of the interventricular septum; often the AV node and bundle of His are spared, but severe damage is done to the bundle branches; complete AV block may develop
   10. Management: Assess patient's clinical status continually, notify physician, and administer atropine I.V. bolus when patient begins to show first signs of decompensation; withhold digoxin or other drugs, if indicated; if patient does not respond to atropine, prepare an isoproterenol drip and prepare for insertion of transvenous pacemaker; if no response to isoproterenol and pacemaker therapy occurs, initiate cardiopulmonary resuscitation; become thoroughly familiar with all drugs that may be administered and closely observe patient for both desired and adverse effects; maintain proficiency in all emergency skills; provide emotional and psychological support to patient and family; document strips, treatment, and patient response

M. Fig. 6-41.
   1. Rate:
      Atrial: 125
      Ventricular: 125
   2. Rhythm:
      Atrial: Regular
      Ventricular: Basically regular, except for abnormal complexes
   3. P wave: Upright but not visible with ectopic complexes
   4. PR interval: 0.14 second
   5. Ratio of P/QRS: 1:1, but not relevant with ectopic complexes
   6. QRS interval: 0.06 second normal complex; 0.12 second in abnormal complexes
   7. QT interval: 0.28 second
   8. Interpretation: Sinus tachycardia with two sequentially occurring PVCs
   9. Common cause(s): Myocardial ischemia or infarction, congestive heart failure (CHF), organic heart disease, prolapsed mitral valve, hypotension, hypoglycemia, anemia, electrolyte imbalance, anoxia, acid-base imbalance, digoxin intoxication, etc.
   10. Management: Observe patient's clinical status and ECG pattern and treat underlying heart disease; withhold digoxin if applicable; administer lidocaine if necessary; closely observe and document

ECG pattern for excessively slow or fast rhythms; closely observe patient's hemodynamic status and notify the physician of any changes in blood pressure, pulse, level of consciousness, etc.; be knowledgeable about drugs possibly used for treatment and be prepared to administer if necessary; maintain skills with emergency equipment should ventricular tachycardia or ventricular fibrillation occur; provide support to the patient and family should the need arise; document strips, treatment, and patient response

N. Fig. 6-42.
1. Rate:
   Atrial: 60
   Ventricular: 80
2. Rhythm:
   Atrial: Regular
   Ventricular: Irregular because of abnormal complexes
3. P waves: Upright
4. PR interval: 0.16 second with normal QRS complexes; 0.20 with abnormal complexes
5. Ratio of P/QRS: 1:1, except no P waves exist before abnormal complexes
6. QRS interval: 0.08 second with normal complexes; 0.12 second with abnormal complexes
7. QT interval: 0.32-0.34 second with normal complexes; not measurable with abnormal complexes
8. Interpretation: Normal sinus rhythm with two interpolated PVCs
9. Common cause(s): Myocardial ischemia or infarction, congestive heart failure (CHF), organic heart disease, prolapsed mitral valve, hypotension, hypoglycemia, anemia, electrolyte imbalance, anoxia, acid-base imbalance, digoxin intoxication, etc.
10. Management: Observe patient's clinical status and ECG pattern and treat underlying heart disease; withhold digoxin if applicable; administer lidocaine if necessary; closely observe and document ECG pattern for excessively slow or fast rhythms; closely observe patient's hemodynamic status and notify the physician of any changes in blood pressure, pulse, level of consciousness, etc.; be knowledgeable about drugs possibly used for treatment and be prepared to administer if necessary; maintain skills with emergency equipment should ventricular tachycardia or ventricular fibrillation occur; provide support to the patient

and family should the need arise; document strips, treatment, and patient response

O. Fig. 6-43.
1. Rate:
   Atrial: 84
   Ventricular: 84
2. Rhythm:
   Atrial: Slightly irregular
   Ventricular: Irregular because of abnormal complexes
3. P waves: Upright, or slightly inverted
4. PR interval: Approximately 0.18-0.20 second, except for post-ectopic P waves
5. Ratio of P/QRS: 1:1 except in abnormal complexes
6. QRS interval: 0.08 second normal complexes; 0.20 second in first abnormal complex; 0.16 second in second abnormal complex
7. QT interval: 0.32 in normal complexes; 0.40 in second abnormal complex; not measurable in first abnormal complex
8. Interpretation: Normal sinus rhythm with two multiformed sequential PVCs
9. Common cause(s): Myocardial ischemia or infarction, CHF, organic heart disease, prolapsed mitral valve, hypotension, hypoglycemia, anemia, electrolyte imbalance, anoxia, acid-base imbalance, digoxin intoxication, etc.
10. Management: Observe patient's clinical status and ECG pattern and treat underlying heart disease; withhold digoxin if applicable; administer lidocaine if necessary; closely observe and document ECG pattern for excessively slow or fast rhythms; closely observe patient's hemodynamic status and notify the physician of any changes in blood pressure, pulse, level of consciousness, etc.; be knowledgeable about drugs possibly used for treatment and be prepared to administer if necessary; maintain skills with emergency equipment should ventricular tachycardia or ventricular fibrillation occur; provide support to the patient and family should the need arise; document strips, treatment, and patient response

P. Matching:
1. c   6. a
2. f   7. g
3. b   8. e
4. h   9. j
5. d   10. i

MODULE

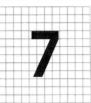

7 Pacemakers

PRETEST (Answers on p. 183)

Directions: Circle one answer to each question unless otherwise indicated.

A. The essential components of any pacemaker system are:
1. Pulse generator and pacing cells
2. Pulse generator and pacing leads
3. Transvenous leads and a grounding wire
4. Pulse generator and a unipolar stimulus

B. Indications for temporary pacing include which of the following? (Circle all that apply.)
1. Atrioventricular block after open heart surgery
2. Dysrhythmias responsive to medical therapy
3. Diagnostic testing
4. Sick sinus syndrome

C. Determining pacing threshold with a temporary pacemaker system can be done by:
1. Manipulating the rate control and determining which rate the patient responds to best
2. Manipulating the sensitivity control to maximum threshold
3. Manipulating the output setting toward 10 mA and observing the ECG monitor to obtain adequate pacing
4. Manipulating the volume to reach threshold

D. Indications for permanent pacing include which of the following? (Circle all that apply.)
1. Complete heart block
2. Mobitz type I
3. Mobitz type II with AV block distal to the bundle of His
4. Increased carotid flow
5. Hypersensitive carotid sinus syndrome

E. A permanent pacemaker system cannot be implanted in the:
1. Subcutaneous tissue
2. Subclavicular area
3. Brachial area
4. Abdomen

F. Electromagnetic interference can inhibit pacemaker function. Some things that can cause this interference are:
1. A malfunctioning auto battery when the patient gets close to the battery
2. Electrocautery, transcutaneous electrical nerve stimulators, and electrical razors
3. Cardiac myopotentials
4. Electrical ovens

G. An example of an asynchronous fixed-rate ventricular pacemaker is:
1. VVI
2. AAT
3. VOO
4. DVI

H. A dual chamber pacing modality is a(n):
1. VVI
2. AAT
3. VOO
4. DVI

I. The advantages of a temporary bipolar electrode include which of the following? (Circle all that apply.)
1. It can be converted to a unipolar electrode
2. The bipoles last longer
3. It does not produce muscle stimulation at the pocket site where the generator is implanted
4. Less electromagnetic interference is picked up

J. When defibrillating a patient who has a permanent pacemaker, the paddles should be placed:
1. To the left of the pulse generator
2. To the right of the pulse generator
3. At least 10 cm from the pulse generator
4. As close to the pulse generator as possible for maximum power

K. DVI pacemakers are indicated for:
1. Atrial fibrillation
2. Atrial dysrhythmias with or without impaired AV conduction
3. Atrial flutter with 2:1 block
4. Diagnostic mapping for reentrant tachydysrhythmias

151

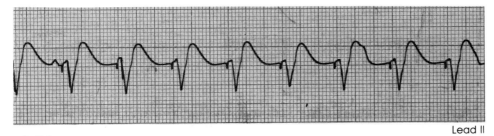

FIG. 7-1

Lead II

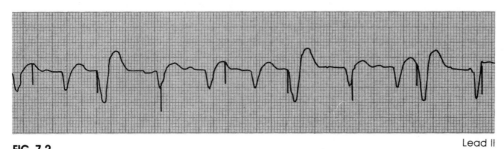

FIG. 7-2

Lead II

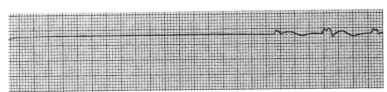

FIG. 7-3

Lead II

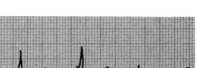

FIG. 7-4

Lead II

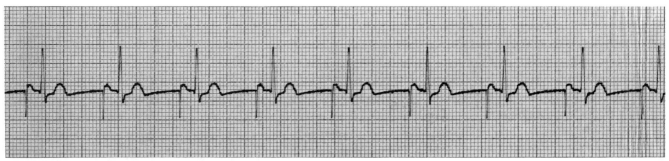

FIG. 7-5

Lead II

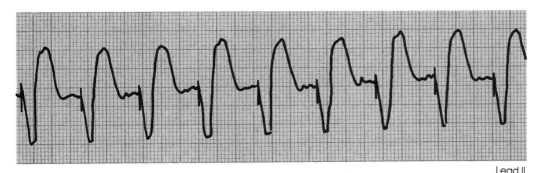

FIG. 7-6

Lead II

L. The strip in Fig. 7-1 demonstrates:
1. The patient's own rhythm with a widened QRS (bundle branch block)
2. A pacer-induced rhythm
3. A noncapturing pacemaker
4. A nonsensing pacemaker

M. If a temporary pacemaker is not capturing properly, the nurse should:
1. Tell the patient to get up and walk around so his/her heart rate will increase
2. Check the pacemaker terminals and increase the mA
3. Decrease the set rate on the pacemaker generator so more energy will be available
4. Call the physician and inform him/her about the malfunctioning pacemaker and be ready to re-charge the pulse generator

N. The strip in Fig. 7-2 is an example of:
1. A continuous paced rhythm
2. A noncapturing pacemaker
3. A sensing pacemaker
4. Asynchronous pacing

O. The strip in Fig. 7-3 is an example of:
1. A continuously paced rhythm
2. A noncapturing pacemaker
3. A nonsensing pacemaker
4. Asynchronous pacing

P. If the ECG shows asystole, as in Fig. 7-4, and the patient is unconscious, which of the following should you do?
1. Call a code and wait for the team to insert a pacemaker
2. Manipulate the battery cable for at least 10 minutes, which may help to dislodge the blockage
3. Initiate CPR
4. Reposition the patient and increase the mA

Q. The strip in Fig. 7-5 is an example of:
1. Atrial pacing
2. AV sequential pacing
3. Intermittent pacing as the ventricles are not being paced
4. A malfunctioning sensing mechanism

R. The strip in Fig. 7-6 is an example of:
1. Atrial pacing
2. Ventricular pacing
3. Complete pacing
4. AV sequential pacing

PURPOSE

The purpose of this module is to provide the learner with information about the following:

A. Artificial pacemaker systems
B. Indications for artificial pacemakers
C. Treatment and nursing care of patients with pacemakers
D. Various ECG patterns manifesting both properly functioning and malfunctioning pacemakers
E. Complications and solutions for malfunctioning pacemakers

BEHAVIORAL OBJECTIVES

Upon completion of this module, the learner should be able to:

A. Define and identify components of temporary and permanent pacemaker therapy
B. List indications for temporary and permanent pacemaker therapy
C. Describe insertion techniques for temporary and permanent pacemakers
D. Discuss the care of the patient receiving pacemaker therapy
E. Recognize on rhythm strips normal and abnormal pacemaker function
F. Define various pacing modalities

VOCABULARY

Aberrant conduction Impulse(s) that is (are) abnormally conducted through the ventricles, producing a change in the QRS morphology.

Afterpotential The spread of delivered electrical current from the pacemaker to the myocardial tissue. This can be of a significant magnitude to cause a lack of firing by the pacemaker.

Anode The positive position of a pacer lead system.

Asynchronous A type of pacemaker that fires despite the heart's own intrinsic rate. It is also considered a fixed rate pacemaker. (See Fixed rate pacemaker.)

AV delay A constant pacemaker timing interval; it begins with an atrially paced or sensed event and ends with a ventricularly paced event. The usual AV delay is 200 ms (0.20 second).

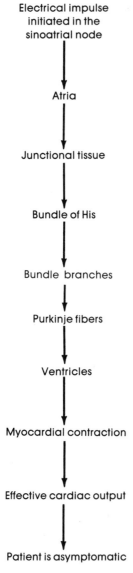

Electrical impulse
initiated in the
sinoatrial node

↓

Atria

↓

Junctional tissue

↓

Bundle of His

↓

Bundle branches

↓

Purkinje fibers

↓

Ventricles

↓

Myocardial contraction

↓

Effective cardiac output

↓

Patient is asymptomatic

FIG. 7-7
Normal conduction producing effective cardiac output.

Cathode The negative portion of a pacer lead system.

Committed sequential pacing The DVI (dual chamber–paced, ventricular chamber–sensed, mode of response is inhibited) pacing modality in which ventricular stimulation is obligated after atrial stimulation.

Demand pacemaker A type of pacemaker that fires only when necessary; that is, when the heart's own intrinsic rate becomes slower than the rate at which the pacemaker is set. It is synchronized to the patient's intrinsic rate.

Escape interval The interval in milliseconds between an intrinsic complex and the subsequent paced complex.

Fixed rate pacemaker A type of pacemaker that fires constantly despite the patient's intrinsic rate. It is said to be asynchronous because it does not synchronize its firing with the patient's own intrinsic rate.

Hysteresis The extended time interval after an intrinsic beat and before the next paced beat.

Microshock Stray electrical current that may result from static electricity or from a short-circuit electrical device. The current enters the pacer leads and elicits myocardial depolarization during the vulnerable period, thereby producing tachydysrhythmias.

Myopotential The electrical current of muscle contraction resembling cardiac potentials that can cause sensitive pulse generators to inhibit or trigger pacemaker activity.

Noncommitted sequential pacing The DVI (dual chamber–paced, ventricular chamber–sensed, mode of response is inhibited) pacing modality in which ventricular output is optional after atrial output.

Overdrive pacing The use of an artificial pacemaker to stimulate the heart's own intrinsic rate in order to suppress an abnormal tachydysrhythmia.

Programmability The ability to change an implantable pacemaker's mode (rate, impulse amplitude, etc.) by noninvasive means. An example of simple programmability is the placement of a magnet over an implanted synchronous pacemaker to change it to the asynchronous mode.

Sensitivity The minimum signal that consistently activates the pacemaker (pulse generator). This is also known as the sensing threshold.

Synchronous See Demand pacemaker

Threshold The lowest amount of electrical energy necessary to cause the heart to contract from a pacemaker stimulus.

CONTENT
Suggested review

Before beginning this module on pacemakers, it is recommended that the learner review the previous modules and successfully complete their pretests and posttests.

Normal human pacemaker

The normal pacing system consists of the initiation of an electrical impulse in the SA node, with depolarization occurring in the atria, through the AV node to the junctional tissue, bundle of His, Purkinje fibers and the ventricles, ultimately producing an effective cardiac output (Fig. 7-7).

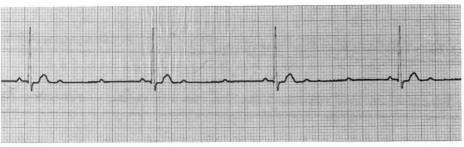

Lead II

FIG. 7-8

3:1 heart block. There are three P waves for every QRS complex.

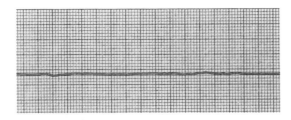

Lead II

FIG. 7-9

Asystole. Complete lack of cardiac electrical activity.

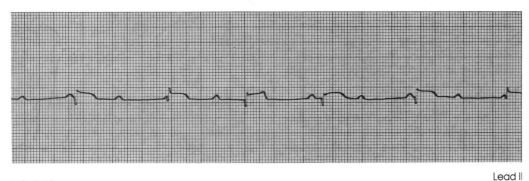

Lead II

FIG. 7-10

Complete heart block.

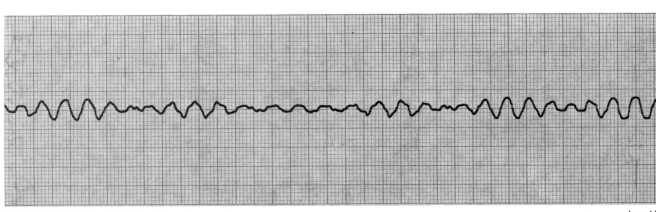

Lead II

FIG. 7-11

Ventricular fibrillation.

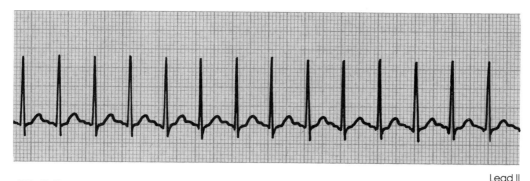

FIG. 7-12   Lead II

Paroxysmal atrial tachycardia (PAT).

Failure of the human pacemaker

The failure of the human pacing system can occur because of acute or chronic circulatory insufficiency, infection, trauma, chemical toxicity, collagen diseases, calcium deposits, or congenital malformations.[34]

Abnormal electrical conduction will be noted on the ECG by a(n):

1. Lack of initiation of an effective impulse, resulting in a block or asystole (Figs. 7-8 and 7-9, p. 155)
2. Inadequate conduction of an impulse as seen with complete heart block or ventricular fibrillation (Figs. 7-10 and 7-11, p. 155)
3. Initiation of a rapid and ineffective rate causing inadequate cardiac output, as seen with paroxysmal atrial tachycardia (Fig. 7-12)

Principles of electrical activity in relation to cardiac pacing

The principles of electrical activity are involved in pacemaker therapy. These principles deal with current, voltage, and resistance, illustrating one of the basic laws of electricity—Ohm's law. Pacemaker therapy involves an electrical circuit that functions as follows:

$$\text{Electrical current flow (amperes)} = \frac{\text{Driving force (voltage)}}{\text{Resistance (ohms)}}$$

There are several factors that produce an electrical circuit.

1. *Current* is measured in amperes and is defined as the flow of electrons. An *electrical circuit* is composed of a power source with an anode (positive) and cathode (negative) terminal connected by an electrically conductive wire.
2. The power source or pulse generator initiates the *voltage* (power) that pushes the current (flow of electrons) through the wire from the cathode

(negative) pole to anode (positive) pole in a circular pattern. In a pacemaker, the power is conducted through the lead from the pulse generator to the heart and the electrical activity is sensed from the heart back to the pulse generator. This makes a complete circuit.

3. The amount of current the heart receives depends on the amount of voltage delivered and the amount of *resistance* in the wire to the current flow. If resistance increases, then the *voltage* will have to be increased to maintain the current flow. Pacemaker therapy is instituted to produce adequate myocardial depolarization (activation of automatic, conductile, and contractile elements from the resting or polarized state to an active or depolarized state) and an effective cardiac output. The pulse generator should sense the intrinsic rhythm and be able to fire an impulse when there is an inadequate intrinsic rhythm. The discharged impulse should produce myocardial depolarization, thereby producing a *captured complex* or a *paced complex* (Fig. 7-13).

Temporary pacemaker therapy

Temporary pacemaker therapy involves the use of a temporary pulse generator. This is worn externally and the leads are in contact with the heart to establish an adequate heart rate and cardiac output.

COMPONENTS OF TEMPORARY PACEMAKER THERAPY

1. There is an external pulse generator, which uses a *non-AV sequential battery,* illustrated in Fig. 7-14. The dials on the generator include:
   a. *On-off switch,* which turns the battery on (activates) and turns the battery off (deactivates).

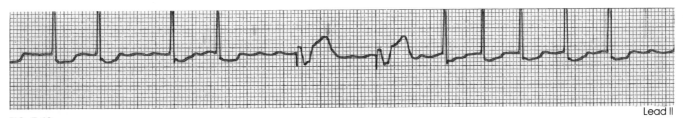

Lead II

FIG. 7-13

Fifth and sixth complex in above strip are captured beats. Pacer spike is seen.

b. *Safety lock* that requires two steps to terminate the energy from the battery and, as a result, assists in preventing accidental deactivation.

c. *Mode,* which may be asynchronous (fixed rate) or synchronous (demand). With the asynchronous mode, the pacemaker fires continuously at a predetermined rate. To attain this mode, the dial is turned completely *counterclockwise.* With the synchronous (demand) mode, the dial is turned completely *clockwise* and the battery will fire only if it has not detected the patient's own electrical impulse after a preset period of time.

d. *Rate* that regulates the number of impulses delivered per minute.

e. *mA dial* that regulates milliamperes or the amount of energy delivered to the electrodes.

f. *Sensitivity dial* that regulates the sensitivity threshold by determining the proper firing rate. The control ranges from 0.5 mV to 20 mV. These numbers represent the millivolt size of amplitude, of a P, R, or T wave that the pacemaker is capable of sensing. A setting of 0.5 mV is most sensitive, whereas a setting of 20 mV makes the unit incapable of sensing any intrinsic configuration and fixed-rate pacing will occur. Sensitivity is important because it allows the pacemaker to avoid competition with the patient's intrinsic rhythm. It is determined by turning the dial just until the patient's R wave is sensed. This is determined by the sense/pace indicator. An ECG lead demonstrating a positively deflected R wave is necessary for determining sensitivity. If a P-QRS-T complex has a tall P or T wave, the sensitivity dial is turned until it senses the R wave only and not the tall P or the T wave. If the pulse generator remained sensitive to a tall P wave, for example, it would not fire an impulse in the case of a 3 : 1 AV block because it would be sensing the three P waves only.

g. *Sense/pace indicator,* which varies with the type of pacemaker used. Each time the patient's own complex (R wave) occurs, a light flashes, or the indicator moves to the "sense" position. When the pacemaker fires, the light flashes, or the indicator moves to the "pace" position.

2. An external *AV sequential pulse generator* is illustrated in Fig. 7-15, p. 158. The dials on the generator include:

a. *Atrial pace indicator light,* which flashes each time an atrial pacing stimulus is emitted by the pulse generator. The flashing of the light only indicates

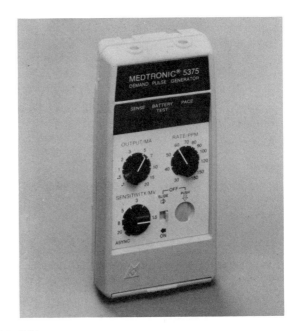

FIG. 7-14

Non-AV sequential temporary pulse generator, Medtronic Demand 5375 (Courtesy Medtronics).

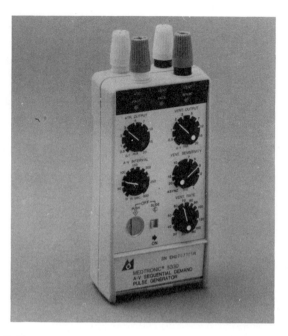

FIG. 7-15

AV sequential temporary pulse generator, Medtronic Demand 5330 (Courtesy Medtronics).

TABLE 7-1. Advantages of unipolar and bipolar leads

Unipolar advantages	Bipolar advantages
Larger pacing artifact eases ECG analysis	Less electromagnetic interference is picked up since both terminals are intracardiac and not in contact with skeletal tissue
Only one electrode on the heart is necessary	It can be converted to an unipolar system if one of the stimulating electrodes is not functioning or if it is fractured*
Possibly lower voltage is needed to maintain threshold because indifferent electrode within pulse generator has low site resistance	There is no muscle stimulation interference where the generator is implanted
Lead is smaller than bipolar one and can be introduced more easily through a small vein	
More sensitive	

*Procedure to convert a bipolar to an unipolar is described on p. 167.

that a stimulus has been emitted and does not indicate capture or myocardial depolarization.

b. *Ventricular pace indicator light,* which flashes each time a ventricular stimulus is emitted by the pulse generator. Once again the flashing of this light does not indicate a capture. When the atrial and ventricular indicator lights are flashing simultaneously, the sequential function of the unit can be noted.

c. *Ventricular output control* that adjusts the pulse amplitude of the stimulus emitted through the ventricular output terminal. Normally, the setting is two or three times the patient's ventricular stimulation threshold.

d. *Atrial output control* that adjusts the pulse amplitude of the stimulus emitted through the atrial terminal. It usually is set at two or three times the patient's atrial stimulation threshold.

e. *AV interval control* that adjusts the time interval between the atrial and ventricular pacing stimuli, thereby allowing atrial and ventricular depolarization to synchronize and improve cardiac output. The usual setting is 150 ms.

f. *Ventricular sensitivity control* that adjusts the sensitivity of the pulse generator to the amplitude of the myocardial R wave signal, which will inhibit the pulse generator during demand pacing.

g. *Ventricular rate control* that regulates the number of ventricular impulses per minute. It also controls the atrial rate when the pacemaker is operating in the AV sequential mode.

3. Electrodes are the other essential components necessary for pacing to occur. Electrodes are wires in contact with the epicardium or endocardium through which the electrical impulse travels from the pulse generator. They can be unipolar or bipolar.

a. A *unipolar* electrode has a negative electrode in contact with the heart and an externally positioned positive electrode (usually the metallic housing of the pulse generator). Pacing with a unipolar electrode produces a large pace spike because the current travels a long distance from the pulse generator to the electrode tip. Therefore a large pacer spike will be seen in a paced rhythm on the ECG (Fig. 7-16).

b. A *bipolar* electrode has a positive and a negative electrode at the tip of wire. The current travels a shorter distance since the electrodes are at the tip of the wire, thereby producing a small spike and sometimes making it difficult to detect the spike on the ECG (Fig. 7-17).

c. There are many types of unipolar or bipolar electrodes or leads that can be inserted. The advantages

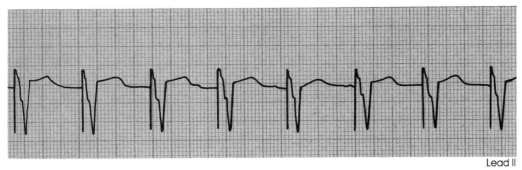

Lead II

FIG. 7-16
Paced rhythm with unipolar electrode in place, thereby causing
large pacer spikes.

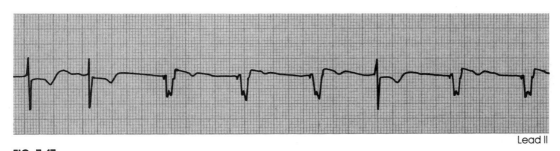

Lead II

FIG. 7-17
Third, fourth, fifth, seventh, and eighth complexes are paced ventricular
complexes with a bipolar electrode. Spike preceding paced complex
is usually small and at times may be difficult to detect.

of the bipolar vs. the unipolar electrodes are listed
in Table 7-1.[12,32,38] Leads are also described according to their area of insertion or contact with
the heart.

(1) For example, *transvenous endocardial lead* may be:

   (a) A balloon-tipped lead, with a balloon at the end
of the electrode. With this type of lead, the
catheter is inserted via a large vein into the right
atrium and the balloon is inflated, allowing the
electrode to float into the right ventricle.

   (b) An endocardial lead that is usually *bipolar* and is
used for atrial, ventricular, or AV sequential
pacing (Fig. 7-18, p. 160).

(2) An *epicardial lead* (pacing wires) is/are inserted during surgery with the wire or wires brought out
through the patient's anterior chest. Each wire is a
unipolar lead. Many times a patient may return from
surgery with only one wire in place in the myocardium; however, if pacing is needed, a wire must be

sutured to the subcutaneous tissue in order to make a
complete circuit. This wire is connected to the
positive terminal and the myocardial wire is connected to the negative terminal.

(3) A *transthoracic or subxiphoid lead* is a *bipolar* J-shaped
lead (Fig. 7-19, p. 160). It is inserted via a needle and
an obturator into the ventricular chamber. The approach allows for easy insertion and removal; however, the lead is less reliable than other temporary
leads and is rarely used.

INDICATIONS FOR A TEMPORARY PACEMAKER

There are a number of indications for use of a
temporary pacemaker. They are:

1. *Atrioventricular blocks* associated with a heart attack or
following open heart surgery until ischemia around the
conduction system subsides or a permanent pacemaker
is implanted (because a permanent block has developed)[11,14,16]

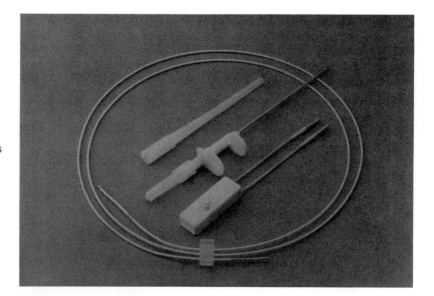

FIG. 7-18
Medtronic Temptron temporary bipolar pacing leads (Courtesy Medtronics).

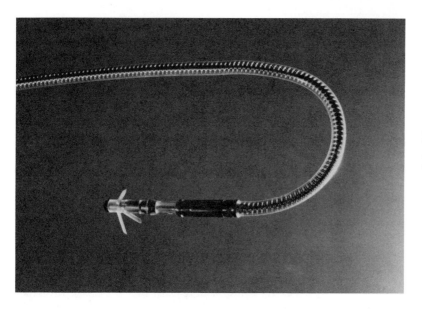

FIG. 7-19
J-shaped pacing lead, Medtronic Target tip Model 4511 (Courtesy Medtronics).

2. *Malfunctioning permanent pacemaker* until another permanent pacemaker can be inserted

3. *Dysrhythmias* unresponsive to medical therapy in which the artificial pacemaker is used to "overdrive" the dysrhythmia by increasing the rate[39]

4. *Pacemaker on standby* when maximal dosages of antidysrhythmic drugs are being administered that could precipitate complete heart block or decreased heart rate

5. *Cardiac arrest* with ventricular asystole

6. *Tachy-brady dysrhythmias* related to sick sinus syndrome[35]

7. *Diagnostic testing,*[35] which assists in defining specific electrophysiological problems and allows for the most appropriate treatment plan

VARIOUS APPROACHES AND COMPLICATIONS IN THE INSERTION OF A TEMPORARY PACEMAKER

1. *Transvenous approach* (Fig. 7-20) involves the pacer wire being inserted percutaneously or by a cutdown into one of the major veins (jugular, subclavian, anticubital, or femoral). It is advanced through the superior or inferior vena cava to the right atrium and is ultimately lodged in the right atrium and/or the right

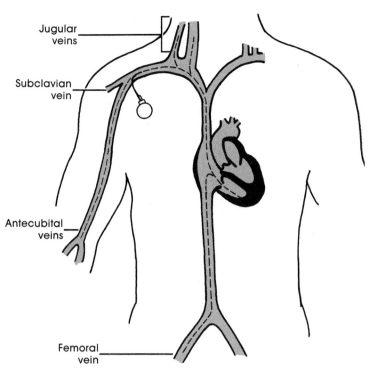

FIG. 7-20

Temporary transvenous electrode insertion sites include internal or external jugular vein, subclavian vein, basilic or cephalic vein or femoral vein.

Labels on figure:
- Jugular veins
- Subclavian vein
- Antecubital veins
- Femoral vein

ventricle. Complications with the transvenous approach may involve:

a. Systemic infection

b. Damage to the tricuspid or pulmonic valve

c. Premature ventricular complexes (PVCs)

d. Loss of electrode contact with the endocardium

e. Septal perforation

2. *Epicardial approach* requires that an epicardial wire be sutured on the myocardial surface. The procedure is generally performed during cardiac surgery. The terminal end of the wire or wire(s) are placed through the abdomen. The disadvantages of this approach are:

a. It requires a thoracotomy

b. It exposes the patient to electrical hazard if the terminal wires are not grounded properly

3. *Transthoracic or subxiphoid approach* may be used during advanced life support. This approach involves the insertion of a needle or an obturator transthoracically through the fourth intercostal space or below the xiphoid bone where the electrode is put in contact with the heart. The disadvantages may include:

a. Pneumothorax

b. Coronary artery damage

c. Cardiac tamponade

d. Ineffective pacing

e. Electrode displacement

f. Decreased cardiac output because of prolonged interruption of chest compression

PATIENT CARE DURING PREINSERTION, POST-INSERTION, OR TERMINATION PHASE OF TEMPORARY PACEMAKER THERAPY

The type of care provided to the patient with a temporary pacemaker depends on the phase involved.

1. *Preinsertion phase* involves preparing the patient and family physically and psychologically for the insertion of the pacemaker. One should:

a. Explain the procedure to the patient and/or family.

b. Obtain a signed permit for the procedure.

c. Start an I.V., if possible, in the patient's arm not being used for pacemaker insertion.

d. Sedate the patient as ordered.

e. Have a defibrillator and emergency drugs available at the bedside.

f. Monitor and record the patient's heart rhythm before and during the insertion.

g. Disconnect the patient from all unnecessary electrical equipment.

h. Ensure that all electrical equipment in use is grounded.

i. Assist the physician using sterile technique.

j. Provide reassurance to the patient and his/her family.

2. *Post-insertion phase* involves constant monitoring and assessment. One should:

a. Connect the distal electrode of the lead to the negative terminal and the proximal electrode to the positive terminal; this electrode position generally lowers thresholds.

b. Determine *pacing threshold* by turning the output setting toward 10 mA and observe the ECG monitor during adequate pacing. After adequate pacing is established, slowly turn down the output control until pacing is lost and then once again slowly turn the output control back toward 10 mA until pacing returns. This is the pacing threshold. Higher thresholds may be needed with epicardial pacing 2 or 3 days after electrode insertion because of fibrosis. The output dial may be turned two and a half times the threshold to accommodate for rising thresholds.[34]

c. Record on the nurse's notes and on the patient care plan:

(1) Date and time of insertion

(2) Name of the physician inserting the pacemaker

(3) Pacemaker settings (mA, rate, and pacing threshold)

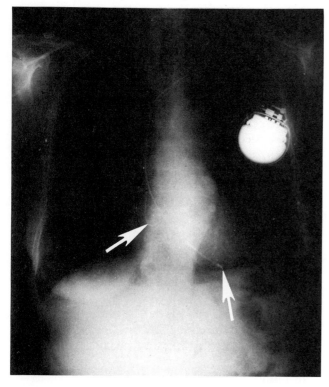

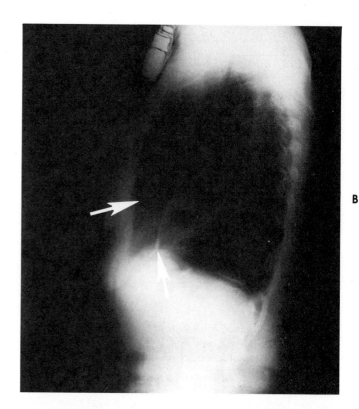

FIG. 7-21

Radiographs illustrating (**A**) anterior-posterior and (**B**) lateral view of implanted AV sequential pacemaker (Courtesy Dr. William Spencer).

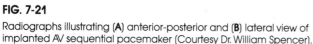

(4) Patient's response to the procedure and the type of rhythm that is being obtained

(5) Patient's rhythm on a ECG strip

d. Monitor cardiac output status by assessing vital signs, neurovital signs, urinary output and observing for signs of angina pectoris, heart failure, and ventricular irritability.

e. Obtain a portable chest radiograph to assess for lead placement and possible pneumothorax if the lead was inserted intravenously. Anteroposterior and lateral chest films should be obtained after insertion of a transvenous lead. With a right ventricular lead, the anteroposterior chest film should show the lead to the left of the sternum, and, in the lateral view, the lead should be directed anteriorly. If the right ventricular lead is pointing upward, it may be in the coronary sinus. Atrial J leads should point anteriorly (Figs. 7-21 and 7-22).

f. Obtain a 12-lead ECG.

g. Prevent infection and phlebitis by providing site care according to hospital policy and procedure. Document site care in the nurse's notes or as indicated by hospital policy and procedure.

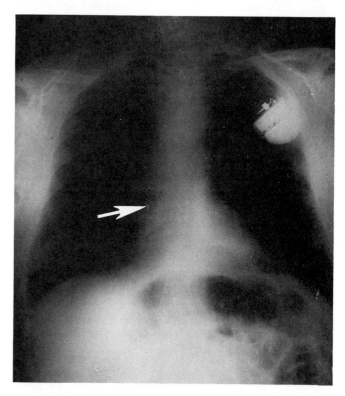

FIG. 7-22

Radiograph illustrating anterior-posterior view with implanted atrial electrode (Courtesy Dr. William Spencer).

h. Check and record the patient's temperature regularly for signs of infection and observe for erythema, edema, and drainage at the insertion site.

i. Observe and record the patient's heart rhythm and document:
   (1) Paced vs. nonpaced rhythms
   (2) Rhythm strips when the patient is symptomatic (e.g., when the patient has complaints of dizziness, weakness, diaphoresis, low blood pressure, or a slow or rapid pulse rate)

j. Prevent catheter displacement by securing the catheter with tape to the skin nearest the insertion site. An antimicrobial ointment may be applied at the insertion site, according to hospital policy and procedure. Apply a sterile dressing and secure with tape. If the pacemaker catheter is inserted via the basilic or cephalic vein, an ace bandage may be wrapped around the arm and the upper torso to help secure the catheter and battery source. An armboard attached to the arm will help provide immobilization.

k. Observe for bleeding at the lead insertion site.

l. Apply manual pressure to the insertion site initially. If bleeding occurs, apply manual pressure initially and then apply a pressure dressing.

m. Check for arterial pulses distal to a transvenously inserted lead and record their status in the nurse's notes.

n. Monitor for signs of interpericardial bleeding and cardiac tamponade (see p. 176).

o. Protect the patient from potential microshock by:
   (1) Insulating all exposed terminals of the pacemaker's electrodes in a rubber glove and securing with tape.
   (2) Following the guidelines of the user's manual for the specific pacemaker.
   (3) Wearing rubber gloves to prevent your body's static electricity from entering the patient through the lead.[40] The rubber gloves should be worn when connecting or disconnecting the pacemaker. Site care is performed under aseptic conditions and sterile gloves may be indicated according to hospital policy and procedure.
   (4) Avoiding use of an electrical bed. If an electrical bed is used, the bed should be checked for proper grounding and the electrical safety should be confirmed. If an electrical bed is malfunctioning, it should be unplugged and inspected by a biomedical engineer or another responsible individual. The patient should be moved to a safe bed.

   (5) Ensuring that all electrical equipment at the patient's bedside is safe for use by checking with the biomedical engineer or by checking for a current safety inspection sticker.
   (6) Using the least amount of electrical devices possible at the patient's bedside.
   (7) Avoiding touching the pacemaker or the terminals while touching an electrical device.

p. Reposition the patient if chest wall twitching or hiccoughs occur. These conditions usually occur because of phrenic nerve stimulation.

q. Use an extension cable so the pulse generator can be attached to an area that causes the patient the least amount of discomfort yet still provides some range of mobility. For example, the pulse generator may be taped to the headboard of the bed.

r. Record in the nurse's notes and on the nursing process record any changes made in the pacemaker setting and the reasons for these changes.

3. *Termination phase* occurs when the patient's conduction system has resumed or when a permanent pacemaker has been inserted. During this phase one should:
   a. Observe and record the patient's heart rhythm when a transvenous catheter is being removed by the physician. The patient may have dysrhythmias at that time.
   b. Apply pressure with a sterile pressure dressing at the insertion site following catheter removal.
   c. Return the pacemaker catheter and the pulse generator to the designated area.
   d. Observe the insertion site for bleeding and check for the pulse, sensation, and movement of the involved extremity. Document the findings.
   e. Record in the nurse's notes and on the nursing process record when the pacemaker is removed and the patient's rhythm and reaction to the removal of the temporary pacemaker.

Permanent pacemaker therapy

Permanent pacemaker therapy is a pacemaker system implanted within the body for long-term use. There are almost a half million people in the United States who have permanent pacemakers.[30] Permanent pacemakers have decreased mortality significantly in people with complete heart block. For instance, before the use of pacemakers, there was a mortality rate of 50% after 1 year and 90% after 5 years.[27] Currently 50% of those patients who received their permanent pacemaker before the age of 65 will survive for more than 10 years. Thirty percent will survive for longer than 10 years, regardless of the age category at the time of implant.[7] Presently 80% of the

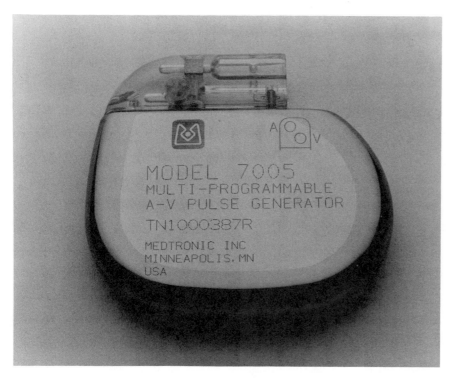

FIG. 7-23
Programmable pulse generator, Medtronic Symbios (Courtesy Medtronics).

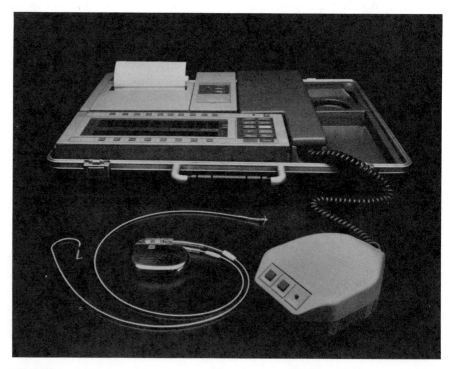

FIG. 7-24
Pulse generator with atrial and ventricular leads and programmer (Courtesy Medtronics).

implanted pacemakers are in patients 70 years old or older.[10,14]

COMPONENTS OF A PERMANENT PACEMAKER SYSTEM

1. Implantable pulse generators have progressed significantly over the years from when the first pacemaker was implanted in 1959 by Senning and Hunter.[17,36]
   a. Some of the earlier implantable pulse generators were *mercury zinc generators,* which were used until the early 1970s. The disadvantages of this type of power source are:
      (1) It is heavy
      (2) Its life span is only 2 to 2½ years
      (3) It cannot be hermetically sealed (i.e., airtight) to protect the generator from the body's fluids.
   b. *Nuclear-powered generators* became popular in the early 1970s. However, because of government regulations, this type of pacemaker is not economically feasible.
   c. *Rechargeable battery generators* depend on the patient or his/her family to maintain the battery charged. As a result, such generators have failed to gain popularity.
   d. Because of the disadvantages mentioned above, the *lithium pulse generator* is the most common type used today. Its lifespan is between 5 to 15 years with an average of 6.8 years.[4]
   e. There are *programmable pulse generators* (Fig. 7-23) that are capable of receiving coded radio frequency impulses from a transmitter outside the body (Fig. 7-24). Features that can be programmed are rate, pulse, pulse width, sensitivity, refractoriness, pulse amplitude, and pacing mode. For example, there is a special type of pulse generator used for tachycardias that the patient can activate when experiencing symptoms of the tachydysrhythmia. With this type, the patient simply puts the battery-operated transmitter over the pulse generator site and presses a button. This energizes the pulse generator stimulator, which sends out short bursts of asynchronous stimuli to terminate the dysrhythmia.
2. Permanent pacing electrodes are illustrated in Figs. 7-25 and 7-26. They can be unipolar or bipolar. The radiograph in Fig. 7-26, p. 166, shows an implanted permanent epicardial electrode.

INDICATIONS FOR A PERMANENT PACEMAKER

There are a number of indications for the use of a permanent pacemaker. They are:
1. *Complete heart block,* which is the most common reason for permanent implants[14]
2. *Sick sinus syndrome*[14]

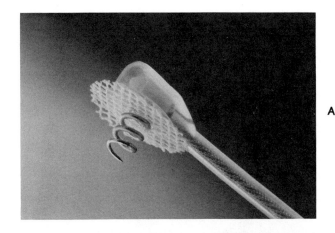

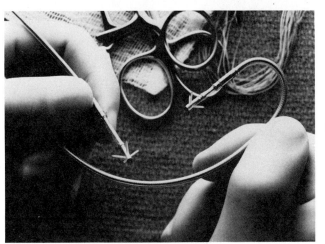

FIG. 7-25

A, Medtronic epicardial ventricular electrode (unipolar). **B,** Medtronic Target Tip leads: left is ventricular bipolar lead; right is atrial bipolar lead (Courtesy Medtronics).

3. *Mobitz type II second-degree AV block* distal to the bundle of His[11]
4. *Symptomatic tachydysrhythmias*[6,8,11] such as in Wolff-Parkinson-White syndrome, paroxysmal atrial tachycardia, and chronic atrial fibrillation with a slow ventricular response
5. *Hypersensitive carotid sinus syndrome*[37]
6. *Ventricular tachycardia,* which is not surgically correctable and is resistant to drug therapy[6,15]

VARIOUS APPROACHES TO THE INSERTION OF A PERMANENT PACEMAKER

1. *Transvenous approach* is the simplest and most commonly used method. Under local anesthesia, a small incision is made above the clavicle on either side of the

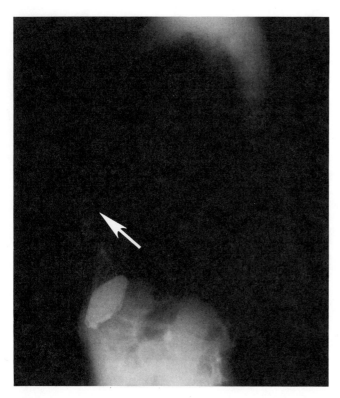

FIG. 7-26
Radiograph illustrating implanted permanent epicardial lead
(Courtesy Dr. William Spencer).

patient's neck. The catheter is threaded through the jugular vein or through an introducer into the subclavian vein and eventually lodged in the apex of the right ventricle.

2. *Transthoracic approach* may require a thoracotomy so the epicardial electrodes can be sutured into the myocardium. This invasive procedure is a disadvantage in treating the elderly and the critically ill since it requires general anesthesia.

3. *Transmediastinal approach* is a method by which electrodes are attached to the myocardium with the chest opened subcostally. (This type of epicardial electrode is illustrated in Fig. 7-26.) The permanent pulse generator can be implanted in a subcutaneous "tissue pocket" either below the clavicle or in a subcutaneous "tissue pocket" in the abdomen (usually above or below the waistline). (This approach is illustrated in Figs. 7-21, 7-22, and 7-26.)

PATIENT CARE DURING PREOPERATIVE OR POSTOPERATIVE PHASE OF PERMANENT PACEMAKER THERAPY

The type of care provided to the patient with a permanent pacemaker depends on phase involved.

1. The *preoperative phase* involves many of the same steps as discussed in care of the patient with a temporary pacemaker. However, this procedure requires more in-depth explanation since it is a permanent implant. In preparing a patient for permanent pacemaker implantation, one should:
   a. Educate the patient and family regarding a permanent pacemaker. Many pacemaker booklets are available through the American Heart Association and through the pacemaker companies. These may be used to supplement teaching done by the nursing staff. A model of a pacemaker may be used.
   b. Explain to the patient and family the follow-up available through pacemaker clinics. Knowledge adds reassurance and security.

2. *Postoperative care* involves the same steps as discussed in the care of a patient with a temporary pacemaker. In addition one should:
   a. Encourage deep breathing and coughing, especially if the patient received a general anesthetic or experienced a thoracotomy.
   b. Prevent catheter displacement, especially with transvenously inserted catheters, by limiting the patient's activity (usually for the first day).
   c. Prevent infection by applying sterile dressings over the operative site. Antibiotics may be prescribed and must be administered as ordered.
   d. Assess and document the patient's and family's response to the permanent pacemaker. Allow adequate time for discussion and questions.
   e. Provide information on the following at the patient's and family's level of understanding:
      (1) Normal heart function and conduction
      (2) Pacemaker function
      (3) The importance of counting the pulse for 1 full minute
      (4) Necessity of having periodic ECGs and follow-up with physician and/or pacemaker clinic
      (5) Recognition of the signs of pacemaker malfunction such as syncope, hiccoughs, dizziness, palpitations, chest pain, or congestive heart failure
      (6) Become certified in Basic Life Support

Special considerations with permanent pacemaker implantation

Some considerations should be taken into account when a pacemaker is implanted:

1. Electromagnetic interference[34] should be avoided. It can be caused by:
   a. External sources, such as:
      (1) Microwave ovens that are operating improperly
      (2) Electric razors if held over the pulse generator

or if used to shave under the arms when the generator is implanted below the clavicle

(3) High-powered transmitting equipment; short-wave citizen band (CB) radios are safe if operated under the rules and regulations of the Federal Communications Commission guidelines and regulations

(4) Transcutaneous electrical nerve stimulators (TENS); the TENS unit is most commonly used during the immediate post-operative phase for pain management and can cause pacing interference; a patient who is being treated with such a device should be monitored with an ECG to determine if interference occurs[21]

(5) Microwave and shortwave diathermy; this should be avoided around the area of the pulse generator as it will cause the metal casing to heat up and will cause damage to the components and tissue burns in the patient

(6) Electrocautery used for cutting and coagulation; this interference can be prevented by using a grounding pad and converting the pulse generator to an asynchronous mode until the surgery is completed

(7) Airport screening devices—metal detectors—may sound the alarm, however, pacemaker interference usually does not occur

b. Internal sources, such as myopotentials, can also cause pacemaker malfunction. A myopotential is the electrical current of muscle contraction that resembles a cardiac potential and can cause sensitive pulse generators to inhibit or trigger with that muscle activity. The risk of this occurring can be measured by isometric exercise.

2. When therapeutic diathermy is used, the unit should not be placed directly over a pulse generator since internal components of the generator may be damaged by the heat.

3. It may be necessary to convert a bipolar lead to a unipolar lead if one of the two wires of a bipolar lead is fractured and until a new lead is inserted or a permanent pacing system is instituted. Converting a bipolar system to an unipolar system is performed by connecting the intact wire to the negative terminal of the pacemaker. In order to have a complete circuit, an ECG electrode plate can be placed on the skin of the extremity nearest to the lead insertion point. A conductive paste or saline-soaked gauze should be applied under the electrode plate. The electrode plate should be secured with tape. The positive pacemaker terminal is then connected to the plate with an alligator clip wire. Using surgical or hypodermic needles instead of

the ECG plate can cause uncomfortable and annoying muscle contraction at the insertion site because of the small needle size and the high current density.[33]

4. When defibrillating or cardioverting a patient with a pacemaker, the paddles should be positioned 10 cm from the pulse generator.[26] A temporary pacemaker should be on hand[25] and the first two countershocks with defibrillation should be at 200 to 300 watt/sec.[23]

Pacing modalities of pulse generators

Many varieties of pacing modes can be identified.[9]

1. When pacemakers were first used, they were the ventricular fixed-rate variety, which fired an impulse at the set rate of the pulse generator. These were considered *asynchronous* pacemakers because they were not synchronized to the patient's intrinsic rate and could be competitive with the patient's rate.

2. Later a *demand* pacemaker was developed. This pulse generator was sensitive to the patient's intrinsic rate and fired an impulse only when the patient's intrinsic rate did not fire. This type was also called a *synchronous* pacemaker. Primarily these pacemakers were used for ventricular pacing and did not allow for atrial contraction.

3. Atrial contraction may be absent in some dysrhythmias, such as atrial fibrillation so that, subsequently, cardiac output is decreased. Because of the loss of the atrial contraction with ventricular pacing, *atrial pacing* became popular in an attempt to improve cardiac output by inducing atrial contraction and increasing ventricular filling. Atrial pacing is accomplished by having a pacing electrode in the atria producing atrial depolarization. Ultimately, the impulse travels to the ventricle causing ventricular depolarization. With atrial pacing, normal AV conduction has to exist; however, this does not ensure synchronization of atrial and ventricular activity.

4. With technological advancement, pacemakers became more complex, yet more specific and refined. In order to simplify their characteristics, the Inter-Society Commission for Heart Disease (ICHD) accepted a three-letter identification pacemaker code that was developed by Parsonnet, Furman, and Smyth.[28] Recently two more letters were added to this code to include programmable and special tachydysrhythmia functions.[29] The *five-letter identification pacemaker code* can be seen in Table 7-2, p. 168. The first letter of the code designates the chamber(s) paced, the second letter designates the chamber(s) sensed, the third letter designates the mode of response(s), the fourth letter designates the programmable functions, and the last letter designates the special tachydysrhythmic func-

TABLE 7-2. Five-letter identification pacemaker code (ICHD)

First letter (Chamber paced)	Second letter (Chamber sensed)	Third letter (Mode of response)	Fourth letter (Programmability)	Fifth letter (Tachydysrhythmia functions)
V = ventricular A = atrium D = atrium and ventricle 0 = none	V = ventricular A = atrium D = atrium and ventricle	I = inhibited T = triggered D = atrial triggered and ventricular inhibited R = reverse 0 = none	P = programmable rate and/or output M = multiprogrammability 0 = none	B = burst N = normal rate C = competition S = scanning E = external

tions. However, this coding system is not used or discussed in this text.

Because the purpose of this module is to explain basic pacemaker functions only, a brief description of the various pacing modalities of the first three letters is given in Table 7-3.

5. Atrioventricular pacing (AV sequential) is the preferred type of pacing. The physiological benefits of AV sequential pacing[18] are increased ventricular filling, which produces an increase in stroke volume,[41] and increased myocardial stretch, which produces a more forceful contraction.[13,24] There is more effective closure of the AV valves so that regurgitation is reduced with early ventricular systole and this ultimately facilitates venous return.[19,24,31] The two most common types of AV pacing are:

   a. DVI, which paces the atria and ventricles (dual-chamber pacing). The ventricles are sensed and there is an inhibitory function.

   b. DDD, which produces dual-chamber pacing and sensing as well as dual responses. This type of pacing functions very similarly to the normal conduction system. It responds to exercise and other physiologic demands, synchronizing the ventricular rate with increasing atrial rates and thus increasing cardiac output as needed.

Detailed explanation of these various pacing modalities and the ECG interpretations can be attained by reading further references.[2,5,8,22]

Considerations in analyzing the electrocardiogram (ECG) for normal pacemaker function

There are several considerations that need to be taken into account in analyzing the ECG for normal pacemaker function:

1. The ECG lead being monitored
2. A determination of whether the pacemaker is temporary or permanent
3. The type of pacing modality being used
4. Whether the leads are bipolar or unipolar
5. Which chamber(s) are being sensed and/or paced
6. The patient's clinical presentation with regard to the cardiac output

Normal pacing electrocardiograms involve the following considerations.

EVALUATION OF A PACING SPIKE

The pacing spike is also termed a *pacing artifact* and is a sharp deflection usually occurring before the cardiac chamber's depolarization (Fig. 7-27).

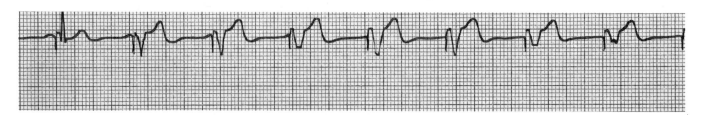

FIG. 7-27   Lead II

In first complex there is a pacer spike that has fused with patient's intrinsic rhythm. Succeeding complexes have a pacer spike preceding ventricular-paced complex.

TABLE 7-3. Summary of pacing modalities[44]

ICHD Chamber paced	Chamber sensed	Mode of response	Description	Indications	Contraindications	Advantages	Disadvantages
A	0	0	Atrial asynchronous; atrial fixed rate	No longer used			
V	0	0	Ventricular asynchronous, ventricular fixed rate	No longer used			
A	A	I	Atrial paced, sensed, and inhibited; P waves inhibited	SSS with normal AV conduction	Atrial in excitability; high atrial threshhold; abnormal AV conduction	Requires only one lead; simplest system providing properly timed sequential AV conduction	If AV block develops, the ventricle will not be paced
V	V	I	Ventricular paced, sensed, and inhibited; R-wave inhibited; demand standby	SSS without retrograde AV conduction	None	Historical inertia; simple	Lacks AV synchronal activity
V	V	T	Ventricular paced, sensed, and triggered; R wave synchronous	SSS with no hemodynamic benefit of atrial pacing; chronic atrial fibrillation or flutter with AV block and a slow ventricular rate	Hemodynamic insufficiency because of loss of AV synchrony	Prevents competitive pacing	Does not alter rate in response to physiological demands
D	0	0	Atrial and ventricular pacing, no sensing function	No longer used			
V	A	T	Atrial synchronous, P-wave synchronous	Normal sinus node functions with required AV conduction	Inappropriate atrial tachycardia or bradycardia; retrograde atrial activation following ventricular stimulation or PVCs	Maintains atrial transport and normal sinus control of ventricular rate when atrial rate is within tracking limits of pacemaker	Since it does not pace the atria, it does not provide synchronous contractions during atrial bradycardia; requires no leads
D	D	D	Atrial and ventricular paced, atrial and ventricular sensed; P and R wave inhibited; fully automatic	Normal sinus rhythm or atrial bradydysrhythmias with or without impaired AV conduction	Retrogrode atrial activation following ventricular stimulation or PVCs Atrial fibrillation/flutter Frequent atrial tachycardias	Maintains sequential AV contraction and sinus control of ventricular rate during sinus bradycardia	Requires two leads
D	V	I	AV sequential demand or bifocal Atrial and ventricular paced, ventricular sensed and response inhibited	Atrial bradydysrhythmias with or without impaired AV conduction and a decreased cardiac output Congestive heart failure ventricular standstill Re-entrant tachydysrhythmia[5, 42]	Extended periods of atrial fibrillation flutter because the electrode senses this atrial activity and pacemaker does not fire	Provides sequential AV contraction during sinus bradycardia. Decreases regurgitation of blood with ventricular systole and increases venous return	Does not alter rate in response to physiological demands Does not maintain AV synchronous contractions during periods of normal sinus Competitive atrial pacing during normal sinus rhythm Requires two leads

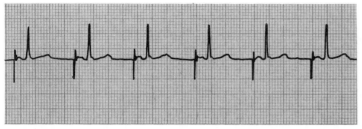

FIG. 7-28

Lead I

The strip illustrates atrial pacing with pacer spike preceding P wave. QRS is within normal limits and is patient's own intrinsic ventricular depolarization.

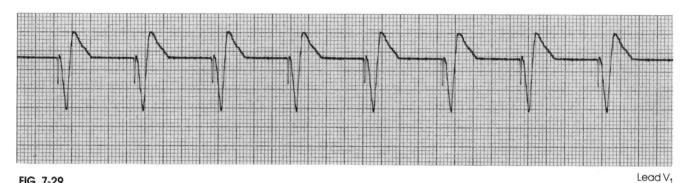

FIG. 7-29

Lead V₁

Ventricular pacing. Pacer spike precedes QRS, and, with capturing QRS becomes widened.

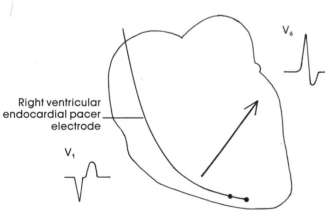

Right ventricular endocardial pacer electrode

V₆

V₁

FIG. 7-30

Left bundle branch block (LBBB) configuration occurs when pacing lead paces from the right ventricle.

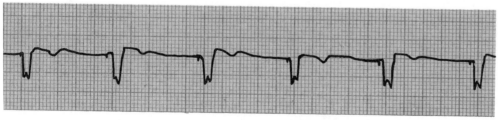

Lead V₁

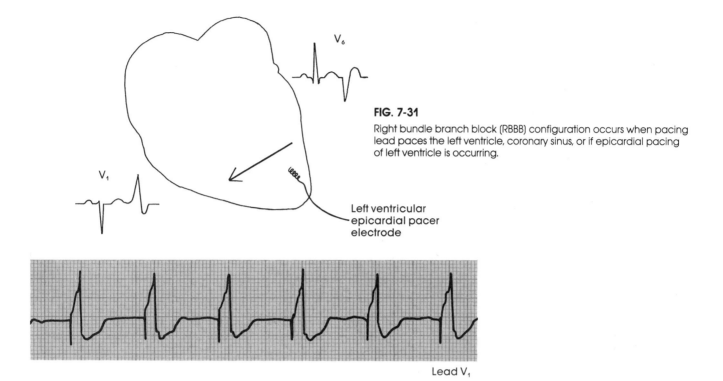

FIG. 7-31

Right bundle branch block (RBBB) configuration occurs when pacing lead paces the left ventricle, coronary sinus, or if epicardial pacing of left ventricle is occurring.

Lead V_1

1. The *size* of the pacing spikes may be small or large, depending on the type of pacer lead in place. A bipolar lead will illicit small spikes on the ECG because the energy travels only between the positive and the negative poles at the tip of the catheter (see Fig. 7-17). A unipolar lead will demonstrate large spikes on the ECG because there is more energy expended and the energy travels a greater distance as compared with a bipolar lead (see Fig. 7-16). With a unipolar lead, the energy travels from the generator to the electrode tip and back to the generator.

2. The pacing spike *position* within the ECG should be considered and usually precedes the chamber it paces. In atrial pacing, the pacing spike precedes the P wave. The best lead to detect the P wave activity is in V_1. The QRS complex will be normal after an atrially paced P wave, provided there is not existing bundle branch block (Fig. 7-28).

3. With ventricular pacing, the pacing artifact precedes the QRS, and the QRS becomes widened (Fig. 7-29).

   a. If a right ventricular endocardial lead is pacing the right ventricle, then a left bundle branch block (LBBB) configuration will appear because the right ventricle is the first chamber to be depolarized and the impulse travels through the septum and ultimately the left ventricle. Deep S waves appear in

leads II, III, V_1, and V_3 with these types of paced complexes (Fig. 7-30).

   b. A right bundle branch block (RBBB) configuration may be seen with epicardial pacing of the left ventricle, when the coronary sinus is being paced or when a right ventricular endocardial lead has perforated the septum and is pacing the left ventricle (Fig. 7-31). If the latter has occurred, a physician should be notified immediately. There are some types of pacemakers in which a pacing artifact occurs within the QRS complex, demonstrating the pacemaker's sensing ability. This pacemaker mode will not be discussed in this module.

EVALUATION OF THE PACEMAKER'S ABILITY TO SENSE, FIRE, AND CAPTURE PROPERLY

The pacemaker must be able to *sense* the patient's intrinsic *rhythm, fire* an impulse when needed, and cause myocardial depolarization and a *captured complex*.

1. A pacemaker's *sensing* ability allows it to depict the patient's intrinsic rhythm and, in the case of a delay or absence of this intrinsic rhythm, relay the message to the pulse generator so an electrical stimulus can occur. If a patient's intrinsic rhythm is adequate, the pacemaker system will sense this and in this case inhibit the artificial stimulus.

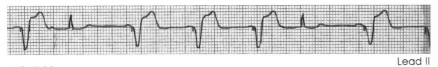

Lead II

FIG. 7-32

First two complexes are paced rhythms. There is a pacer spike
before ventricular depolarization. Third and seventh complexes are
patient's own intrinsic complexes. Pacemaker senses these complexes and does not fire a stimulus. However, there is a significant
delay after third and seventh complexes that the pacemaker senses
and it fires a stimulus to cause ventricular myocardial depolarization.

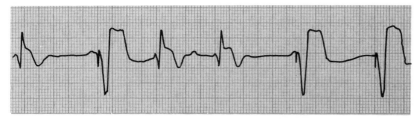

Lead II

FIG. 7-33

VVI pacing. Ventricle is paced and sensed and pacemaker is
inhibited by a ventricular complex. Second, fifth, and sixth complexes
are paced. First, third, and fourth complexes are patient's own
intrinsic complexes.

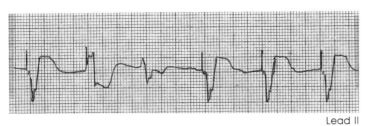

Lead II

FIG. 7-34

Fusion complex is seen in second complex. Paced complexes are
seen in first, fourth, fifth, and sixth complexes. Patient's own intrinsic
complex is seen in third complex. Fusion complex is combination of
patient's own intrinsic complex with a paced complex.

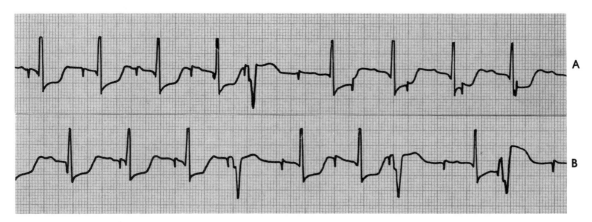

A

B

FIG. 7-35

VVO pacing. Ventricle is paced and there is no sensing. Pacer fires
continuously and is not sensitive to patient's own intrinsic rhythm.

2. A pacemaker's *firing* ability allows the pulse generator to initiate an adequate electrical stimulus to cause myocardial depolarization.

3. *Capturing* allows the delivered electrical stimulus to cause myocardial depolarization. An example of a properly functioning pacemaker is seen in Fig. 7-32.

EVALUATION OF THE PACEMAKER'S PACING MODALITY

Several modalities were discussed earlier. The type of modality will determine the ECG expectations. For example:

1. VVI pacing (ventricular paced, ventricular sensed, inhibited by ventricular complex) is commonly used. This type of pacemaker has a preset rate and a firing and sensing circuit. The sensing circuit detects a patient's own ventricular rhythm and inhibits (or blocks) a pacing stimulus during this rhythm. When a patient's rate slows below the preset pacing rate, the pacemaker then fires (Fig. 7-33).

   This is considered a *synchronous* or *demand* pacemaker because it senses the patient's own rhythm and fires only when necessary, thereby eliminating competition between a pacing rhythm and a patient's own rhythm. However, a patient's own complex may occur too late to prevent the pacemaker from firing. This will produce a *fusion complex*. The complex is a combination of a paced rhythm and the patient's own rhythm (Fig. 7-34).

2. VOO pacing (ventricular paced, no sensing, and no response) is considered to be *asynchronous* or a *fixed-rate pacemaker*. It continuously discharges an electrical stimulus regardless of the patient's spontaneous cardiac rate or rhythm. If a patient has no ventricular rhythm, this type of pacemaker may be indicated (Fig. 7-35).

The disadvantage of this type of pacing occurs if a patient has a periodic ventricular rhythm that occurs intermittently or if the patient's rhythm resumes. The pacemaker can fire during the vulnerable period of the patient's own cycle and cause ventricular tachycardia or fibrillation. This is why this modality is no longer used.

3. The DVI (dual chamber–paced, ventricular sensed, and response inhibited) pacemaker can be a temporary or permanent pacemaker. It protects the patient from heart block. The DVI has the ability to attain two modes: uncommitted or committed.

   a. In the *uncommitted* mode, the ventricular pacing ability is optional and the pacemaker only fires if the patient's PR interval is longer than the atrioventricular (AV) delay. This delay is programmed into the pulse generator. In the uncommitted mode, there may be one, two, or no pacing spikes (Fig. 7-36).

   b. In the *committed* mode, the ventricular pacemaker fires regardless whether the patient's PR interval is shorter or longer than the pacer's AV delay (Fig. 7-37, p. 174).

      In the *committed* mode there will be either two pacing spikes or none. This is an "all or none effect"; either the maximum number of pacing spikes is presented or none are.

Considerations in analyzing electrocardiograms (ECGs) for abnormal pacemaker function

Analyzing ECGs for abnormal pacemaker functions necessitates knowing the ECG lead being monitored as well as the type of pacing system being used. The various types of pacemaker malfunctions, their causes, diagnosis and solutions are discussed.

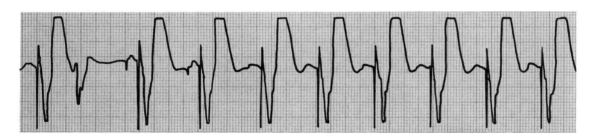

FIG. 7-36

Uncommitted DVI pacing. First and fifth through the tenth complexes have one spike. Atrial mode is inhibited secondary to patient's own intrinsic P waves. Only ventricular mode is activated with these complexes. Second complex is patient's own intrinsic activity, thereby inhibiting both atrial-ventricular modes so no pacer spikes are demonstrated. In third and fourth complexes, there are two spikes in each complex because both atrial-ventricular modes were activated.

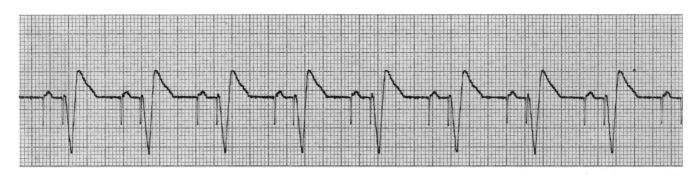

FIG. 7-37   Lead II

Committed DVI pacing. Paced atrial activity is *always* followed by a
ventricular spike. Therefore, there will either be no pacing spikes or
two pacing spikes. Strip demonstrates two spikes per complex.

Abnormal pacemaker function involves the following considerations:

PACEMAKER NOT SENSING PROPERLY

With an improper sensing malfunction, the pacemaker fires without detecting (sensing) the patient's intrinsic rhythm (Fig. 7-38). If it is a ventricular-placed electrode, it can cause competitive complexes to fall during the vulnerable period of the cardiac cycle and cause tachydysrhythmias that can be life-threatening. If it is an atrial-placed electrode, then atrial dysrhythmias may occur.

1. Causes for nonsensing are:
   a. Lead dislodgment or inappropriate placement
   b. Fibrosis of the myocardium where the electrode is implanted
   c. Myocardial infarction (MI)
   d. Myocardial depressant drugs
   e. Electrolyte disturbances
   f. Inappropriate programming of amplifier sensitivity
   g. Lengthened refractory periods, causing pacemaker insensitivity to patient's intrinsic rhythm or to extrasystoles
   h. AOO and VOO pacing modalities that do not have sensing abilities
   i. Lead fracture or insulation defect
   j. Connector defect
   k. Pulse generator failure
   l. After-potential sensing[34]
2. The diagnosis of a nonsensing pacemaker is suggested when there are paced complexes despite the patient's intrinsic rhythm. However, misdiagnosing nonsensing can occur when:
   a. There are fusion beats (Fig. 7-39). This can occur when the pacemaker stimulus initiates its impulse at the same time the patient's own conduction system initiates an impulse, therefore, causing a "fusing"

with each other in the ventricles. This produces a complex lower in voltage than the voltage of the normal pacemaker complex.
   b. The pacemaker reverts to the asynchronous mode because of electromagnetic interference (EMI) (Fig. 7-40). EMI can be ruled out as a cause of nonsensing if a 12-lead ECG shows no signs of electrical interference.
   c. With certain AV sequential (DVI-committed) pacemakers, closely coupled intracardiac signals occurring within the pacemaker's refractory period may cause nonsensing.
3. The action to take when loss of sensing occurs involves:
   a. Ensuring the pulse generator's sensitivity setting is at its maximum
   b. Repositioning the patient to the left lateral recumbent position or a position that may institute proper sensing once again
   c. Increasing the pacing rate to override the intrinsic rhythm
   d. Turning off the pacemaker if the patient can tolerate it
   e. Suppressing the PVCs with ordered antidysrhythmic drugs
   f. Decreasing the pacemaker's output if tolerated; for example, the less current used, the less danger of causing a dysrhythmia
   g. Converting electrode to unipolar (if bipolar) because a unipolar lead is more sensitive than a bipolar one
   h. Being prepared for loss of capture
   i. Assessing patient for electrolyte imbalances, ischemia, hypoxia, and/or digoxin toxicity since these may potentiate the loss of sensing

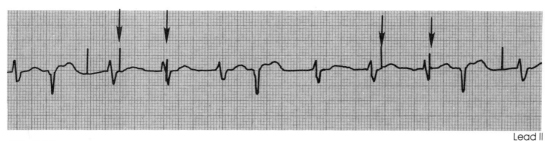

FIG. 7-38
Non-sensing pacemaker. Second, third, fourth, and fifth pacing spikes are not sensing patient's own electrical activity that immediately precedes these spikes. Pacemaker does not sense this activity and continues to fire.

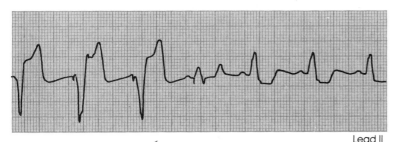

FIG. 7-39
Fusion complex. Fourth complex is combination of paced complex with patient's own intrinsic complex.

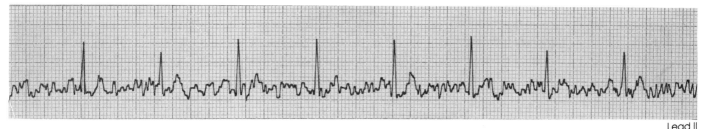

FIG. 7-40
ECG tracing, illustrating electromagnetic interference (EMI).

FAILURE TO PACE[34]

With this malfunction, the pacemaker system fails either to deliver an adequate stimulus (Fig. 7-41, p. 176) or to capture adequately (Fig. 7-42, p. 176).

1. The causes for inadequate pacing are:
   a. Lead displacement
   b. Loose or broken connections
   c. Lead fractures
   d. Inadequate threshold
   e. Inhibition of the pulse generator
   f. Battery exhaustion
2. Diagnosing a pulse generator's failure to pace depends on determining such causes as:

a. Lead displacement, which may be detected by:
   (1) A 12-lead ECG, which illustrates intermittent capture or axis shifts from superior to inferior axis.
   (2) Paced P waves with an initially placed ventricular lead, which demonstrates migration of the lead to the atrium. If AV conduction is absent, a ventricular escape rhythm or asytole may occur. If an initially placed atrial lead is displaced, there may be loss of P waves and QRS complexes.
   (3) Chest radiographs.

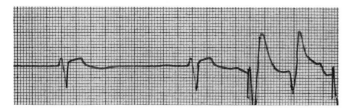

FIG. 7-41   Lead II

Failure to pace. There is a long pause preceding and succeeding
first complex in which the pacemaker should have fired a complex
but did not. After second complex, there is a pause; however, the
pacemaker does fire a stimulus and produces an appropriately
paced complex (also seen in fifth complex).

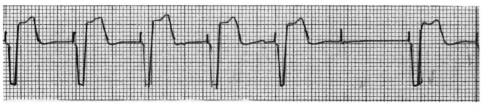

FIG. 7-42   Lead II

Failure to capture. First five complexes have a pacer stimulus
preceding ventricular complex, illustrating appropriate capturing.
Spike after the fifth complex does not cause ventricular depolarization, and a ventricular complex is absent because of failure to
capture.

(4) Chest wall or diaphragmatic pacing, which
occurs if the electrode perforates the myocardium, causing muscle twitching in the chest or
diaphragmatic area at the rate set on the
pacemaker. The patient may complain of chest
discomfort or hiccoughs.

(5) Pericardial rub, dull chest pain, and signs of
cardiac tamponade, which will be indicated on
the ECG by a positive R wave and loss of the
elevated ST segment. An intracardiac electro-
gram from a distal electrode may occur because
of electrode perforation into the pericardial sac.
Signs of cardia tamponade are:
(a) Elevated venous pressures (central venous
and pulmonary capillary wedge)
(b) Rising jugular venous distension
(c) Positive Kussmaul's sign
(d) Fall in the arterial blood pressure
(e) Sinus tachycardia
(f) Pulsus paradoxus
(g) Distant heart sounds
(h) Low voltage ECG tracing
(i) Signs and symptoms of decreased cardiac
output

b. Loose or broken connections, which are the most
common cause of failure to pace. There may be
intermittent pacer spikes noted, especially with
manipulation of an external pacing system. These
may be prevented by routine checks of the terminals
and connections.

c. Lead fracture, which will be demonstrated on the
ECG with continuous or interminnent loss of pacer
spikes. A chest radiograph or an intracavitary or
epicardial ECG recording may diagnose a lead
fracture. If the fractured lead is a bipolar lead, it can
be converted to a unipolar one.

d. Inadequate threshold; a higher than normal threshold may be needed to pace the myocardial tissue for
one of the following reasons:
(1) The electrode may be in contact with fibrosed,
ischemic, or infarcted myocardium.
(2) It may be the first sign of lead displacement
and may be diagnosed by a lack of pacing.
(3) Temporary epicardial wires require higher
thresholds as compared to endocardial leads
and may rise beyond the pulse generator's
capability after 7 to 10 days. Scar tissue development around the suture and epicardial

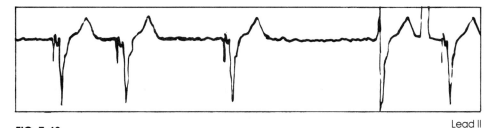

Lead II

FIG. 7-43

Oversensing. This is demonstrated in the strips when there are pacing pauses without causes (Courtesy Intermedics, Inc.).

wire insertion sites may be the explanation for this occurrence.[43]

e. Inhibition of the pulse generator, which causes failure to pace. Examples of factors causing inhibition of the pulse generator are:
   (1) Oscillating magnetic fields
   (2) Sixty-cycle interference from electrical equipment
   (3) Electrocautery
   (4) A ventricular endocardial lead displaced in the atrium or in the coronary sinus in which it senses the P waves
   (5) DVI pacing, when the endotracheal atrial electrode has migrated to the ventricle and the ventricular electrode senses the electrical activity of the atrial electrode, thereby inhibiting ventricular pacing
   (6) PVCs
   (7) Oversensing

f. Battery exhaustion, which rarely occurs with the temporary units, but should be checked for routinely. Signs of battery exhaustion may initially be demonstrated by intermittent pacing followed by the complete absence of pacing spikes.

3. Actions which may be taken if a pacemaker system is not pacing adequately include:
   a. Repositioning the patient or having the physician reposition the electrode
   b. Checking and securing all connections of the pacemaker system
   c. Converting a bipolar lead into a unipolar lead if a fractured bipolar lead is the cause
   d. Increasing threshold as needed
   e. Removing factors causing the pacemaker to be inhibited
   f. Administering ordered drugs to suppress PVCs
   g. Turning the pacemaker to the asynchronous mode if electrocautery is necessary
   h. Replacing the battery

i. Checking actions to take under "oversensing" in the section that follows

A more extensive discussion of pacemaker-induced dysrhythmias is given in various references.[20,34]

OVERSENSING

This occurs when the pacemaker is sensing other electrical intracardiac or extracardiac activity:
1. One cause for oversensing is that the pacemaker's sensitivity is too high and is detecting:
   a. The magnitude of P or T waves and after-potentials or myopotentials
   b. Electromagnetic interference
2. Oversensing is diagnosed by:
   a. Intermittent pauses without causes and no pacing (Fig. 7-43).
   b. The pacemaker rate falling below the set rate of control.[1,3]
3. Actions to be taken when oversensing occurs are to:
   a. Decrease the sensitivity until the pauses cease
   b. Place the permanent pacemaker in an asynchronous mode by applying a magnet over the pulse generator. Then turn off the sensitivity[34] if it is a temporary external pacemaker

RUNAWAY PACEMAKER

This occurs when there is a failure within the circuitry of the pulse generator:
1. The cause is pulse generator malfunction
2. A runaway pacemaker is diagnosed when there is a rapidly paced rate, usually in the upper rate limit of the pulse generator, despite the setting on the rate control (Fig. 7-44, p. 178)
3. The action to be taken with a runaway pacemaker is to replace the pulse generator

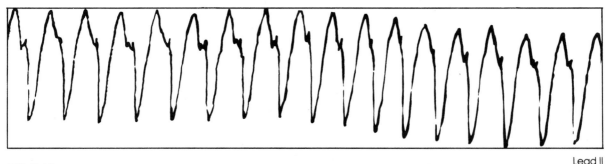

Lead II

FIG. 7-44

Runaway pacemaker. Tiny pacing spikes are seen within the ventricular tachycardia (Courtesy Intermedics, Inc.).

REFERENCES

1. Barold, S., and Gaidula J.: Evaluation of normal and abnormal sensing functions of demand pacemakers, Am. J. Cardiol, **28**:201, 1971.
2. Barold, S.S. et al.: Characterization of pacemaker-induced arrhythmias due to normal functioning AV demand (DVI) pulse generators, PACE **3**:712, 1980.
3. Berman, N.: T-wave sensing with a programmable pacemaker, PACE **3**:657, 1980.
4. Bilitch, M., et al.: Performance of cardiac pacemaker pulse generators, PACE **4**(4):479, 1981.
5. Bognalo, D.: Practical approach to physiologic cardiac pacing, Tarpon Springs, 1983, Tampa Tracings.
6. Citron, P. and Duffin, E.: Implantable pacemakers for management of tachyarrhythmias, Herz **4**(3):269, 1979.
7. Conover, M.B.: Understanding electrocardiography: arrhythmias and the 12-lead ECG, ed. 4, St. Louis, 1984, The C.V. Mosby Co.
8. Cooper, T., et al.: Overdrive pacing for supraventricular tachyarrhythmia: review of theoretical implications and therapeutic techniques, PACE **1**(2):196, 1978.
9. Duffin, E.G. and Zipes, D.P.: Artificial cardiac pacemaker. In Andreoli, K.G., et al., editors: Comprehensive cardiac care: a textbook for nurses, physicians, and other health care practitioners, ed. 5, St. Louis, 1983, The C.V. Mosby Co.
10. Elmquist, R., and Senning, A.: An implantable pacemaker for the heart, Proceedings of the Second International Conference Medical Electrical Engineering, London, Iliffe and Sons, Ltd., 1959.
11. Furman, S.: Cardiac pacing and pacemakers: I. Indications for pacing bradyarrhythmias, Am. Heart J. **93**(4):523, 1977.
12. Furman, S., Hurzeler, P., and Mehra, R.: Cardiac pacing and pacemakers: IV. Threshold of cardiac stimulation, Am. Heart J. **93**(1):118, 1977.
13. Gilmore, J. et al.: Synchronicity of ventricular contraction: observations comparing hemodynamic effects of ventricular and atrial pacing, Brit. Heart J. **25**:299, 1963.
14. Goldman, B.S., and Parsonnet, V.: World survey on cardiac pacing, PACE **2**(5):W1, 1979.
15. Hartzler, G.: Treatment of recurrent ventricular tachycardia by patient-activated radiofrequency ventricular stimulation, Mayo Clin. Proc. **54**:75, 1979.
16. Hindman, M.C., et al.: The clinical significance of bundle branch block complicating acute myocardial infarction: II. Indications for temporary and permanent pacemaker therapy, Circulation **58**:689, 1978.
17. Hunter, S.W., et al.: A bipolar myocardial electrode for complete heart block, Lancet **79**:506, 1959.
18. Klein, L.,: Temporary AV sequential pacing, Crit. Care Nurse **36**:36, 1983.
19. Little, R.C.: Effect of atrial systole on ventricular pressure of AV valves, Am. J. Physiol. **166**:289, 1951.
20. Mandel, W. J.: Pacemaker-induced arrhythmias. In Mandel, W.J., editor: Cardiac arrhythmias: their mechanisms, diagnosis, and management, Philadelphia and Toronto, 1980, J.B. Lippincott Co.
21. Mannheimer, J., and Lampe, S.: Clinical transcutaneous electrical nerve stimulation, Philadelphia, 1982, F.A. Davis Co.
22. Maytin, O. et al.: Pacemaker-induced arrhythmias. In Mandel, W.J., editor: Cardiac arrhythmias: their mechanisms, diagnosis, and management, Philadelphia and Toronto, 1980, J.B. Lippincott Co.
23. McIntyre, K.M., and Lewis, A.J., editors: Textbook of advanced cardiac life support, Dallas, 1981, American Heart Association, Section VIII, p.4.
24. Medtronics, Inc.: Atrial and AV pacing: an overview, 1979.
25. Owen, P.M.: The effects of external defibrillation on permanent pacemakers, Heart Lung **12**:274, 1983.
26. Owen, P.M.: Defibrillating pacemaker patients, Am. J. Nurs. **84**:1129, 1984.
27. Parsonnet, V.: Permanent pacing of the heart: 1952 to 1976, Am. J. Cardiol. **39**:250, 1977.
28. Parsonnet, V., et al.: Implantable cardiac pacemakers: status report and resource guideline, Circulation **50**:A-21, 1974.
29. Parsonnet, V., et al.: A revised code for pacemaker identification, PACE **4**(4):400, 1981.

30. Parsonnet, V., et al.: Dual-chamber pacing for cardiac arrhythmias: controversies in cloning the conduction system, Tex. Heart Instit. J. **11**:208, 1984.

31. Perry, M.,: Current AV sequential pacing, Paper presented at Midlands Area AACN Conference, Columbia, S.C., March, 1982.

32. Principles of pacing: Vol. 1. In Troubleshooting pacing problems, St. Paul, 1980, Cardiac Pacemakers, Inc.

33. Proctor, D., et al.: Temporary cardiac pacing: causes, recognition, and management of failure to pace, Nurse Clin. North Am. **13**:409, 1978.

34. Sager, D.P.: The person requiring cardiac pacing. In Guzzetta, C., and Dossey, B.M., editors,: Cardiovascular nursing: bodymind tapestry, St. Louis, 1984, The C.V. Mosby Co.

35. Scheinman, M., et al.: Electrophysiologic testing for patients with sinus node dysfunction, J. Electrocardiol. **12**(2):211, 1979.

36. Senning, A.: Discussion of Stephenson, S.E., Jr.; Edwards, W.H.; Jolly, P.C.; and Scott, W.H., Jr.: Physiologic P-wave cardiac stimulator, J. Thorac. Cardiovasc. Surg. **38**:369, 1959.

37. Sutton, R., et al.: Physiological cardiac pacing, PACE **3**(2):207, 1980.

38. Thalen, H.J.T.: Electrode design and new developments: Boston colloquium on cardiac pacing, 1951-53. In Harthorne, J.W., and Thalen, H.J.T. editors, The Hague, Netherlands, 1977, Martinis Nijhoff Medical Division.

39. Waldo, A., et al.: Temporary cardiac pacing: applications and techniques in the treatment of cardiac arrhythmias, Prog. Cardiovasc. Dis. **23**(6):451, 1981.

40. Whalen, R., and Starmer, C.: Electric shock hazards in clinical cardiology, Mod. Con. Cardiovasc. Dis. **26**:7, 1967.

41. Wirtzfeld, A., et al.: Atrial and ventricular pacing in patients with the sick sinus syndrome (Abstract), The Sixth World Symposium on Cardiac Pacing, Montreal, 1979.

42. Yashar, J., et al.: Atrioventricular sequential pacemakers: indications, complications, and long-term follow-up, Ann. Thorac. Surg. **29**(1):91, 1980.

43. Young, D.: Pacemaker implant in children and adolescents, Impulse **10**:3, 1978.

44. Zipes, D.P. and Duffin, E.O.: Cardiac pacemakers. In Brunwald, E., editor: Heart disease: a textbook of cardiovascular medicine, Part II, Philadelphia, 1984, W.B. Saunders Co.

SUGGESTED LEARNING ACTIVITIES AND EXPERIENCES

A. Interpret ECG strips of patients with pacemakers in the coronary care unit

B. Visit a coronary care unit or a pacemaker clinic to become more familiar with the various pacing modalities

C. Observe the insertion and termination of temporary pacemaker therapy and the insertion of a permanent pacemaker

POSTTEST (Answers on p. 183)

Directions: Circle one answer to each question unless otherwise indicated.

A. The "funny-looking" beat delineated by the arrow in Fig. 7-45 is a:
1. PVC (premature ventricular complex)
2. PAC (premature atrial complex)
3. Nonsensing complex
4. Fusion complex

B. Indications for temporary pacemaker therapy include which of the following? (Circle all that apply.)
1. Atrioventricular blocks
2. Malfunctioning permanent pacemaker
3. Dysrhythmias unresponsive to medical therapy
4. Chronic atrial fibrillation

C. If a temporary pacemaker is not functioning properly and the patient becomes unconscious, you should:
1. Immediately notify the physician, set up for a new pacemaker to be inserted, and wait until the physician arrives
2. Initiate CPR

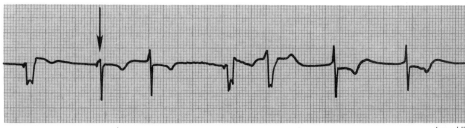

FIG. 7-45

Lead II

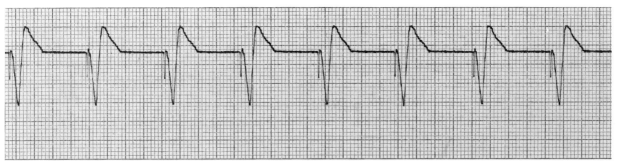

FIG. 7-46

Lead II

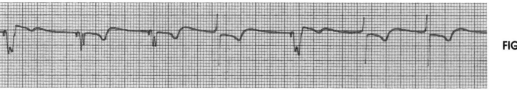

FIG. 7-47

Lead II

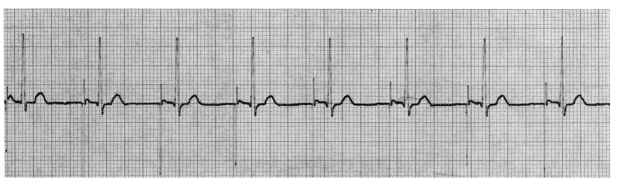

FIG. 7-48

Lead II

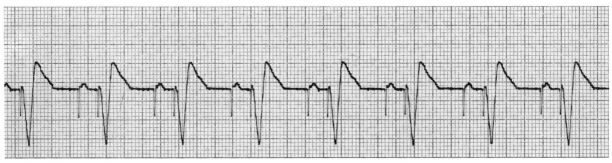

FIG. 7-49

Lead II

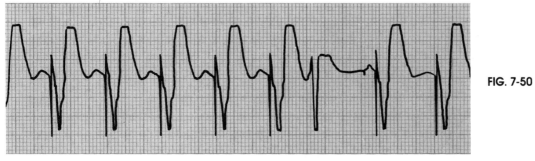

FIG. 7-50

Lead II

3. Administer propranolol to increase the patient's heart rate
4. Turn up the mA

D. The following are complications that may arise with pacemaker insertion (circle all that apply):
   1. Myocardial perforation and tamponade
   2. Local infection and/or septicemia
   3. Thrombosis and/or embolization
   4. Electrocution and/or cardiac arrest
   5. Continuous pacing

E. The strip in Fig. 7-46 is an example of:
   1. A patient's own rhythm with a widened QRS (bundle branch block)
   2. A pacer-induced rhythm
   3. A noncapturing pacemaker
   4. A nonsensing pacemaker

F. After a temporary pacemaker is inserted:
   1. The patient should be on bedrest for 4 days or more
   2. An ECG and chest radiograph should be obtained
   3. The dressing at the insertion site should be left undisturbed for 72 hours to prevent electrical hazards
   4. Preparation for a permanent pacemaker should be made

G. The strip in Fig. 7-47 is an example of:
   1. A continuous-paced rhythm
   2. A noncapturing pacemaker
   3. A nonsensing pacemaker
   4. A synchronous pacemaker

H. Indications for permanent pacing include which of the following? (Circle all that apply.)
   1. Complete heart block
   2. Stokes-Adams attacks and/or sick sinus syndrome (SSS)
   3. Tachydysrhythmias
   4. Mobitz type I with AV block

I. The strip in Fig. 7-48 is an example of:
   1. An atrial pacemaker

2. A pacer-induced rhythm
   3. A noncapturing pacemaker
   4. A nonsensing pacemaker

J. The strip in Fig. 7-49 is an example of:
   1. A malfunctioning pacemaker
   2. A ventricular pacemaker
   3. An atrial pacemaker
   4. A DVI-committed pacemaker

K. The strip in Fig. 7-50 is an example of:
   1. An uncommitted AV sequential pacemaker
   2. A committed AV sequential pacemaker
   3. A nonsensing pacemaker
   4. A noncapturing pacemaker

L. A pulse generator's failure to pace may be caused by:
   1. Intact electrodes and battery
   2. Lead displacement, inadequate threshold, or battery exhaustion
   3. Lead displacement, lead fracture, or patient's exhaustion
   4. Inhibition of the pulse generator by chest radiographs

M. Temporary epicardial wires may require:
   1. Oversensing abilities
   2. An extra grounding wire
   3. Higher thresholds
   4. Less electrical precautions

N. The strip in Fig. 7-51 is an example of:
   1. VOO pacing
   2. AOO pacing
   3. VVI pacing
   4. AAI pacing

O. The strip in Fig. 7-52, p. 182 is an example of:
   1. VOO pacing
   2. AOO pacing
   3. VVI pacing
   4. AAI pacing

P. The strip in Fig. 7-53, p. 182 is an example of:
   1. A noncapturing pacemaker
   2. Nonsensing

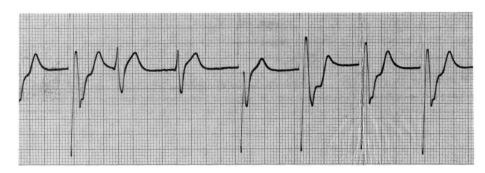

FIG. 7-51

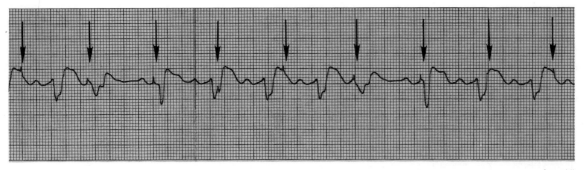

FIG. 7-52

Lead II

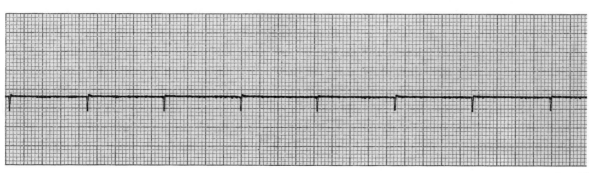

FIG. 7-53

Lead II

3. An intermittent atrial pacer
4. Intermittent fusion complexes

Q. Matching: Match the term in Column A with the definition in Column B.

Column A Term	Column B Definition	
___ 1. Anode	a. DVI pacing modality in which ventricular output is optional after atrial output	g. The lowest amount of electrical energy necessary to cause the heart to contract
___ 2. Committed sequential pacing		h. Stray electrical current or static electricity, eliciting myocardial depolarization during the vulnerable period and producing tachydysrhythmias
___ 3. Non-committed sequential pacing	b. Ability to depict the patient's intrinsic rate	
___ 4. Sensitivity	c. Minimum signal that consistently activates the pulse generator	
___ 5. Synchronous		
___ 6. Threshold	d. DVI pacing modality in which ventricular output is obligated	i. Pulse generator initiating adequate electrical stimulus to cause myocardial depolarization
___ 7. Firing	e. VVI pacing	
___ 8. Asynchronous	f. The positive portion of a pacer-lead system	j. VVO pacing
___ 9. Sensing		
___ 10. Microshock		

ANSWERS TO PRETEST AND POSTTEST

Pretest

A. 2
B. 1, 3, 4
C. 3
D. 1, 3, 5
E. 3
F. 2
G. 3
H. 4
I. 1, 3, 4
J. 3
K. 4
L. 2
M. 2
N. 4
O. 2
P. 3
Q. 1
R. 2

Posttest

A. 4
B. 1, 2, 3
C. 2
D. 1, 2, 3, 4
E. 2
F. 2
G. 4
H. 1, 2, 3
I. 1
J. 4
K. 1
L. 2
M. 3
N. 3
O. 1
P. 1
Q. 1. f
   2. d
   3. a
   4. c
   5. e
   6. g
   7. i
   8. j
   9. b
   10. h

MODULE 8

Antidysrhythmic drugs and electrolytes

PRETEST (Answers on p. 229)

Directions: Circle one answer to each question unless otherwise indicated.

A. Which of the following are side effects of lidocaine? (Circle all that apply.)
1. Paresthesias
2. Slurred speech
3. Hypertension
4. Bradycardia

B. The drug of choice for the treatment of ventricular extra-systoles in digoxin intoxication is:
1. Lidocaine
2. Procainamide
3. Phenytoin
4. Quinidine

C. Which of the following drugs would be contraindicated in a person with known hypersensitivity to local anesthetics? (Circle all that apply.)
1. Propranolol (Inderal)
2. Procainamide
3. Lidocaine
4. Phenytoin

D. Monitoring the QT interval should be done on which of the following drugs? (Circle all that apply.)
1. Procainamide
2. Quinidine
3. Disopyramide
4. Lidocaine

E. Which of the following drugs is most likely to induce or potentiate digoxin intoxication?
1. Lidocaine
2. Procainamide
3. Phenytoin
4. Quinidine

F. The most common side effect of quinidine is:
1. AV block
2. Diarrhea
3. Ventricular tachycardia
4. Heart failure

G. Phenytoin I.V. is compatible with which of the following solutions?
1. D_5W
2. $D_5\frac{1}{2}NS$
3. NS (normal saline)
4. Lactated Ringer's

H. An antidysrhythmic drug associated with producing a lupus-like condition is:
1. Bretylium
2. Propranolol
3. Quinidine
4. Procainamide

I. Which of the following drugs is most useful in suppressing supraventricular dysrhythmias?
1. Lidocaine
2. Quinidine
3. Bretylium
4. Procainamide

J. The physician writes an order for propranolol 20 mg qid. You would most likely schedule the drug to be given:
1. 9AM—1PM—5PM—9PM
2. 8AM—12 noon—4PM—8PM
3. 12 noon—6PM—12 midnight—6AM

K. A peak serum level of a drug is drawn:
1. 30 minutes before the next dose
2. Immediately after a dose is given
3. 30 minutes to 1 hour after a dose is given
4. 6 hours after a dose is given

L. Of the following drugs, which should be taken with meals or milk to decrease GI irritation?
1. Digoxin
2. Quinidine, procainamide
3. Phenytoin
4. Propranolol
5. All of the above
6. 2 and 3

M. A drug commonly used to correct supraventricular tachycardia is:

1. Atropine
2. Nifedipine
3. Verapamil
4. Quinidine

N. Cinchonism is a side effect related to which of the following?
   1. Lidocaine
   2. Propranolol
   3. Quinidine
   4. Bretylium

O. Side effects such as dry mouth, urinary retention, blurred vision are usually associated with the anticholinergic properties of which drug?
   1. Lidocaine
   2. Phenytoin
   3. Disopyramide
   4. Propranolol

C. Identify the major actions, indications for use, and side effects of the following investigational drugs:
   1. Tocainide
   2. Flecainide
   3. Encainide
   4. Lorcainide
   5. Mexiletine
   6. Ethmozine
   7. Cibenzoline

D. State the etiology, ECG effects, clinical features, and nursing observations concerning the following:
   1. Hyperkalemia
   2. Hypokalemia
   3. Alterations in magnesium
   4. Hypercalcemia
   5. Hypocalcemia
   6. Hypothermia

PURPOSE

The purpose of this module is to familiarize the learner with the action, indications for use, preparation and dosage in administration, normal effects, side effects, toxic effects, and nursing management of a variety of drugs used in the treatment of cardiac dysrhythmias and cardiovascular disease.

It is *imperative* that health care providers assume responsibility and accountability in familiarizing themselves with drugs *before* their administration.

BEHAVIORAL OBJECTIVES

Upon completion of this module, the learner should be able to:

A. Identify at least six major principles of drug administration

B. State the actions; indications for use; contraindications; preparation, dosage, and administration; absorption and excretion; serum levels; side effects; nursing implications; and special precautions for the following drugs:
   1. Digoxin
   2. Quinidine
   3. Procainamide
   4. Disopyramide
   5. Lidocaine
   6. Phenytoin
   7. Bretylium
   8. Propranolol
   9. Amiodarone
   10. Verapamil
   11. Isoproterenol
   12. Atropine

VOCABULARY

Accessory pathway An "extra" pathway through which impulses may be conducted to bypass the normal delay in the AV junction.

Adrenergic A term used to describe the fibers that release and the receptors that respond to catecholamines.

Afterdepolarizations Rapid, repetitive, weak depolarizations that occur toward the end of normal repolarization or after normal repolarization is complete. Under normal conditions, the cells do not respond to these efforts to depolarize. However, if the cell environment is vulnerable because of hypoxia, catecholamines, etc., it can respond and set up a rapid tachycardia, either atrial, junctional, or ventricular. Also known as "triggered activity."[10]

Afterload Refers to resistance in the systemic vasculature. Vasoconstriction *increases* afterload or the workload of the myocardium and vasodilation *decreases* afterload or the workload of the myocardium.

Antiadrenergic A term applied to nerve fibers that at their endings, when stimulated, block epinephrine or other catecholamines.

Anion A negatively charged electrolyte.

Asystole Lack of cardiac contraction and/or electrical cardiac activity, usually denoted as a straight line on the ECG.

Automaticity Electrical property of cells that permits spontaneous initiation of the cardiac impulse.

Atrioventricular (AV) block Refers to atrioventricular block or the alteration of an impulse initiated in the sinoatrial (SA) node or atrium in conduction to the ventricles.

Beta-adrenergic receptor Beta receptors are found mainly in the heart (beta$_1$) and lungs (beta$_2$).
   1. Stimulation of these receptors results in:
      a. ↑ heart rate
      b. ↑ AV conduction (velocity/time)
      c. ↑ myocardial contractility
      d. ↑ bronchial dilation
   2. Blocking of these receptors results in:
      a. ↓ heart rate
      b. ↓ AV conduction
      c. ↓ myocardial contractility
      d. ↑ bronchial constriction

Bigeminy A rhythm composed of pairs of complexes.[10]

Bioavailability A means of expressing the overall efficiency of drug absorption. It is the amount of drug available systemically after oral ingestion divided by the amount of drug available following I.V. administration.[22]

Bradycardia A heart rate below 60 beats per minute.

Cardiac output (CO) The volume of blood the heart pumps per minute. CO = stroke volume (SV) × heart rate (HR). SV determines the amount of blood pumped from the left ventricle with each heart beat (approximately 70 ml). The normal CO is between 4 to 8 liters per minute.

Cardioversion A direct electrical current synchronized to be delivered on the R wave of the ECG via paddles applied to the chest in order to terminate a tachycardia.

Catecholamines A group of neurohormones (epinephrine and norepinephrine) produced largely by the adrenal medulla and adrenergic nerve endings, which have a stimulating (sympathetic) effect of the autonomic nervous system, resulting in:
1. ↑ heart rate
2. ↑ AV conduction
3. ↑ myocardial contractility

Cation A positively charged electrolyte.

Cholinergic A term applied to nerve endings that liberate acetylcholine, such as the vagus nerve.

Chronotropic Refers to automaticity from the SA node:
1. Positive chronotropic effect = ↑ heart rate
2. Negative chronotropic effect = ↓ heart rate

Cinchonism The toxic effects produced from overingestion of cinchona bark from which quinidine is extracted. Effects are usually headaches, tinnitus, deafness, and blurred vision.

Conduction time Refers to the amount of time it takes for an impulse to travel through any part of the conduction system.

Dromotropic Refers to AV conduction:
1. A positive dromotropic effect accelerates AV conduction
2. A negative dromotropic effect slows AV conduction

Escape complex/rhythm A complex or rhythm that is initiated by a lower pacemaker when the sinus node slows or fails. Usually preceded by a pause in the normal heart rhythm, it is also known as "passive rhythm" or "rhythm by default."

Excitability The ability of the heart to respond to a stimulus.

Excitation-contraction-coupling A complex mechanism involving calcium and muscle proteins whereby the myofibrils in the myocardium shorten and contract in response to a stimulus.[25]

Extrasystole A premature impulse from a focus other than the SA node.

Fibrillation Rapid, chaotic, unsynchronized quivering or twitching in the myocardium during which no effective pumping occurs.

Half-life The time it takes for an amount of drug dose in the blood to be reduced by one half.

Heart sound (third) (S$_3$) A low-pitched sound heard with the bell of the stethoscope, occurring immediately after the second heart sound (S$_2$) or the "dub" of the "lub-dub" sequence. It indicates heart failure in the adult.

Hyper- Refers to greater than normal.

Hypo- Refers to less than normal.

Idiopathic hypertrophic subaortic stenosis (IHSS) A congenital heart defect characterized by enlargement (hypertrophy) of the muscle of the left ventricular wall and ventricular septum. During systole, obstruction occurs beneath the aortic valve, which may decrease stroke volume and cardiac output. Also known as hypertrophic obstructive cardiomyopathy (HOCM).

Inotropic Refers to contractility of the myocardium:
1. A positive inotropic effect = ↑ contractility.
2. A negative inotropic effect = ↓ contractility.

Preload Refers to the volume of blood in the left ventricle before contraction.

Reentry The circus movement of an impulse traveling two pathways that have a disparity (imbalance) in their response time to the impulse. This sets up a rapid tachycardia that may originate in the atrium, AV junction, Purkinje fibers, ventricular muscle, or accessory pathways.

Refractory period (absolute or effective) The interval of total unexcitability wherein a cell cannot respond to a stimulus. This correlates to the beginning of the QRS and the beginning of the T wave on the ECG, including the ST segment.

Serum levels A method that assays drug levels in the serum. There is a standard that indicates whether a drug level is "therapeutic" (whether enough drug is in the serum to be beneficial to the patient) or the drug level is too high and may produce toxic effects.

Serum levels must be drawn *before* a dose of the drug. At times, the physician may want to determine the drug level *before* a dose and then *after* a dose is administered to determine if the drug level is therapeutic. This, when it is requested, is called a "trough and a peak drug level." Trough means "low": therefore, the trough level is drawn *before* the next drug dose. Peak means "high": therefore, the peak level is drawn approximately 30 minutes to 1 hour *after* a drug dose is given. Both samples are sent to the laboratory together and must be labeled with the patient's name, time drawn, bed number, and whether it is the trough or peak specimen.

Steady state The timing and dosage required for a drug to reach a therapeutic serum level in a patient. It takes approximately five dosing intervals or five "half-lives" of a drug for this to occur.[22]

Supraventricular dysrhythmias Refers to abnormal impulse formation originating above the ventricle, which may be from the SA node, atrial muscle, or AV node. This also refers to abnormal impulse conduction, such as occurs in the circus-type reentry movement in atrial tissue, the AV junction, or in accessory pathways.

Systemic vascular resistance (SVR) Resistance to the flow of blood from the left ventricle, which is determined by vascular muscle tone and the diameter of the vessel, usually the arterioles. Also known as "peripheral vascular resistance."

Torsade de pointes A term used to describe a paroxysmal type of ventricular fibrillation and/or tachycardia, characterized by alterations in voltage that appear to be twisting around an isoelectric line. It is usually precipitated by lengthening of the QT interval. Refer to Ventricular Dysrhythmias module.

Weight Most drug dosages are based on a patient's weight in kilograms (kg) (2.2 pounds = 1 kg). Example: A person weighing 132 pounds would weigh 60 kg.

Wolff-Parkinson-White syndrome The presence of an accessory pathway, formerly known as a Kent bundle, which allows impulses to prematurely activate a portion of the ventricle before the normal impulse has time to arrive. This is characterized on the ECG as a short PR interval and a widened QRS interval. This may also precipitate a circus reentry through the dual pathways.

CONTENT
Suggested review

Before beginning this module on antidysrhythmic drugs and electrolytes, it is recommended that the learner review the following:

1. Anatomy and physiology of the heart and conduction system (Module I)
2. Basic principles of electrophysiology (Module I)
3. Administration of medications (refer to policy and procedure in your place of employment)

Principles of drug administration

1. Before the administration of drug therapy, familiarize yourself with the patient's diagnosis, information about the drug, (including the reason it is being given), actions, usual dose, side effects, expected clinical response, and necessary nursing observations.
2. Assure a 12-lead ECG as a baseline on the patient's chart *before* drug therapy is initiated. Measure intervals (PR, QRS, QT) before drug administration and record on the nurse's notes.
3. Assess the patient's renal, hepatic, and GI function before and during drug administration (note urinary output, BUN, creatinine, liver enzymes and liver size, appetite, GI bleeding, etc.)
4. Observe the patient's electrolyte values before and during drug administration.
5. If you have *any* question regarding the drug, dosage, ordered route of administration or rationale for giving, refer to the original order or question the physician and/or pharmacist *before* administration of the drug.
6. *Always* check the patient's nameband and ask the patient (if conscious) to state his/her name to you before a drug is given.
7. Administer drugs *on time*. All drugs given for dysrhythmia control *must* be equally divided over a 24-hour period. If the drug is ordered qid, it *must be* scheduled every 6 hours.
8. Whenever possible, inform the patient and/or his/her family of the name of the drug, why it is being given, and the frequency of administration. Patients need to be informed and, by doing so, you may decrease their level of anxiety, fear of the unknown, and promote cooperation for long-term compliance with drug therapy. In addition, if the drug dosage is changed (either increased or decreased) during the course of therapy, *always* inform the patient and/or family of this fact.

Cardiac glycosides

Cardiac glycosides have been used in the treatment of heart disease, especially heart failure, for many years. More recently they have been used for their antidysrhythmic effects. Most preparations are obtained from the foxglove plant: *digitalis purpurea* (digitoxin) and *digitalis lanata* (digoxin). Since digoxin is the most commonly used, the following discussion will be limited to this preparation.

Treatment with digoxin provides a narrow margin of safety between therapeutic and toxic and between toxic and lethal doses. When a desired therapeutic response is attained, it is usually the case that approximately 60% of a toxic dose has been administered, and, when toxic symptoms appear, approximately 50% of a lethal dose has been given. Therefore, digoxin is a drug to be used with caution and with careful consideration of the risk/benefit ratio.[48]

ACTIONS
Cardiac

1. Positive inotropic effect
   Digoxin increases the force of myocardial contraction and, in the failing heart, increases cardiac output. The mechanism is assumed to be related to the direct effect of increasing the availability of calcium to the contractile elements at the time of excitation-contraction-coupling.[48] Digoxin binds at receptor sites on the myocardial cell membrane, specifically at the sodium and potassium membrane pump.
2. Negative chronotropic effect
   a. Digoxin slows the heart rate by direct vagal stimulation of the SA node and by indirect vagal stimulation as a result of increased cardiac output.
   b. Digoxin shortens the refractory period of the atrial and ventricular muscle tissue. This may convert atrial flutter to atrial fibrillation or may accelerate the fibrillatory rate. This action may also cause rapid ventricular dysrhythmias to occur such as premature ventricular complexes, ventricular tachycardia, or fibrillation.
3. Negative dromotropic effect:
   Digoxin slows AV conduction by prolonging the absolute refractory period of the AV node, both by a direct and indirect vagal effect.[48] This action slows the ventricular response in atrial flutter and fibrillation and in other supraventricular tachydysrhythmias such as paroxysmal atrial tachycardia or junctional tachycardia.
4. Digoxin decreases heart size in the failing heart by decreasing preload (as a result of hepatic venous constriction) and decreasing ventricular wall tension.[20] This decreases myocardial oxygen demands and improves cardiac output. Other effects produced by this action include relief of edema and diuresis because of improved renal perfusion and inhibition of tubular reabsorption of sodium.[48]

Extracardiac

When digoxin is given rapidly I.V., arterial vasoconstriction occurs, increasing systemic vascular resistance, increasing blood pressure, and increasing myocardial oxygen demands. It is for this reason that the use of digoxin is highly controversial in the presence of acute myocardial infarction with sinus rhythm. When given slowly I.V. or by the oral route, arterial vasoconstriction is minimized.

Venous constriction occurs with resultant pooling of blood in the splanchnic bed, resulting in decreased venous return and preload, although this effect is minimal.

INDICATIONS FOR USE

1. Digoxin is used in the treatment of heart failure or other states characterized by decreased myocardial contractility. Recent evidence suggests that digoxin has major clinical effects in patients with congestive heart failure who have an associated third heart sound (S_3).[31] Other patients in heart failure, however, without an S_3, do as well with diuretic and vasodilator therapy alone.[18,31]

    Heart failure, resulting from pressure or volume overload because of hypertension, mitral, and/or aortic regurgitation, responds more favorably to positive inotropic action than does heart failure resulting from coronary artery disease.[2,18]

2. Digoxin is used in the treatment of atrial flutter, atrial fibrillation, paroxysmal atrial tachycardia, or junctional tachycardia to slow the ventricular response. Although digoxin tends to aggravate atrial fibrillation, conversion to normal sinus rhythm presumably occurs by slowing the ventricular response, increasing cardiac output, and increasing myocardial oxygenation.[48]

3. Digoxin may be used in atrial reentrant dysrhythmias since the shortening of the refractory period in atrial muscle may interrupt a reentry circuit.[25]

4. Digoxin is used in the prophylactic control of atrial tachydysrhythmias, such as in mitral valve prolapse or before coronary artery bypass surgery, although some controversy exists in relation to this use.[48]

CONTRAINDICATIONS

1. Digoxin is contraindicated in digoxin toxicity and in idiopathic hypertrophic subaortic stenosis (IHSS), a form of obstructive cardiomyopathy. In IHSS, the ventricular muscle wall and septum have an abnormally large muscle mass, which on ventricular contraction, comes together below the aortic valve to cause obstruction to flow. The positive inotropic effect of digoxin enhances this obstruction during systole, reducing stroke volume, and, ultimately, cardiac output from the left ventricle. This disorder is also known as hypertrophic obstructive cardiomyopathy (HOCM).

2. Digoxin is contraindicated in patients with acute myocardial infarction with sinus rhythm because increased afterload and increased force of contraction may increase infarct size.[18]

3. Digoxin should be used with caution in patients with acute myocardial infarction with atrial fibrillation, incomplete AV block, chronic constrictive pericarditis, severe pulmonary disease with right ventricular hypertrophy, and in renal insufficiency and hypothyroidism because of the decreased clearance of the drug.[39]

PREPARATION, DOSAGE, AND ADMINISTRATION

1. Digoxin is available in both the oral and parenteral form. The parenteral form is used to rapidly digitalize a patient or to achieve rapid inotropic action as needed for treatment of congestive heart failure with acute pulmonary edema.

    The oral form is used for slowly digitalizing a patient where it is not necessary to correct the myocardial function so immediately and as a maintenance form of digoxin therapy. See Table 8-1 for usual dosing schedules.

2. The parenteral form of digoxin should be administered diluted in a normal saline solution and given gradually I.V. (over 10 to 15 minutes) to prevent peripheral vasoconstriction, elevation of blood pressure, and increased myocardial oxygen demands.[48]

3. The oral form is administered before meals to enhance absorption.

ABSORPTION AND EXCRETION

1. Digoxin is incompletely absorbed from the gastrointestinal tract, and, if administered after meals or with antacids, is likely to decrease peak serum levels.[48] Absorption does not seem to be affected by malabsorption disorders [39] but does *decrease* if given with drugs increasing gastrointestinal motility and/or *increases* if given with drugs that decrease motility.[48]

2. Eighty to ninety percent of digoxin is absorbed with very little bound to protein, yielding a bioavailability of approximately 67%.

3. Digoxin is excreted unchanged in the urine and frequently there is excretion of a relatively inactive metabolite, dihydrodigoxin.

    Renal excretion is proportional to the glomerular filtration rate (GFR). With normal renal function, there is a loss of approximately one third of body stores daily. A steady state is reached when daily losses are matched by daily intake. This takes four to five half-lives or about 7 days in those receiving digoxin without a loading dose. In renal failure, there is increased tissue binding, and digoxin is not effectively removed by hemo or peritoneal dialysis.[48] In renal failure, the half-life is prolonged to approximately 4 days, and the period required to reach a steady state is up to 3 weeks.[48]

TABLE 8-1. Digitalizing schedule for digoxin compounds*

Generic name	Trade name	Absorption	Excretion	Average dose for digitalization and maintenance	Onset of action	Peak	Half-life
Digoxin	Lanoxin Novodigin	55-75% from GI tract	Renal	*I.V.* 0.75-1.0 mg in divided doses over 12-24 hours at 6-8 hour intervals *Available* 2-ml ampules of 0.5 mg (1 ml = 0.25 mg)	10-15 minutes	$\frac{1}{2}$-4 hours	3-5 days
				Oral 1.25-1.5 mg in divided doses over 12-24 hours at 6-8 hour intervals *Available* 0.125 mg and 0.25 mg tablets *Maintenance dose* 0.125-0.5 mg daily, depending on clinical status	15-30 minutes	$1\frac{1}{2}$-5 hours	36-48 hours
	Lanoxicaps (encapsulated gel form)	GI tract	Renal	*Average digitalizing dose* Should be lowered 20% *Available* 0.05, 0.10, and 0.20 mg capsules			

*Modified from Smith, T.W., and Braunwald, E.: The management of heart failure. In Braunwald, E., editor: Heart disease—a textbook of cardiovascular medicine, vol. 1, ed. 2, Philadelphia, 1984, W.B. Saunders Co.

4. Drugs affecting distribution and excretion of digoxin are:

a. Amiodarone

The addition of amiodarone to existing digoxin therapy causes sharp increases in serum digoxin concentrations. This mechanism is thought to occur in the adult because of displacement of digoxin from its binding sites since no evidence of digoxin toxicity is noted,[14] while in children it appears to be a mechanism of decreased tubular secretion and a decrease in the volume of distribution of digoxin by amiodarone.[28] It is suggested the digoxin dose be decreased.

b. Antibiotic therapy

Antibiotic therapy instituted concurrently with digoxin therapy may decrease the amount of degradation of digoxin for which the gastrointestinal organisms are responsible. This leads to more digoxin being absorbed in active form and thereby will alter the digoxin requirement.[11]

c. Quinidine

If quinidine is added to the medical regimen of a patient on a stable digoxin dose, the serum digoxin level may increase two-fold, predisposing the patient to the effects of digoxin toxicity. This mechanism is related to a change in the volume of distribution and to interference in renal clearance of digoxin by quinidine; it is not one of interfering with active receptor sites in the myocardium. The digoxin dose, consequently, requires an adjustment downward.[46,48,57]

d. Rifampin

When rifampin is added to combined quinidine/digoxin therapy, the metabolism of quinidine greatly increases in the liver. This, in turn, creates a drop in serum digoxin concentrations by accelerating renal clearance. Patients must be carefully monitored whenever rifampin is added to or discontinued from a combination of quinidine/digoxin therapy.[8]

e. Verapamil/nifedipine

In verapamil/digoxin combination therapy for atrial fibrillation, serum digoxin concentrations increase. The mechanism is thought to be a reduction in renal tubular secretion, in metabolic clearance, and in the volume of distribution of digoxin.[47] Patients are prone to gastrointestinal effects rather than dysrhythmia effects.

Nifedipine-digoxin combinations elevate serum digoxin concentrations in a similar fashion. It is recommended patients be observed closely for signs of digoxin toxicity.[48]

SERUM LEVELS

The therapeutic digoxin serum level is 0.6 to 2.0 ng/ml. The serum level is a tool to measure possible toxicity; however, digoxin therapy is often administered to elicit a clinical response with close observation of side effects and dosage is not based exclusively on serum levels alone.

SIDE EFFECTS

1. Normal digoxin effects on the ECG

a. Digoxin may prolong the PR interval and slow the sinus rate.

b. Shortening of the QT interval occurs because of shortening of the refractory period in ventricular muscle, which results in a rapid recovery time.[16]

c. A slurring or "sagging" of the ST segment can be seen that is the result of alterations in ionic exchange across the myocardial cell membrane, leaving intracellular potassium decreased. It may be

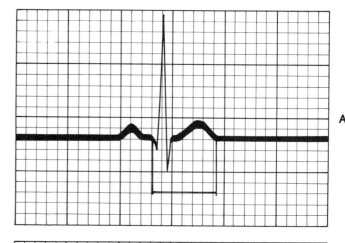

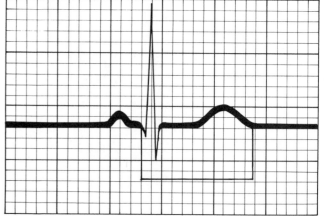

FIG. 8-1

Shortening of QT interval. **A,** QT interval of 0.24 second. **B,** Normal QT interval.

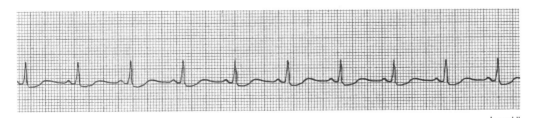

FIG. 8-2

Sagging of ST segment.

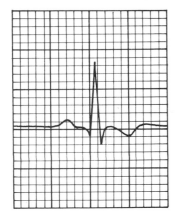

FIG. 8-3

T wave inversion.

difficult to differentiate this effect from that produced by other causes, such as myocardial ischemia. The effect may also be exaggerated by myocardial disease, tachydysrhythmias, and increased amplitude of QRS complexes. However, if the QT interval is also shortened, digoxin is the likely cause.[16] It is suggested digoxin be discontinued at least 1 week before elective exercise testing because of this effect.[16]

d. The T wave may be inverted or decreased in amplitude. If T wave inversion is present, it is rarely symmetrical as in pericarditis or ischemia. A shortened QT may also be a clue to digoxin effect.[16]

e. These alterations in the ECG may frequently be seen on the standard limb leads (I, II, III) and on the anterior lateral chest leads (V_3 to V_6)[2] (Figs. 8-1 to 8-3).

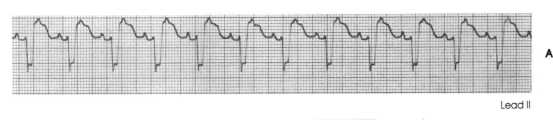

A

Lead II

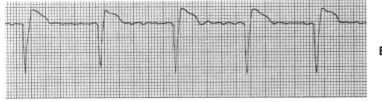

B

Lead II

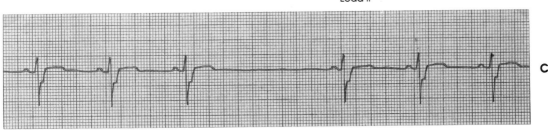

C

Lead III

FIG. 8-4

Rhythms associated with digoxin toxicity: **A,** PAT with block (2:1), **B,** atrial fibrillation with a regular ventricular response, and **C,** sinoatrial block.

2. Toxic effects
   a. Patients on digoxin therapy may develop any dysrhythmia associated with toxic levels but especially marked sinus bradycardia, sinoatrial block, paroxysmal atrial tachycardia (PAT) with block, atrial fibrillation with a regular ventricular response, nonparoxysmal junctional tachycardia, AV block (first degree, second degree [type I], or third degree), AV dissociation, premature ventricular complexes (bigeminal or multifocal), ventricular tachycardia, and ventricular fibrillation (Fig. 8-4, p. 191).

   These dysrhythmias are forms of alterations of impulse formation and conduction and can be explained both in terms of altered refractory periods and automaticity of cardiac tissue and in alterations of sympathetic activity and vagal tone.

   b. Factors predisposing a patient to digoxin toxicity include:
   (1) Administration of sympathetic blocking agents such as reserpine and quanethidine sulfate (Ismelin)
   (2) Electrolyte imbalances
       (a) Hyperkalemia
           The myocardial concentration of digoxin is decreased
       (b) Hypokalemia
           1) The absolute refractory period of Purkinje cells is decreased, shortening the coupling interval for premature ventricular complexes
           2) Low potassium is accentuated with diuretic therapy, insulin therapy, corticosteroid therapy, and renal disease
       (c) Hypercalcemia
           1) Hypercalcemia occurs in hyperparathyroidism, multiple myeloma, and with the I.V. administration of calcium salts
           2) Calcium shortens the refractory period in Purkinje cells, as well as enhancing the force of contraction, which, with additive effects to digoxin, may result in rapid ventricular dysrhythmias
       (d) Hypomagnesemia
           1) Hypomagnesemia enhances potassium loss from the cell, shortens the refractory period through the AV node and bundle branches, and increases excitability of ventricular muscle
           2) Hypomagnesemia is seen in patients on chronic diuretic therapy, with gastrointestinal disease, diabetes mellitus, poor nutritional states, and in chronic congestive heart failure
   (3) Pulmonary disease
       (a) Digoxin toxicity may be seen at normal serum digoxin concentrations
       (b) Factors related to toxicity are hypoxemia, diuretic therapy, metabolic alkalosis, and increased sympathetic tone
   (4) Aging
       Patients with advanced age are susceptable to digoxin toxicity because of many associated factors in this group:
       (a) Increased severity of heart disease
       (b) Decreased glomerular filtration rate with resultant increase in the half-life of digoxin
       (c) Associated renal, neurological, and pulmonary impairment
       (d) Combination therapy of many drugs
   (5) Renal function
       With decreased renal function, digoxin levels tend to increase
   (6) Thyroid function
       (a) Hyperthyroidism, which increases renal clearance and decreases half-life of digoxin; larger doses are needed to treat the dysrhythmia
       (b) Hypothyroidism, which decreases renal clearance and lengthens the half-life of digoxin[39,48]

3. Other side effects
   a. Gastrointestinal side effects include anorexia, nausea, vomiting, and diarrhea; these may occur by a direct irritant effect on the gastrointestinal mucosa and by a direct central nervous system effect[48]
   b. Neurological side effects include mental depression; personality changes; visual disturbances, including color halos around objects (yellow, green, brown), blurred vision, and scotomas; cerebral excitation, including headache, vertigo, increased irritability, and convulsions; and generalized muscular weakness
   c. Other side effects include gynecomastia (enlargement of breast tissue in males and females) and allergic reactions, such as skin rash[2,48]

4. It becomes important to assess digoxin therapy in relation to the clinical diagnosis(es) and observe closely for the therapeutic/toxic balance.

5. Treatment of toxic effects
   Treatment of digoxin toxicity takes many forms, the most frequently used being:
   a. Withholding digoxin until the symptoms subside
   b. Carotid sinus massage, which can provide a useful bedside clue to impending digoxin toxicity; this maneuver can elicit second-degree AV block, accelerated junctional rhythm, premature ventricular

complexes, including bigeminy before they spontaneously occur[48]

c. Giving magnesium salts, which:
(1) Reduces intracellular potassium loss
(2) Lengthens the refractory period in the AV junction and in ventricular muscle

d. Giving phenytoin, which:
(1) Increases the speed of AV conduction
(2) Decreases automaticity in Purkinje cells and ventricular muscle
(3) Suppresses delayed afterdepolarizations in the Purkinje fibers that have been induced by digoxin[10]

e. Lidocaine, which decreases automaticity and excitability in the Purkinje fibers and in ventricular muscle

f. Initiating a temporary pacemaker until dysrhythmias resolve[48]

g. Administering digoxin-specific antibodies
(1) Digoxin-specific antibodies are reserved for those who either accidentally or with suicidal intent receive an overdose of digoxin, such as children finding a bottle of tablets or an elderly person who may forget what and how many medicines have been taken.
(2) Healthy hearts can tolerate serum digoxin levels as high as 10-15 ng/ml. Primary ECG manifestations without cardiac disease may be sinus bradycardia, sinoatrial block (first, second, or third degree). Atropine and/or temporary pacing may or may not be effective.[48]
(3) The I.V. infusion of digoxin-specific Fab fragments (a form of digoxin antibody) is effective in binding the digoxin molecule to the Fab fragments, which are then excreted rapidly in the urine. This is a very effective method of reversing life-threatening dysrhythmias.[50]

NURSING MANAGEMENT

1. The nursing observations for patients receiving digoxin therapy are many and include:
a. Being aware of the clinical diagnosis and the rationale for digoxin therapy
b. Observing ECG strips and recording and measuring intervals (PR, QRS, QT) daily
c. Assessing renal function and potassium levels since renal failure and hypokalemia predispose to digoxin toxicity
d. Observing for dysrhythmias and recording on nurse's notes if they occur as well as notifying the physician, and administering digoxin I.V. with caution, especially in the presence of acute myocardial infarction

2. Nurses should also be aware of drug interactions with digoxin that raise the serum digoxin concentration (amiodarone, antibiotics, nifedipine, quinidine, rifampin, verapamil).

3. Other nursing observations:
a. Take the patient's heart rate before administration of digoxin. If it is below 60 per minute, question the physician to assure that he/she wants the medication given. Otherwise, question at what heart rate the physician wants the digoxin to be withheld. Remember that administering calcium salts to the patient receiving digoxin is contraindicated since calcium affects contractility, excitability, and automaticity of the myocardium as much as digoxin and may lead to serious dysrhythmias.
b. If a patient is to be transferred to an intensive care unit for elective cardioversion of a tachydysrhythmia, be aware if the patient is receiving digoxin and also if a recent serum potassium level is documented on the patient record. Digoxin may precipitate a very serious ventricular dysrhythmia with electrical shock, which is aggravated further in the presence of hypokalemia. Usually the digoxin is withheld 48 hours before electrical cardioversion if possible. Alert the physician if the patient has received a digoxin dose before cardioversion.

Classification of antidysrhythmic drugs

Drug therapy is the primary treatment for most cardiac dysrhythmias. For this reason, a great variety of pharmacological agents have been produced for similar rhythm disturbances. Many of these drugs share a common mechanism of action, and, because of this, a classification system for antidysrhythmic agents has developed. There is more than one classification system. The one that will be used in this text is that of Vaughn Williams.[56] This system classifies drugs according to their electrophysiological action on isolated myocardial fibers. Because this system uses advanced concepts of electrophysiological principles to classify drugs, for this level, the classification system will be listed with a brief description of the distinguishing features of each class[56] (Table 8-2, p. 194).

Specific drugs
QUINIDINE
Actions

1. Quinidine decreases the automaticity of all pacemaker cells, prolongs the effective refractory period of both atrial and ventricular muscle, and prolongs conduction time throughout the conduction system and cardiac muscle tissue.

2. Quinidine depresses myocardial excitability and, thus, decreases the risk of ventricular fibrillation. It also has

TABLE 8-2. Vaughn Williams' drug classification of antidysrhythmic agents[56]

Class	Action
MEMBRANE STABILIZING AGENTS (I)	
Quinidine Procainamide Disopyramide	Lengthens refractory period and slows conduction
Lidocaine Phenytoin	Shortens refractory period and speeds conduction
Flecainide Lorcainide	Refractory period and conduction unchanged
BALANCED BETA-ADRENERGIC AGONISTS (II)	
Bretylium Propranolol	Beta blockade
III	
Amiodarone Disopyramide	Lengthens absolute refractory period
CALCIUM CHANNEL BLOCKERS (IV)	
Verapamil (Nifedipine) (Diltiazem)	Blocks slow channel calcium

a negative inotropic effect that decreases the force of myocardial contractility.

3. Quinidine has a vagolytic effect that can actually increase sinus impulse formation and conduction through the AV junction.

Indications for use

1. Quinidine is used for both atrial and ventricular dysrhythmias. It can convert atrial fibrillation or flutter to normal sinus rhythm or maintain normal sinus rhythm after electrical cardioversion is performed. Because of its vagolytic effect and the possibility of inducing rapid 1:1 conduction through the AV junction, quinidine is frequently used in combination with digoxin or beta blockers to slow AV conduction in atrial dysrhythmias.
2. Quinidine is effective in controlling ventricular tachycardia and fibrillation in long-term therapy.[13]
3. Quinidine is also useful in the treatment of supraventricular tachycardia associated with the Wolff-Parkinson-White syndrome. It prolongs the refractory time of the accessory pathway and reduces the number of premature atrial complexes that usually perpetuate the tachycardia.[59]

Contraindications

Quinidine should not be given to a patient who has the following: history of thrombocytopenia purpura,

digoxin toxicity, complete heart block, junctional or idioventricular escape rhythms, hypokalemia, congestive heart failure, hypovolemic states, congenital QT prolongation, or *torsade de pointes*.

Preparation, dosage, and administration

Quinidine is available in the sulfate and gluconate form. Oral preparations come packaged in 200- and 300-mg tablets and in time-delayed capsules, while parenteral quinidine comes packaged in the gluconate form in 10 cc vials of 80 mg per ml. Quinidine can be given orally (p.o.), intramuscularly (IM), or intravenously (I.V.).
1. Oral
   a. The dosage range is 200 to 400 mg four to six times a day. The total daily dose should not exceed 3 to 4 gm. All doses must be titrated to clinical response and serum levels and must be divided equally over 24 hours.
   b. Longer acting compounds, such as Quinidex Extentabs are available in 200- to 300-mg tablets and the frequency of dosing is decreased to every 8 to 12 hours. There is more available quinidine in the sulfate than in the gluconate form. Therefore the gluconate dosage may be higher than sulfate. The gluconate form is less rapidly absorbed; therefore the frequency of dosing is less.[10]
2. Parenteral
   a. IM: The dosage range is 200 mg every 4 to 6 hours. The IM route, however, is painful, may increase creatine phosphokinase (CK) enzyme activity as much as seven-fold with a single injection, and is generally not recommended.[20,34]
   b. I.V.: The intravenous route is reserved for life-threatening ventricular dysrhythmias. A range of 300 to 750 mg may be required to terminate the dysrhythmia. Before administration, the patient must be monitored and the drug infused via a controlled infusion pump. One vial of 800 mg is diluted in 50 ml D5W and given no faster than 16 mg (1 ml) per minute. The blood pressure and length of the QRS and QT intervals must be monitored continuously during infusion for toxic effects of the drug (hypotension and lengthening of the QRS and QT intervals).

Absorption and excretion

Quinidine is rapidly absorbed from the gastrointestinal tract and peaks in 1 to 4 hours. The activity lasts for 6 to 8 hours and a steady state is reached in 1 to 3 days. It is highly protein bound—80% to 90%. The half-life is 4 to 8 hours.

Quinidine is metabolized in the liver and excreted in the kidney. Up to 50% of the drug is excreted unchanged

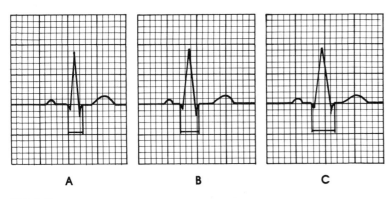

FIG. 8-5
Prolongation of QT interval: **A,** normal (0.10 second), **B,** effect (0.13 second), and **C,** toxicity: over 50% of baseline (0.16 second).

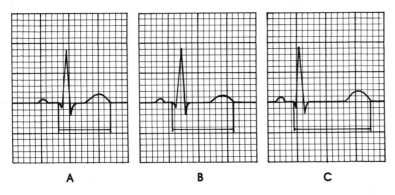

FIG. 8-6
Prolongation of QT interval: **A,** baseline (0.36 second), **B,** effect (0.42 second), and **C,** toxicity: almost up to 50% of baseline (0.52 second).

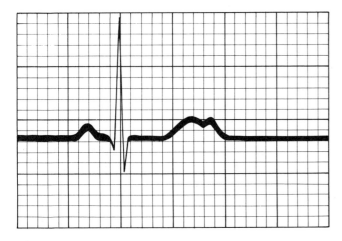

FIG. 8-7
TU fusion.

in the urine; the remainder is excreted as metabolites. Urine pH affects elimination since alkalotic urine *decreases* excretion while acidotic urine *increases* excretion. In renal failure, quinidine and its metabolites are cleared by dialysis.[37]

Serum Levels

The therapeutic serum levels range from 2 to 5 μg/ml with toxic effects in the range of 8 μg/ml.

Side effects

1. Normal ECG effects of quinidine are related to therapeutic quinidine levels and include:
   a. Prolongation of the QRS interval (a function of the slowing of conduction)
   b. Prolongation of the QT interval because of prolongation of the effective refractory period and repolarization changes in Purkinje and ventricular muscle fibers
   c. Enlarged U wave that encroaches upon the terminal portion of the T wave, creating a TU fusion, mimicking hypokalemia, especially when quinidine is combined with digoxin therapy[54] (Figs. 8-5 to 8-7)

2. Toxic effects
   a. Widening of the QRS interval to 25% of baseline is cause for concern and a warning to discontinue the drug (see Fig. 8-5, p. 195)
   b. Widening of the QT interval up to 50% of baseline (see Fig. 8-6, p. 195)
3. Other side effects
   a. Cinchonism
      This usually occurs in patients on a full dosing schedule or on chronic therapy and is associated with a cluster of symptoms (in its mildest form) of tinnitus, headache, nausea, and blurred vision
   b. Central nervous system reactions
      Decreased auditory acuity and vertigo (eighth cranial nerve involvement); visual changes including diplopia, photophobia, altered color perception and night blindness; restlessness, apprehension, tremors, excitement, and delerium
   c. Gastrointestinal reactions
      Anorexia, nausea, vomiting, diarrhea (by far, the most common complaint), abdominal cramping, and/or pain
   d. Skin reactions
      Cutaneous flushing, intense pruritis, exfoliative dermatitis, and sweating
   e. Cardiovascular symptoms
      (1) Quinidine syncope
         Develops from a rapid ventricular dysrhythmia—either ventricular tachycardia or nonsustained ventricular fibrillation—and a form of *torsade de pointes* that usually occurs from prolongation of the QT interval[49]
      (2) Hypotension
         Often seen with I.V. administration or as a combination of peripheral vasodilation (alpha-adrenergic blockade) and myocardial depression
      (3) Heart block
         Because of prolongation of refractory period
      (4) Congestive heart failure
   f. Hypersensitivity
      Fever may be the only symptom experienced and disappears when the drug is discontinued; anaphylactic reactions are rare; other symptoms include urticaria, angioedema, polyarthralgias, dyspnea, exacerbation of asthma, and respiratory depression and/or arrest; if hypersensitivity occurs, it is always immediate and not observed in chronic quinidine therapy
   g. Hematological effects
      Acute hemolytic anemia, hypoprothrombin-

emia, thrombocytopenia, leukopenia, and agranulocytosis
   h. Electrolyte imbalance
      Hypokalemia will decrease the action of quinidine, whereas hyperkalemia will potentiate depressant effects of quinidine on pacemaker cells[13,34,46]

Nursing management

1. Monitor and record QRS and QT intervals before drug administration and follow through with monitoring during drug therapy.
2. Administering quinidine with meals may reduce gastrointestinal side effects or the gluconate form may be substituted to minimize these effects. Diarrhea is very common when quinidine therapy is first instituted; therefore, monitoring intake and output, electrolytes (especially potassium), and acid-base balance is important. Diarrhea may be a limiting consideration in the use of quinidine even though the condition can be treated with anticholinergic agents such as Lomotil.
3. Inform the patient to notify the physician for syncopal episodes or symptoms of tinnitus, vertigo, headache, and/or blurred vision.
4. If quinidine is given I.V., it *must* be given by controlled infusion pump to avoid rapid influx of drug. Continuous ECG and blood pressure monitoring must be done. Emergency resuscitation equipment must be readily available. Because of toxicity, the I.V. route is reserved for emergency situations.

Special considerations

1. Quinidine added to a patient's medical regimen on a stable digoxin dose can predispose the patient to digoxin toxicity. The mechanism is thought to be one of interference with renal clearance and alterations in volume of distribution of digoxin by quinidine.[46,48,57]
2. When the serum level of quinidine approaches 8 μg/ml, signs of toxicity appear, including prolongation of the QRS or QT intervals up to 50% or greater of baseline and the disappearance of P waves, which may predispose the patient to *torsade de pointes*.
3. Quinidine potentiates the hypoprothrombinemia effects of coumarin. It also can potentiate vagolytic effects if given with anticholinergic agents, such as atropine, belladonna, and propanthaline. Drugs that alkalinize the urine, such a acetazolamide or Diamox, can predispose the patient to quinidine toxicity because of enhanced reabsorption of the drug in the renal tubules.[20,37]
4. Other drug interactions include: barbiturates and phenytoin, which act as hepatic enzyme inducers and increase the elimination of quinidine (shortening its

half-life), and cimetidine, which acts as a hepatic enzyme inhibitor, lengthens the drug's half-life, interferes with elimination, and increases quinidine serum levels.

PROCAINAMIDE
Actions

1. Procainamide depresses the excitability of both ventricular and atrial muscle fibers. The refractory period of the atrial and ventricular muscles is also prolonged.
2. Procainamide prolongs conduction time in the cardiac muscle, Purkinje fibers, and the AV junction.
3. Procainamide decreases automaticity of all pacemaker cells and slows the rate of repolarization, thus decreasing the risk of fibrillation in both the atria and the ventricles.
4. Procainamide has a negative inotropic effect, but to a lesser degree than quinidine.
5. Procainamide produces pulmonary and systemic vasodilation, most probably from its effect of producing autonomic ganglionic blockade.[20]

Indications for use

1. Procainamide is used in the treatment of acute premature ventricular complexes and ventricular tachycardia. It can be used as the primary agent when an oral route is desired or it can be used parenterally for control of ventricular rhythms not suppressed by lidocaine.
2. Procainamide is also used for atrial flutter or fibrillation, paroxysmal atrial tachycardia, and preexcitation syndromes such as Wolff-Parkinson-White. In these situations, procainamide will not only slow the ventricular rate by slowing conduction through the AV junction, but it will also decrease automaticity and the rate of repolarization in the atrial muscle cells.
3. In preexcitation syndromes, procainamide can terminate tachycardia by breaking the circus movement of the impulse in either the AV junction or assessory pathway through lengthening the refractory period and/or speed of conduction.[59]

Contraindications

1. Procainamide is contraindicated in patients with:
   a. Hypersensitivity to procainamide or to any procaine-related drugs
   b. Myasthenia gravis, although not absolutely; it may also potentiate the effects of the drugs used to treat myasthenia
   c. Second-degree, type II, or complete AV block in the absence of a pacemaker
   d. Sinus node dysfunction, because procainamide

abolishes more of the essential subsequent pacemaker sites, resulting in slow rates or even asystole
2. Procainamide should be used with extreme caution in patients with:
   a. Congestive heart failure
   b. Ventricular dysrhythmias associated with digoxin toxicity
   c. Electrolyte disturbances, especially hyperkalemia, which enhances the cardiodepressant effects of procainamide
   d. Hepatic or renal insufficiency[20]

Preparation, dosage, and administration

1. Procainamide is available orally in tablets and/or capsules of 250 mg, 375 mg, 500 mg, and 750 mg, in sustained release capsules of 500 mg, and for parenteral administration, in doses of 100 mg/ml (10-ml vials) or 500 mg/ml (2-ml vials).
   a. Oral administration is the preferred route to control dysrhythmias that do not require immediate suppression, or for maintenance therapy after control of a serious dysrhythmia has been achieved by parenteral administration.
      (1) The usual oral dose is 50 mg/kg/day in divided doses for a total of 3 to 6 gm per day. General dosing is 250 to 500 mg every 3 to 6 hours or 500 mg to 1 gm every 4 to 6 hours. Intervals will very with the desired therapeutic serum levels.
      (2) If sustained release capsules are used, dosing can be decreased to every 6 to 8 hours. The advantages of this preparation include: prolonged absorption, avoidance of toxic peak levels, and unchanged availability of the drug that allows maintenance of therapeutic levels with larger, less frequent doses.[7]
   b. For parenteral intravenous use, 25 to 50 mg of procainamide can be given per minute at 5-minute intervals under closely monitored conditions (blood pressure, heart rate and rhythm, and measurement of QRS and QT intervals). At no time should the dose exceed 50 mg/min. Dosing should continue until the dysrhythmia is suppressed, 1 gm is given, hypotension occurs, or QRS widening greater than 50% of baseline occurs. After control of the dysrhythmia is achieved by I.V. bolus infusion, a continuous infusion of 2 to 6 mg per minute is required to maintain therapeutic serum levels. This is achieved by diluting 1 gm of procainamide in 250 ml D_5W or normal saline (NS), producing a 4% solution or a 4 mg per ml concentration. Using the above doses, the flow rate is 30 to 90 ml per hour.

c. Procainamide may be given intramuscularly (IM) in a dose of 500 mg to 1 gm every 4 to 8 hours until oral therapy is instituted.[17]

Absorption and excretion

1. Procainamide is almost completely absorbed orally from the gastrointestinal tract when the patient is fasting and is rapidly distributed to most body tissues except the brain. It is minimally bound to plasma proteins, yielding a high concentration of the drug at its binding sites. Absorption varies when it is taken with meals. With capsules, levels peak in 1 hour with a steady state reached in 24 hours. With sustained release preparations, levels peak in 1 to 2 hours with a steady state reached within 48 hours. Parenteral administration peaks in 15 minutes or less and a steady state is reached within 2 to 15 hours.

2. Twenty to forty percent of a procainamide dose is metabolized in the liver where acetylation occurs. This results in a pharmacologically active metabolite, N-acetylprocainamide (NAPA). Sixty to eighty percent of the parent drug and its metabolites are excreted unchanged in the urine.[20]

3. The half-life of procainamide is 3 to 4 hours in the presence of normal renal and liver function, while the half-life of NAPA is 6 to 8 hours. In individuals with poor renal function, the half-lives can increase to 3 to 8 hours and 6 to 30 hours, respectively.

Serum levels

Therapeutic serum levels vary from 4 to 10 µg/ml for procainamide and up to 22 µg/ml for the active metabolite, NAPA. It is recommended by some authorities that both serum levels of procainamide and NAPA be monitored and used in combination as a guideline for effective therapy. Combined levels should be between 5 to 30 µg/ml although 20 µg/ml may be associated with toxicity.[3,37]

Side effects

1. Normal ECG effects of procainamide include:
   (a) Widening of the QRS interval
   (b) Widening of the QT interval
   (c) Less frequently prolongation of the PR interval and/or loss of voltage in the QRS complex and T wave (Fig. 8-8)
2. Toxic ECG effects include:
   (a) Widening of the QRS up to 50% of baseline (see Figs. 8-5 and 8-6, p. 195)
3. Other adverse reactions:
   (a) Hypotension
       This may be transient but severe and occurs more frequently with I.V. administration; it may lead to cardiovascular collapse, convulsions, or coronary insufficiency and is probably caused more by peripheral vasodilation and resultant afterload reduction than by actual myocardial depressant effects
   (b) Gastrointestinal
       Nausea, vomiting, abdominal pain, diarrhea, and bitter taste
   (c) Central nervous system
       Flushing, weakness, giddiness, insomnia, mental depression, psychosis with hallucinations, and seizures
   (d) Hypersensitivity reaction
       Eosinophilia, urticaria, rash, pruritis, fever, changes in hair color, angioedema, myalgias, digital vasculitis, and Raynaud's phenomenon
   (e) Systemic lupus erythematosus–type syndrome
       This syndrome is characterized by polyarthralgias, arthritis, pleuritic pain, and, less frequently, by myalgias, skin lesions, pleural effusions or pericarditis; these symptoms reverse on discontinuation of procainamide
   (f) Impotence
       This may occur as a result of depression
   (g) Agranulocytosis
       Reported symptoms include oral lesions, fever, and infection[3,7,17,20]

Nursing management

1. When procainamide is administered orally, the patient should be instructed to take it with meals to reduce gastrointestinal effects. If the form is sustained release, inform the patient that he/she may find the orange

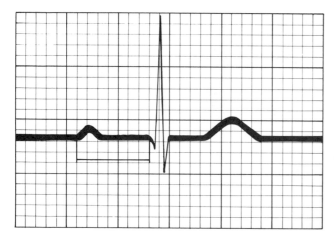

FIG. 8-8
Prolongation of PR interval.

capsule in the stool. The drug is absorbed in the gastrointestinal tract but the capsule does not absorb; it passes through.

2. Measure the QRS and QT intervals before drug therapy and continue through administration, noting lengthening of one or both, which would indicate possible toxicity. During I.V. administration, continuous ECG and blood pressure monitoring is mandatory. The drug must be administered through a controlled infusion pump, and a vasopressor, such as norepinephine or dopamine, should be readily available to counteract hypotensive espisodes. Observe for the development of *torsades de pointes*.[49]

3. If there is a change from I.V. to oral therapy, wait one half-life (approximately 4 hours) after I.V. therapy is discontinued to begin the first oral dose. This avoids peak and potentially toxic levels after the first dose.[7,20]

4. In patients treated for atrial dysrhythmias, it is important to observe for embolic events caused by dislodgement of an atrial thrombus. Also observe for the development of a tachycardia because of slowing of the atrial rate to one that can be conducted on a 1:1 ratio through the AV junction.

5. Instruct the patient to report any signs of lightheadedness, syncope, and signs of systemic lupus erythematosus to the physician.

Special considerations

1. Individuals with renal or liver disease should have loading and maintenance doses of procainamide reduced 25% to 50%.[3]

2. Use with caution for ventricular dysrhythmias in the presence of acute myocardial infarction, as absorption is unpredictable.

3. In the presence of first-degree, second-degree, type II, or complete AV block, procainamide may precipitate complete heart block, ventricular fibrillation, or asystole.

4. A 24-hour Holter monitor plus serum levels are used for evaluating the effectiveness of the therapy.[3,17,20]

5. Do not combine I.V. procainamide with any other drug since the following procainamide-drug interactions may occur:
   a. Propranolol, narcotics, and barbituates may have additive cardiodepressant effects
   b. Anticholinergic agents may have additive vagolytic actions
   c. Cholinergic agents may be antagonized by procainamide
   d. Antihypertensive agents may cause additive hypotensive effects
   e. Antibiotics, such as the aminoglycosides, may be potentiated with neuromuscular action

   f. There may be additive cardiodepressant effects with drugs such as lidocaine and quinidine
   g. Muscle relaxants used in surgery and in intensive care units, such as curare and succinylcholine, may be potentiated by procainamide, causing accentuation of respiratory depression with possible apnea; caution should be used postoperatively until the effects of these agents have been eliminated[6,17,20]

DISOPYRAMIDE (NORPACE)
Actions

1. Disopyramide decreases automaticity, prolongs the effective refractory period, and prolongs conduction time in the Purkinje fibers.

2. Disopyramide's action on conduction through the AV junction is not consistent. Because of a significant anticholinergic effect, disopyramide can *increase* sinus node impulse formation and *decrease* conduction time through the AV junction, especially if cholinergic activity is present.

3. Disopyramide *increases* the conduction time and effective refractory period of the accessory pathways seen in the Wolff-Parkinson-White syndrome.

4. Disopyramide has a negative inotropic effect.

Indications for use

1. Disopyramide is used for the control of ventricular dysrhythmias, such as premature ventricular complexes and ventricular tachycardia, and for reentrant tachycardia seen in such preexcitation syndromes as Wolff-Parkinson-White.

2. Disopyramide equals quinidine in suppressing ventricular dysrhythmias, but it has fewer gastrointestinal side effects.[12]

Contraindications

Disopyramide is contraindicated in patients with uncontrolled congestive heart failure, acute pulmonary edema, cardiogenic shock,[41] glaucoma, urinary retention, sinus node dysfunction, and advanced degrees of AV block.

Preparation, dosage, and administration

1. Disopyramide is available in 100- and 150-mg capsules and in a sustained-release form. There is a parenteral form, but it is not yet approved for general use by the U.S. Federal Drug Administration.

2. The usual adult oral dose ranges from 400 to 800 mg daily given in four equally divided doses. The maximum daily dose should not exceed 1600 mg. For adults weighing less than 50 kg, it is recommended

that 100 mg be given every 6 hours. Usually, a loading dose of 300 mg is given. Frequency of the sustained release form is decreased to every 8 to 12 hours.

Absorption and excretion

Disopyramide is almost completely absorbed from the gastrointestinal tract. Peak serum levels are usually reached within 2 to 3 hours after ingestion. The drug is primarily excreted in the urine. In the presence of renal failure, clearance is delayed and elevated serum levels will result. The dosage must be reduced depending on the severity of the clinical situation.[12,20,34]

Serum levels

Therapeutic serum levels range from 2 to 4 µg/ml with toxic levels at 9 µg/ml. This drug is less protein-bound than quinidine, ranging from 50% to 65%. The half-life of disopyramide ranges from 4 to 10 hours with a mean of 7 hours.

Side effects

1. ECG changes manifested by disopyramide include widening of the QRS and QT intervals. If these intervals widen to 25% to 50% of baseline, toxicity may occur (see Figs. 8-5 and 8-6, p. 195).
2. Most of the side effects of disopyramide therapy are associated with its anticholinergic effects, which come from one of its active metabolites. The common effects seen are dry mouth; urinary hesitancy, frequency or retention; blurred vision; dizziness; muscle weakness; headache; malaise; anorexia; diarrhea; vomiting; hypotension; shortness of breath; syncope; and congestive heart failure because of the negative inotropic effect.

Nursing management

1. Measure and record QRS and QT intervals before and during drug therapy; observe for a 25% to 50% increase or more over baseline as an indicator of toxicity and notify the physician if this occurs
2. Prolongation of the QT interval may induce ventricular tachycardia and/or fibrillation (torsade de pointes), so monitor the ECG closely during institution of drug therapy
3. Monitor laboratory values, especially potassium, as it potentiates the effects of disopyramide if values are high
4. Instruct the patient with benign prostatic hypertrophy or diabetic bladder regarding the possibility of urinary retention
5. If signs of toxicity occur, have emergency equipment available to treat cardiodepressant effects[12,20]

Special considerations

1. Precautionary measures should be used when the patient is in atrial flutter or fibrillation as the reduction in atrial rate may allow a rapid 1:1 conduction to the ventricles.
2. Renal or hepatic disease may easily precipitate overdosage and toxicity. Hyperkalemia should be treated very early as this potentiates the effects of disopyramide toxicity.
3. Excretion of disopyramide is not greatly affected by urine pH as is quinidine.
4. Blood pressure should be monitored frequently and observations made for signs of congestive heart failure since disopyramide has a profound negative inotropic effect.[41]
5. Because of significant and uncomfortable anticholinergic effects, disopyramide is not widely used.

LIDOCAINE
Actions

1. Lidocaine depresses the automaticity of the His-Purkinje system by slowing the rate of depolarization. In Purkinje fibers and ventricular muscle there is a selective slowing of conduction and lengthening of the refractory period in ischemic tissue but not in normal tissue, thereby creating a block for a circus movement reentry tachycardia, such as ventricular tachycardia. The risk of ventricular fibrillation is decreased.
2. There is no significant effect of lidocaine on shortening or lengthening the refractory period in accessory pathways, and it is therefore not recommended in preexcitation syndromes.[10]
3. Lidocaine has little, if any, effect in the sinus node and atrial tissue and is not effective in treating sinus or atrial dysrhythmias. However, there may be increased sensitivity to a diseased or ischemic sinus node, in which sinus arrest may occur.[38]
4. Lidocaine has little effect on the conduction time of the AV junction. However, there have been reports of accelerated AV conduction in response to rapid atrial dysrhythmias and of markedly depressed AV conduction in the presence of AV junctional disease.[38]

Indications for use

1. Lidocaine is the acute treatment of choice for both automatic and reentrant ventricular dysrhythmias, such as premature ventricular complexes; ventricular tachycardia or fibrillation resulting from acute myocardial infarction, surgical procedures, cardiac catheterization, digoxin toxicity; or other drug therapy such as dopamine or catecholamines.[3,44]

2. Lidocaine is also used prophylactically in the coronary care unit to prevent ventricular tachycardia and primary ventricular fibrillation from occurring in acute myocardial infarction.

3. Lidocaine has little effect in the treatment of atrial or junctional dysrhythmias and is not recommended.[3]

Contraindications

1. Lidocaine is contraindicated in the individual with known hypersensitivity to local anesthetics.

2. It should be used with caution in the presence of bradycardias since the rhythm may be of a passive nature, which lidocaine may further depress or abolish. In many instances the heart rate is accelerated by using a drug such as atropine before administration of lidocaine. If the ventricular dysrhythmia still persists, then lidocaine may be given.

3. Lidocaine is contraindicated in second-degree AV block, type II, and complete heart block, especially in the absence of a temporary or permanent pacemaker.

4. Caution should be used in individuals with impaired hepatic and renal function, congestive heart failure, or the elderly since metabolism and excretion of the drug occur in the liver and kidney, respectively. Typically, a reduction in dosage and frequent monitoring is required.

Preparation, dosage, and administration

1. Lidocaine comes prepared in 100-mg prefilled syringes ready for direct I.V. administration, 1000-mg (1 gm) prefilled syringes ready for dilution into an I.V. bag for continuous infusion, and in premixed I.V. bags of a 4% solution (1 gm lidocaine in 250 ml D_5W) for continuous I.V. infusion.

2. Only lidocaine hydrochloride injection without preservatives or catecholamines and clearly labeled for I.V. use should be used.

3. Dosing with lidocaine is a combination of using I.V. bolus injections and a continuous I.V. infusion. The usual initial dose is 1 mg/kg of body weight or 50- to 100-mg I.V. bolus. This should be infused at a rate not to exceed 25 mg per minute in order to prevent toxic symptoms from occurring. This bolus may be repeated every 5 to 10 minutes until suppression is achieved or a maximum of 225 mg is administered. Following bolus therapy, a continuous infusion of 2 to 4 mg per minute is necessary to maintain a steady state blood level because of lidocaine's rapid distribution, metabolism, and short half-life. A 4% solution (1 gm lidocaine in 250 ml D_5W) will yield a 4 mg/ml concentration.[3,61] Lidocaine is chemically stable for a minimum of 24 hours after dilution in D_5W.[20,24]

4. Lidocaine is absorbed poorly and irregularly from the gastrointestinal tract; therefore, oral forms are not available.

Absorption and excretion

1. Lidocaine is rapidly metabolized by the liver and has two pharmacologically active metabolites. Less than 10% of lidocaine is excreted in the urine unchanged.

2. Lidocaine is 70% to 80% protein bound and exerts its effects rapidly by direct action on target organs.

3. Therapeutic steady-state concentrations of lidocaine are related to infusion rate and elimination clearance, with variables relating to cardiac output, plasma volume, age, hepatic blood flow and function (direct relationship), total body weight, active metabolites, and to a lesser extent, renal function.[3]

    After a single I.V. bolus, the distribution half-life (to target organs) is 8 minutes, while the elimination half-life is 1½ hours in normal subjects. After prolonged infusion (over 48 hours), the half-life may rise to 4 hours.

4. The presence of metabolites may have additive effects on lidocaine's antidysrhythmic and convulsant properties and may become more pronounced in the presence of congestive heart failure.[3]

Serum levels

The desired or therapeutic plasma concentration is between 2 to 5 μg/ml. Toxic effects have been reported between 6 to 10 μg/ml, and 20 μg/ml has been reported as the seizure threshold.[3]

Side effects

1. Most side effects are dose related and affect the cardiovascular or central nervous systems: such as hypotension (at serum levels of 6 to 10 μg/ml); drowsiness; lightheadedness; dizziness; numbness of the lips, tongue, pharynx and/or face; dysphagia; dysarthria (difficulty in speaking); slurred speech; tinnitus; decreased hearing acuity; blurred or double vision; paresthesias, including sensations of heat or cold, excitement, and euphoria (at serum levels above 10 μg/ml); muscle tremors; altered mental status or confusion, hallucinations, and psychosis (at serum levels of 20 μg/ml); coma; and seizures. The seizure threshold is lowered by respiratory acidosis and/or alkalosis and may be followed by respiratory arrest.[3]

2. Other side effects include allergic reactions (urticaria, rash, edema, and anaphylactoid reaction), nausea, vomiting, anorexia, excessive perspiration, or local thrombophlebitis, usually after prolonged I.V. administration.

3. ECG effects of toxicity include: prolonged PR or QRS interval (rare), complete heart block, AV dissociation, bradycardia, sinus arrest (especially with sinus node dysfunction), and increased frequency of premature ventricular complexes or ventricular tachycardia.

Nursing management

1. Use only lidocaine without preservatives or epinephrine that is specifically labeled for intravenous use
2. Assess the patient before lidocaine administration for baseline vital sign parameters (blood pressure, heart rate and rhythm, respiratory status, neurological assessment, presence of a third heart sound, and pulmonary rales)
3. Monitor for and observe continuously for signs of toxicity. If they occur:
   a. Stop the infusion and stay with the patient, observing vital signs and neurological vital signs frequently; signs and symptoms will usually subside within 15 to 20 minutes, depending upon the duration of the infusion, age, and the presence of liver disease or congestive heart failure
   b. Monitor ECG and blood pressure continuously
   c. Have drugs and equipment available to treat adverse reactions such as hypotension, bradycardia, and seizures; avoid use of agents that will increase ventricular irritability
   d. Monitor respiratory status; maintain an open airway and oxygenation
4. Use a controlled infusion pump; if there is not one available, a microdrip tubing must be used (60 microdrops = 1 ml; microdrops per minute = ml/hr); record the dosage on the nurse's notes in mg/minute and the total dosage of lidocaine the patient has received in an 8- and 24-hour period
5. Never inject a bolus more rapidly than 25 to 50 mg/minute to avoid toxic central nervous system effects
6. Always infuse the least amount of drug that adequately controls the dysrhythmia; monitor the ECG continuously and the blood pressure every 10 to 15 minutes until the infusion rate is stabilized, then every hour; if the blood pressure falls, slow the infusion rate or discontinue, notify the physician, and increase the frequency of vital signs
7. Assess frequently for pulmonary rales and an S$_3$, especially in older patients and those with hepatic or severe cardiac disease who tend to metabolize the drug slowly[2,3,10]

Special considerations

Use lidocaine with caution in the following situations:
1. In patients receiving propranolol, a single large I.V. bolus of lidocaine may potentiate myocardial depression because of the abolition of compensatory sympathetic reflexes by beta blockade
2. In patients with severe liver or renal impairment, accumulation of plasma concentration of lidocaine may lead to toxic effects
3. Lidocaine should be avoided in patients with hypovolemic shock and congestive heart failure
4. Administration for PVCs in the presence of sinus bradycardia without prior acceleration of the sinus rate by atropine, isoproterenol, or pacing, may increase the frequency of the PVCs and possibly lead to ventricular tachycardia
5. While controlling immediate PVCs with lidocaine, other factors that can produce PVCs should be searched for and treated, such as hypoxia, pain, stimulants, digoxin toxicity, hypotension, or other drugs
6. Combined use of phenytoin and quinidine with lidocaine may have additive cardiodepressant effects
7. Older people may develop toxic symptoms more readily and the dosage should be decreased. If lidocaine toxicity develops, these people will continue to have symptoms for a longer period of time after the infusion is discontinued
8. Lidocaine should be discontinued with signs of prolonged conduction (prolongation of PR or QRS intervals) since the severity of the AV block may be increased
9. Lidocaine should be discontinued if a dysrhythmia appears or increases with drug therapy; the ventricular rate may increase in the presence of atrial fibrillation
10. Since lidocaine crosses the placental barrier, safety for use in pregnancy is not established
11. Knowledge of the effect of lidocaine dosage in children is limited[3,7,20,34]

PHENYTOIN
Actions

1. Phenytoin shortens the effective refractory period and decreases automaticity of the Purkinje fibers.
2. Phenytoin also reduces automaticity and suppresses afterdepolarizations caused by catecholamines or digoxin.[10]
3. Phenytoin decreases activity of sympathetic nerve fibers within the heart.[19]

Indications for use

1. Phenytoin is indicated in the treatment of dysrhythmias associated with digoxin toxicity, especially premature ventricular complexes and/or ventricular tachycar-

dia. It is also effective in the treatment of ventricular dysrhythmias associated with acute myocardial infarction, especially when they are nonresponsive to other drug therapy.[10,15]

2. Because of the potential for serious toxic effects with I.V. therapy and the bothersome effects of long-term oral therapy, phenytoin is mainly limited to the control of digoxin-induced dysrhythmias.

Contraindications

1. Phenytoin is contraindicated in patients with bradycardia and SA or AV blocks.
2. Precautions must be taken when administering the drug I.V. It may precipitate hypotension, bradycardia, asystole, or respiratory arrest.
3. Phenytoin is also extremely alkaline and readily causes irritation at the I.V. site that can lead to phlebitis.

Preparation, dosage, and administration

1. Phenytoin is available orally in 30-mg, 50-mg, and 100-mg capsules and in a 125-mg/5 ml suspension. For parenteral administration, it is supplied in a 100-mg prefilled syringe.
2. Phenytoin requires a loading dose to achieve therapeutic levels, otherwise it may take 5 to 15 days to achieve a therapeutic range. The loading dose for I.V. administration is 100 mg every 5 minutes until the dysrhythmia is suppressed or until 1 gm is given. Usually, 700 to 1000 mg is necessary. If given orally, 1 gm is given on the first day and 500 mg on the second and third day. After this dosing schedule, a maintenance dose of 300 to 400 mg daily is sufficient.
3. When giving phenytoin I.V., the rate should not exceed 50 mg per minute. It must be given in a normal saline solution and as close to the I.V. site as possible as a glucose solution causes precipitation of the drug and it readily binds to plastic tubing. The I.V. route is reserved for those situations when it is urgent to terminate the dysrhythmia.
4. The dosage for intramuscular (IM) administration is 100 to 150 mg every 8 hours although this is not a recommended route of administration because it causes pain and erratic absorption.[10,15,20]

Absorption and excretion

1. Phenytoin is readily absorbed by the gastrointestinal tract and is slowly absorbed IM because of poor solubility. Steady-state plasma levels are achieved in 3 to 7 days after initiation of oral therapy
2. To achieve rapid therapeutic serum levels, the I.V. route is necessary.
3. The plasma half-life of phenytoin ranges from 7 to 42 hours with an average of 22 hours. Phenytoin is

metabolized by the liver and is then excreted in the bile, where its active metabolites are reabsorbed and excreted by the kidney.[15]

Serum levels

The therapeutic serum level is 10 to 20 μg/ml.

Side effects

The side effects of phenytoin therapy affect the central nervous system primarily.

1. Following are some of the possible side effects: nystagmus, dizziness, confusion, visual disturbances, ataxia, neuropathy, somnolence, behavioral changes, nausea, vomiting, and gingivitis
2. Serious side effects usually associated with toxicity are hypotension, bradycardia, asystole, and respiratory depression

Nursing management

1. Administer oral preparations before or after meals to reduce gastrointestinal distress; inform the patient that the medication produces a harmless pink to reddish-brown discoloration of the urine
2. Instruct the patient to report central nervous system symptoms: nystagmus (at serum levels of 20 μg/ml or higher); ataxic gait (about 30 μg/ml); and constant lethargy (at 40 μg/ml)
3. Observe for signs of phlebitis and rotate I.V. site if giving the drug I.V.
4. If phenytoin is being given I.V. and the blood pressure decreases by more than 10 to 15 mm Hg, stop infusing until the blood pressure stabilizes
5. Only administer the drug I.V. if the patient is monitored and emergency resuscitation equipment is readily available
6. Monitor blood glucose levels since phenytoin inhibits insulin release and may result in hyperglycemia
7. Monitor the complete blood count since phenytoin has a depressant effect on the hematopoietic system
8. Instruct the patient to practice good oral hygiene to reduce the risk of gingivitis and to notify the physician if a rash develops[15,20]

Special considerations

1. Patients with liver disease or on medication that affects liver enzymes, such as oral anticoagulants, chloramphenicol, isoniazid, should be observed closely for signs of toxicity. It is recommended to maintain these patients at subtherapeutic plasma levels.
2. In elderly individuals with associated congestive heart failure, the I.V. administration of phenytoin is contraindicated.[10,15]

BRETYLIUM
Actions

1. Bretylium is described as a ganglionic blocking agent. It initially releases norepinephrine from the sympathetic nerve endings and then prevents the release of norepinephrine from the same nerve endings. It does this without depleting the site or decreasing the responsiveness of the adrenergic receptors to norepinephrine. This action can be described as a chemical sympathectomy.
2. Bretylium prolongs the effective refractory period of atrial and ventricular muscle fibers and of Purkinje fibers, which decreases the possible incidence of ventricular fibrillation.
3. Bretylium has a positive inotopic effect, the mechanism not being clear.
4. There is an initial increase in automaticity during bretylium administration because of the release of norepinephrine before blockade. This may initially increase the heart rate and/or blood pressure and resolves when norepinephrine stores are depleted. This effect may be prevented by the administration of a beta blocker before bretylium administration.[7,9,10]

Indications for use

1. Bretylium is indicated for the control of life-threatening ventricular dysrhythmias, especially ventricular fibrillation.
2. It is recommended as a first-line drug but is more commonly used in the treatment of ventricular tachycardia when lidocaine or procainamide fail to terminate the dysrhythmia.[35]

Contraindications

1. Bretylium is contraindicated in digoxin-induced dysrhythmias and in the presence of pheochromocytoma because there is an initial increase in automaticity as a result of catecholamine release.[35]
2. Bretylium is contraindicated in individuals with a fixed cardiac output, such as severe aortic stenosis, pulmonary hypertension, or right ventricular infarction, because of the profound vasodilatory action of the drug. This decreased afterload without the ability to compensate by increasing cardiac output is hazardous.[9,35]

Preparation, dosage, and administration

1. Bretylium is available in 500 mg/10 ml ampules for parenteral use only. The oral form is not currently approved for use in the United States.
2. The dose for life-threatening dysrhythmias is 5 mg/kg of body weight by I.V. bolus injection followed by DC countershock. If this is ineffective, the dose should be repeated at 10 mg/kg of body weight, again followed by DC countershock.
3. For recurrent or refractory ventricular tachycardia, 500 mg of bretylium diluted in 50 ml D_5W or normal saline solution may be infused over 10 to 20 minutes. If the dysrhythmia is not suppressed, the dose may be repeated up to 10 mg/kg. The total daily dose should not exceed 30 mg/kg.
4. To maintain therapeutic levels, a continuous infusion should be delivered at a range of 0.5 to 2.0 mg per minute.
5. Bretylium may be given as an undiluted IM injection of 5 to 10 mg/kg every 1 to 2 hours until the dysrhythmia is suppressed and then every 6 hours. A maximum of 5 ml per injection site is recommended. This route is not recommended for life-threatening situations.

Absorption and excretion

1. The oral form of bretylium (under investigation) is poorly absorbed with only 50% bioavailability.
2. Bretylium is minimally metabolized in the liver and is excreted essentially unchanged in the urine. Renal dysfunction may predispose to toxicity.[10,22] The half-life ranges from 8 to 10 hours.[22]

Serum levels

Therapeutic serum levels have not been ascertained as therapeutic levels are not correlated with antidysrhythmic effects.

Side effects

1. Cardiovascular
   a. Initial increase in heart rate, blood pressure, and the dysrhythmia may occur because of the initial release of norepinephrine. This persists until blockade occurs or for up to 30 minutes. This may be magnified in patients with digoxin-induced dysrhythmias.[35]
   b. Hypotension may occur as a result of sympathetic blockade. This hypotension is orthostatic in nature because of peripheral vasodilation and may be lessened if the patient remains supine. Patients with compromised cardiac function may experience hypotension even in the supine position and it may persist even with the administration of fluids and pressor agents.
2. Gastrointestinal
   a. Nausea and vomiting occur most commonly with rapid I.V. administration and may be minimized by giving the drug over a 10- to 30-minute period.

3. Central nervous system
   a. Vertigo, dizziness, lightheadedness, and syncope may occur as a result of hypotension.

Nursing management

1. Monitor heart rate, blood pressure, and rhythm every 5 minutes during initial I.V. therapy and notify the physician immediately of any change; do not leave the patient's bedside
2. If the systolic blood pressure falls below 70, notify the physician who may order vasopressors or volume expanders; maintain the patient in a supine position until a tolerance to sympathetic blockade develops
3. Angina may occur with initial administration; inform the physician if this occurs and await further orders; administer bretylium by a controlled infusion pump if giving a continuous I.V. drip
4. Administer I.V. injections undiluted as rapidly as possible under constant observation for the control of ventricular fibrillation
5. Observe the patient's response carefully as the correction of other ventricular dysrhythmias occurs less rapidly than does ventricular fibrillation; bretylium may be used with other resuscitative measures
6. Avoid subtherapeutic doses (less than 5 mg/kg) as lower doses seem to precipitate hypotension

Special considerations

1. Bretylium is usually reserved for patients who do not respond to other types of therapy, even though it is now accepted as a first-line drug.
2. Bretylium should be administered with caution in digoxin intoxication. Use with caution in patients with fixed cardiac output such as aortic stenosis since they may not be able to compensate for the peripheral vasodilation.
3. Catecholamines should be administered with caution since they will have a significantly pronounced effect. The dosage of bretylium should be decreased in patients with renal failure, as the main route of excretion is through the kidney.

BETA-BLOCKING AGENTS

Currently in the United States there are six beta-blocking agents approved for use. They are propranolol, metoprolol, atenolol, nadolol, timolol, pindolol. They currently are approved for many uses but this discussion will be limited to antidysrhythmic indications. The original beta blocker, propranolol, will be discussed in detail and the remaining five drugs will be compared and contrasted accordingly.

Propranolol (Inderal)
Actions

1. Propranolol produces nonselective $beta_1$ and $beta_2$ adrenergic–receptor blockade. $Beta_1$ blockade causes a negative inotropic, chronotropic, and dromotropic effect that results in oxygen sparing. $Beta_2$ blockade causes increased airway resistance to the point of bronchoconstriction.
2. Propranolol decreases automaticity in sinus and ectopic pacemaker cells and prolongs the refractory period in the AV junction.
3. Propranolol and the other beta-blocking agents do not effect ventricular conduction.

Indications for use

1. Propranolol is indicated for the treatment of supraventricular tachydysrhythmias, including atrial flutter and fibrillation.
2. However, the treatment of atrial flutter is often more effective when propranolol is combined with digoxin.[10]
3. Beta-blocking agents such as propranolol rarely convert an atrial dysrhythmia to normal sinus rhythm.
4. Propranolol may terminate or prevent a reentrant tachycardia such as occurs with the AV junction and an accessory pathway in Wolff-Parkinson-White syndrome.
5. Propranolol is used in treating dysrhythmias induced by digoxin, prolonged QT intervals, and catecholamines.
6. Beta blockers such as propranolol are useful in treating exertional angina by reducing the heart's response to catecholamines, preventing an increase in heart rate and cardiac output, and preventing an increase in oxygen demand.
7. Beta blockers are also used in prophylactic treatment to prevent sudden cardiac death after myocardial infarction.[4]

Contraindications

1. Propranolol should be used with caution in patients with bronchial asthma, emphysema, Raynaud's disease, sinus bradycardia, second-degree or complete AV block, or in combination with other myocardial depressants, including amiodarone.
2. Caution should be used in diabetic patients or persons with hyperthyroidism, as beta blockers can mask symptoms. For example, a diabetic with hypoglycemia may not show heart rate or blood pressure changes or diaphoresis.[20,24,27]

Preparation, dosage, and administration

1. Propranolol is available in oral and parenteral forms. The dosage is individualized to clinical response. A significant percentage of the drug is metabolized by the liver via portal circulation after oral ingestion; thus, there is significant dosage variation between the oral and parenteral routes.
2. In the treatment of cardiac dysrhythmias, a dose of 10 to 30 mg orally every 6 to 8 hours should be given. Parenteral therapy is reserved for those who become symptomatic or are seriously compromised hemodynamically from the dysrhythmia.
3. The I.V. dose is 0.5 to 3 mg. Propranolol administered parenterally comes packaged in 1 mg/1 ml ampules. Each mg is given over 3- to 5-minute intervals under closely monitored conditions until the dysrhythmia is terminated.
4. The oral dosage for the treatment of angina ranges from 10 to 80 mg every 6 to 8 hours and from 160 to 480 mg daily in the treatment of hypertension.[20,24]

Absorption and excretion

1. Propranolol is almost completely absorbed from the gastrointestinal tract but undergoes an extensive metabolism in the liver, significantly reducing bioavailability.
2. The onset of action occurs after approximately 30 minutes with oral administration and 2 minutes with I.V. administration. The peak serum concentration is 60 to 90 minutes oral and 15 minutes I.V. with duration of action 6 hours and 3 to 6 hours, respectively.
3. The half-life ranges from 1 to 8 hours, the average being 4 hours.
4. Propranolol is largely metabolized in the liver and excreted in the kidney.

Serum levels

The therapeutic serum level ranges from 50 to 100 mg/ml. A high degree of effective beta blockade is considered achieved at 100 mg/ml. However, a heart rate response of 50 to 55 beats per minute is a more reliable indicator since there is individual patient variance in metabolism.

Side effects

1. The most significant side effects include depressed myocardial contractility, sinus bradycardia, bronchospasm, nausea, vomiting, fatigue, sleep disturbance, depression, and impotence.
2. Signs and symptoms of hypoglycemia and thyrotoxicosis may be masked.

3. Occasionally bradycardia may be severe and associated with hypotension, shock, and angina. This is usually associated with I.V. use in the patient who is relying on significant catecholamine stimulation for compensation. Profound bradycardia can also be seen with combination beta blocker–amiodarone therapy.
4. A short-lived eosinophilia, as well as thrombocytopenia, may occur as a response to beta blockade. When withdrawal of beta blockade is abrupt, there may be a sympathetic rebound effect such as increase in angina or a worsening of the dysrhythmia because of a sudden increase in sensitivity to catecholamines. Because of this, drug therapy should be tapered over 2 weeks.[20,24]

Nursing management

1. Carefully assess and monitor the patient receiving propranolol for the following: heart rate and rhythm, blood pressure (hypotension), signs of congestive heart failure, signs of bronchial constriction (assess lung sounds before therapy and note any wheezing that may develop during therapy), AV blocks, and decreased urine output.
2. If the physician writes an order to discontinue propranolol, question how the patient is to be weaned. Always *wean* the patient from propranolol therapy to decrease a rebound sympathetic response.
3. Have atropine available (for severe bradycardia), vasopressors (for hypotension), and isoproterenol and aminophylline (for bronchospasm). Cardiac failure is usually treated with digoxin and diuretics.
4. Caution patients that propranolol will interfere with the body's adaptive response to exercise and stress. Lightheadedness, weakness, fatigue, and dyspnea may be experienced when the patient exercises or is stressed.
5. Follow intake and output and daily weights on all patients for signs of congestive heart failure. Monitor the diabetic patient closely for hypoglycemia.

Special considerations

See Nursing management.

Metoprolol (Lopressor)

Metoprolol is different from propranolol in that it is cardioselective or only inhibits beta$_1$ responses; therefore, it is less likely to produce bronchospasm. It is used more frequently in the control of hypertension, afterload reduction, or angina rather than for control of dysrhythmias.

The half-life is 3 to 4 hours with oral doses ranging from 50 to 100 mg twice daily.

Antenolol (Tenormin)

Atenolol is very similar to metoprolol. It is a beta$_1$-selective adrenergic blocker. Similarly, it is used in the treatment of hypertension and angina. Many clinicians prefer metoprolol and atenolol for the treatment of angina and hypertension since lower doses can be used. There is also greater safety in using atenolol in the treatment of patients with diabetes and chronic obstructive pulmonary disease because of the absence of the beta$_2$ effect.

Nadolol (Corgard)

1. Nadolol is similar to propranolol and is a nonselective adrenergic blocking agent. It differs from propranolol in that the negative inotropic effects are significantly less, although there are negative chronotropic and dromotropic effects.
2. Nadolol has a half-life of 20 to 24 hours as it is metabolized very little and is excreted unchanged in the urine. This allows a one-time daily dose that ranges from 40 to 240 mg orally.[10,27]
3. Nadolol is most effective in the treatment of supraventricular dysrhythmias since it slows conduction velocity in the atrial muscle and the AV junction. It has little or no effect in ventricular muscle or Purkinje fibers and is not recommended for the treatment of ventricular dysrhythmias. A decreased dosage is required for persons with renal failure.

Timolol (Blockadren)

1. Timolol is a nonselective adrenergic blocker very similar to nadolol in pharmacological effects. It is similar to propranolol in metabolism and excretion.
2. Timolol is used in the treatment of hypertension, chronic angina, and chronic supraventricular dysrhythmias.

Pindolol (Visken)

1. Pindolol is a nonselective adrenergic blocker similar to propranolol. Unlike other beta blockers, pindolol exerts an intrinsic sympathetic agonist activity that significantly decreases resting effects on heart rate, AV conduction, myocardial contractility, and airway resistance, while still blocking the exercise- or stress-induced changes mediated by catecholamines.
2. Currently, pindolol is recommended for the treatment of hypertension and chronic angina. Studies have not confirmed its effectiveness in the treatment of chronic atrial or ventricular dysrhythmias. Table 8-3, p. 208, gives a comparison of the beta-blocking agents.[20,24,27]

AMIODARONE*
Actions

1. Amiodarone increases the effective refractory period of the atrial and ventricular muscle, the AV junction, His-Purkinje system, and in accessory pathways such as are seen in the Wolff-Parkinson-White syndrome. Automaticity of the sinus node is decreased.
2. Amiodarone exerts a noncompetitive antiadrenergic action on both alpha and beta receptors,[40] thereby decreasing coronary and peripheral vascular resistance and myocardial oxygen consumption; it is minimally negatively inotropic.[30,63]
3. These actions may produce the following ECG changes: prolongation of PR and QT intervals and sinus bradycardia. The bradycardia, which may be atropine resistant, can be pronounced if amiodarone is given in combination with beta-blocking agents.[30,40]

Indications for use

1. Amiodarone is indicated in the treatment of complex ventricular dysrhythmias unresponsive to conventional therapy.
2. It is successful in the treatment of supraventricular tachycardias, especially those caused by AV junctional or accessory pathway reentry (see Junctional Dysrhythmias module).

Contraindications

Currently, no contraindications are identified in the patient population experiencing life-threatening dysrhythmias refractory to conventional therapy.

1. In patients with a high degree of AV block and second-degree, type II, or complete heart block, pacemaker therapy must be initiated before drug administration.[42]
2. Caution should be used in persons with iodine allergies or sensitivity as each 200-mg tablet contains 75 mg of iodine. These patients must be monitored closely for allergic responses.[30,40]

Serum levels

Effective levels range from 0.5 to 2.5 µg/ml. Some studies show efficacy in levels as low as 0.1 µg/ml or as high as 11.9 µg/ml. It is reported that supraventricular dysrhythmias respond with lower serum concentrations compared to ventricular dysrhythmias.[63]

Absorption and excretion

1. Amiodarone is absorbed erratically and unpredictably, which results in a bioavailability of 22% to 86%.

---

*As of this printing, amiodarone is still on investigational status.

TABLE 8-3. Comparison of beta-adrenergic blocking agents[10,27]

Beta-blocking agent	Activity		Intrinsic sympathetic agonist	Absorption	Metabolism and excretion	Half-life (hour)	Dosage
	Beta₁	Beta₂					
Propranolol	✓	✓		90%	Hepatic Excreted in the urine	3.4-6	*Oral* Hypertension: 160-480 mg/day in divided doses Angina: 40-240 mg/day in divided doses Dysrhythmias: 10-30 mg every 6 to 8 hours *IV* Acute dysrhythmias: 0.5-3 mg
Metoprolol	✓			95%	Hepatic Excreted in the urine	3-4	*Oral* Hypertension: 100-450 mg/day Angina: 50-100 mg/day (Divide every 8 to 12 hours)
Atenolol	✓			50%	Excreted in the urine	16-27	*Oral* Hypertension: 50-100 mg/day Angina: 100 mg/day (One dose daily)
Nadolol	✓	✓		30%	Excreted in the urine unchanged	10-24	*Oral* Hypertension: 80-320 mg/day Angina: 40-240 mg/day (One dose daily)
Timolol	✓	✓		90%	Hepatic Renal	3-4	*Oral* Hypertension: 20-40 mg/day Angina: 15-45 mg/day (Divide every 6 to 8 hours)
Pindolol	✓	✓	✓	50-95% 60%	Low hepatic Excreted in the urine unchanged	3-4	*Oral* Hypertension: 5 mg every 12 hours Angina: 15-40 mg daily (One dose daily)

Achieving therapeutic levels following oral therapy may take between 2 to 30 days. Amiodarone is highly lipophilic (fat soluble) and is distributed extensively throughout body tissues. This high distribution prolongs the half-life from 13 to 100 days following long-term oral therapy.

2. Amiodarone may still be detectable in the serum up to 6 months or in the urine up to 1 year after therapy is discontinued.[40,42,63]

3. Amiodarone is metabolized in the liver, resulting in an active metabolite, desethyl amiodarone. Studies have shown that no unchanged drug is found in the urine. Amiodarone may also be excreted in the bile, only to be reabsorbed again.[22,63]

Preparation, dosage, and administration

1. Amiodarone is available for oral and I.V. therapy. The oral dose is 200 to 800 mg daily as a loading dose for 8 to 15 days or until a therapeutic clinical response is achieved. The maintenance dose is adjusted to the minimal amount of drug needed to maintain rhythm control and may vary from 200 mg per week to 300 mg daily for supraventricular tachycardias and to 400 to 800 mg daily for complex, life-threatening ventricular dysrhythmias.[42,63]

2. The I.V. dose is 5 to 10 mg/kg, diluted in 20 ml D_5W and administered over 10 minutes. The effect should be evident immediately when the drug is infused and continues for 20 minutes to 4 hours. A second I.V. dose may be repeated but only after 15 minutes have elapsed. If administered too rapidly, tachycardia may occur, which can be related to the form of diluent used, particularly one containing benzylic alcohol. Hypotension, AV block, hot flashes, or complete cardiovascular collapse may also occur; thus, I.V. administration requires continuous monitoring.[63]

Side effects

1. The most serious side effect is the development of pulmonary fibrosis. With careful clinical follow-up, however, this effect has been limited to an incidence of less than 5% in the United States.[22,33,42]

2. Other side effects include anorexia, nausea, vomiting, weakness, thyroid function abnormalities, hepatic insufficiency, corneal microdeposits, bluish skin discoloration, insomnia, nightmares, tremor, headache, and rare neuropathy.[6,22,40,42,63]

3. Amiodarone potentiates the effects of warfarin and elevates serum digoxin concentrations to the point of toxicity.[14,22,28,42]

4. Amiodarone also potentiates effects of vasodilators, beta blockers, and class I antidysrhythmic agents.[22,42,63]

Nursing management

1. Establish and follow closely baseline thyroid function (T_3, T_4, and TSH), pulmonary function, and liver function as well as conducting an eye examination before amiodarone therapy is initiated

2. Give emotional support to the patient and family because of the life-threatening nature of ventricular dysrhythmias

3. Monitor the patient closely during I.V. and oral therapy for side effects, especially bradycardia, hypotension, and cardiovascular collapse

4. Be aware of interactions with other drugs (see Side effects)

5. Instruct the patient to report visual changes, symptoms of thyroid dysfunction, or excessively slow heart rates to the physician

6. Instruct the patient to use a sunscreen if prolonged exposure to sunlight is anticipated; many patients will be discharged with a telephone monitoring device and must be instructed as to its use

VERAPAMIL

Verapamil is included in a classification of drugs known as calcium antagonists or calcium-channel blockers. There are currently two other drugs in this class, nifedipine and diltiazem. The latter two drugs are not used as frequently as antidysrhythmic agents but they do have electrophysiological effects.

Actions

1. Verapamil is known to inhibit the cell membrane influx of the calcium ion in myocardial and vascular smooth muscle. Calcium is used in the cell for two purposes: electrical impulse transmission and myofibril contraction. As a result of reducing the influx of calcium, the following will result:
   a. Decrease in automaticity of the pacemaker cells of the sinus node and AV junction
   b. Decrease in speed of conduction through the AV junction (a negative dromotropic effect)
   c. A negative inotropic effect
   d. Systemic arterial vasodilation
   e. The possibility of reducing the area of necrosis during coronary occlusion[26,47]

2. Verapamil has no effect on the refractory period of accessory pathways.[10]

Indications for use

1. Verapamil is indicated in the treatment of supraventricular tachycardias and atrial flutter and fibrillation, especially those related to circus movement reentry in the AV junction. The ventricular response to atrial

flutter and fibrillation is slowed but the flutter and fibrillation may not be terminated.

2. Verapamil may be used in the Wolff-Parkinson-White syndrome to interrupt a reentry circuit by prolonging the refractory period through the AV node only. It has no effect on the accessory pathway.[10]

3. Verapamil has been used in idiopathic hypertrophic subaortic stenosis (IHSS) with some success. Its effect seems to be related to the improvement in diastolic compliance (stretch) rather than by decreasing myocardial contractility; however, it is not the drug of choice for this condition.[26]

4. Verapamil is also used in controlling exertional angina by its effect of decreasing myocardial oxygen demands; however, large doses are frequently required to maintain this effect.[20,26]

Contraindications

1. Verapamil is contraindicated in the presence of second-degree, type II, or complete AV block in the absence of pacemaker therapy.

2. Extreme caution should be used in hypotension, congestive heart failure, SA node dysfunction, shock, or with concurrent use of I.V. beta blockade, as this may result in profound hypotension or asystole.

3. Verapamil should also be used with caution in patients with liver disease because of its high hepatic metabolism rate.

4. Verapamil will elevate serum digoxin levels but usually not enough to produce toxic effects.[10,26,47]

Preparation, dosage, and administration

1. Verapamil is available in oral and parenteral preparations. The oral dose ranges from 80 to 120 mg every 6 to 8 hours. The onset of action is within 1 hour, with peak serum levels achieved in 3 to 4 hours.

2. The I.V. preparation is packaged in a 2-ml ampule, 5 mg/ml. The usual dose is 0.1 mg/kg given over 1 to 2 minutes. The peak effect occurs within 2 to 5 minutes and the duration of action is less than 1 hour. The dose may be repeated in 30 minutes if the desired clinical response is not achieved.

Absorption and excretion

1. Verapamil is 90% absorbed via the oral route and is highly metabolized in the liver on its first pass through. This is well demonstrated by the variance between the oral and parenteral dose. It is highly protein bound and has an active metabolite.

2. Fifteen percent of verapamil is excreted in the feces within 5 days and 70% is excreted in the urine, 3% to 4% as unchanged drug.[20,26]

3. The oral half-life is 3 to 7 hours and the I.V. half-life is 2 to 8 hours.

Serum levels

A serum level of 125 mg/ml has been reported to accurately terminate a rapid supraventricular dysrhythmia. This is achieved by I.V. administration between 0.075 mg/kg to 0.150 mg/kg.[20,44]

Side effects

1. Side effects are usually dose related and not limiting and include gastrointestinal upset, constipation because of decreased intestinal motility, vertigo, headache, and nervousness. These may occur as a result of hypotension. Administering verapamil with or after meals may decrease the gastrointestinal symptoms.

2. After I.V. administration, observe for hypotension, AV blocks, bradycardia, or signs of heart failure.

3. Because of vasodilation, peripheral edema may result from venous compliance; however, it is not related to heart failure.[26]

4. When verapamil and digoxin are given concurrently to control the ventricular response in atrial fibrillation, the serum digoxin concentrations increase. This mechanism is related to reduction in renal tubular secretion, in metabolic clearance, and in the volume of distribution of digoxin. Patients are prone to gastrointestinal effects rather than dysrhythmia effects.[47]

Nursing management

1. When administering verapamil I.V., monitor heart rate, rhythm, and blood pressure continuously and maintain the patient in the supine position, if possible, to prevent hypotension

2. Observe for signs of congestive heart failure (shortness of breath, increased heart rate, dizziness, presence of a third heart sound)

3. Monitor closely for side effects when giving verapamil concurrently with digoxin, vasodilators, or beta blockers

4. Administer oral verapamil with or after meals to minimize the gastrointestinal side effects

5. Monitor neurovital signs if conversion from atrial fibrillation to normal sinus rhythm is achieved

6. Monitor drug administration closely in the elderly and in patients with sinus node dysfunction (NOTE: Nifedipine and diltiazem are not discussed in this text as their major use is not antidysrhythmic. Table 8-4 gives a brief comparison of these drugs and verapamil.)

TABLE 8-4. Comparison of calcium channel blockers[20,24,26]

Drug	Indications for use	Metabolism and excretion	Dose	Half-life	Serum level	Actions					Side effects
						Heart rate	AV conduction	Coronary vasodilation	Peripheral vasodilation	Contractility	
Verapamil	Supraventricular tachycardias (reentrant) Atrial flutter and fibrillation Coronary artery spasm Not recommended for accessory pathways Use investigationally in IHSS and hypertension	90% absorbed after oral dose Metabolized in liver with 10-20% bioavailability Excreted in feces and urine	*Oral* 80-120 mg. every 6 to 8 hours OOA-1 hr *I.V.* 5-10 mg over 1-2 minutes OOA = 1-2 minutes Peak = 1 hr May repeat in 15-30 minutes if no response	3-7 hours (5) 2-8 hours	200-600 ng/ml	± Reflex ↑ by ↓ afterload	↓ ↓	++ ↓ coronary resistance ↑ coronary blood flow	++ ↓ preload and afterload ↓ myocardial oxygen demands	↓ ↓ Most pronounced in patients with existing left ventricular dysfunction	Usually dose related and not limiting GI upset Constipation ++. Vertigo Headache Nervousness Hypotension (especially after I.V. administration) may exacerbate congestive heart failure (CHF) Contraindicated in AV block; may increase serum digoxin levels
Nifedipine	Coronary artery spasm Hypertension Cerebral artery spasm Suggested for Raynaud's disease	90% absorbed after oral dose Metabolized in liver with 10-20% bioavailability Excreted in feces and urine	*Oral* 10-30 mg. every 8 hours OOA = less than 20 minutes *Sublingual* 10 mg. must puncture capsule OOA = less than 3 minutes Peak (oral) 1-2 hours	3-5 hours (4)	25-100 ng/ml	↑ reflex only by ↓ afterload		+++	+++	± Reflex ↑ cardiac output by ↓ afterload	Hypotension +++ Headache +++ Peripheral Edema +++ Can be used safely with beta blockers but observe for AV block; may increase serum digoxin levels
Diltiazem	Coronary artery spasm Angina Exertional angina Hypertension Preservation of myocardium on heart-lung bypass machine After myocardial infarction (drug of choice for elderly)	90% absorbed 80% protein bound Metabolized in liver with 20-50% bioavailability Excreted in urine	*Oral* 30-90 mg. every 6 to 8 hours OOA = 30 minutes Peak = 30 minutes to 2 hrs *I.V.* Investigational, 75-150 µg/ml	2-6 hours (4) Up to 10 hours in elderly	50-200 ng/ml	↓	↓	+++	+	-	Fewest side effects Hypotension + Peripheral edema ++ AV block + Can be safely used with beta blockers

↑ = increase, ↓ = decrease, OOA = onset of action. (+) = small, (++) = moderate, (+++) = severe, ± = no change.

ISOPROTERENOL
Actions

Isoproterenol is an adrenergic stimulant, having both $beta_1$ and $beta_2$ effects.

1. Beta$_1$ stimulation results in an increase in contractility and heart rate. Electrophysiological effects include increased automaticity of all pacemaker cells, increased speed of conduction through the AV junction, and shortening of the effective refractory period in ventricular muscle and Purkinje fibers.
2. Beta$_2$ stimulation results in dilation of the bronchioles and of the peripheral vasculature.

Indications for use

1. Isoproterenol is indicated in the treatment of symptomatic bradycardia or sinoatrial block unresponsive to atropine, high degrees of AV block (to increase rate while the patient awaits pacemaker insertion), and in the treatment of cardiogenic shock and *torsade de pointes*.[10,35,49]
2. It is also considered a useful agent to stimulate the myocardium in asystole.[35]

Contraindications

1. Isoproterenol is contraindicated in the presence of tachydysrhythmias, especially if they are digoxin-induced.
2. It is also contraindicated in the presence of hypovolemia, hypoxia, or hypokalemia until the abnormality has been corrected.[35]
3. Isoproterenol is not recommended and/or should be used with extreme caution in acute myocardial infarction because of the positive inotropic effect and resultant significant increase in myocardial oxygen demand, both of which increase the risk of extending the infarct.[35]

Preparation, dosage, and administration

Isoproterenol is available for I.V. use in a 1:5000 solution and in 0.2 mg/ml and 1.0 mg/5 ml ampules. The usual concentration is 1 mg of isoproterenol diluted in 250 ml D$_5$W, yielding 4 μg/ml, or 1 mg in 500 ml D$_5$W, yielding 2 μg/ml. The dosage ranges from 2 to 20 μg/min titrated to heart rate and rhythm response.[20,24,35]

Absorption and excretion

1. Intravenous isoproterenol is completely absorbed, metabolized mainly in the liver, and is excreted in the urine.
2. When given I.V. 75% of the dose is excreted in the urine within 22 hours.[20]

Serum levels

Not established.

Side effects

1. The major side effects of isoproterenol are related to its tachycardic and dysrhythmic properties, which may precipitate ventricular tachycardia and/or fibrillation.[35]
2. Other side effects include anxiety, restlessness, sweating, flushing, nausea, and vomiting.

Nursing management

1. Give isoproterenol only under carefully monitored conditions and by controlled infusion pump
2. If the heart rate exceeds 230 beats per minute, serious ventricular dysrhythmias may occur; observe the patient for angina and notify the physician immediately if it occurs
3. Observe for drug interactions:
   a. Combined use with other sympathetic stimulant drugs may precipitate cardiotoxicity
   b. Propranolol is antagonistic to isoproterenol and concomitant use should be avoided
4. Monitor arterial blood gases in low cardiac output states
5. Monitor blood glucose levels as isoproterenol stimulates insulin secretion and glycogenolysis.[20,24]

Special considerations

See Nursing management.

ATROPINE
Actions

Atropine sulfate is a vagolytic agent that inhibits the action of acetylcholine, the neurotransmitter of the parasympathetic nervous system. This action results in increased automaticity of the SA node and increased speed of conduction through the AV junction.[35]

Indications for use

1. Atropine is indicated for the treatment of symptomatic bradyrhythms, such as sinus bradycardia, sinus arrest, and sinoatrial block, especially when associated with hypotension or frequent ventricular ectopic complexes.[35] It is of benefit in first-degree and second-degree, type I, AV blocks. It may be used for second degree, type II, or complete AV block but usually is ineffective as excessive vagal tone is not the primary cause of such blocks.
2. Atropine is also used to counteract the bradycardia associated with morphine or edrophonium (Tensilon).[20]

3. Atropine is also used in cardiac emergencies in the presence of ventricular asystole.[35]

Contraindications

1. Atropine is contraindicated in acute myocardial infarction since it increases oxygen demand and may precipitate ventricular tachycardia and/or fibrillation. It is only used if there is bradycardia associated with low cardiac output and/or frequent ventricular ectopic complexes.[35]
2. Atropine is also contraindicated in patients with narrow-angle glaucoma and adhesions.

Preparation, dosage and administration

1. Atropine comes packaged in three forms: 10-ml (0.1 mg/ml) and 5-ml (0.1 mg/ml) prefilled syringes and in 20-ml (0.4 mg/ml) or (0.5 mg/ml) multidose vials, all for parenteral use.
2. The usual dosage is 0.5 to 1.0 mg I.V. given over a period of 30 seconds to 1 minute.
   a. This may be repeated in 0.5-mg doses every 5 minutes until a described rate is established, usually above 60 beats per minute, or until a total of 2.0 mg is given, which is thought to be a complete vagolytic dose.[35]
   b. Doses less than 0.5 mg may slow the heart rate via a central vagal stimulating or peripheral parasympathomimetic effects.[35] This may also occur if the dose is administered too slowly.
3. Atropine may be given IM but this is not usually recommended since a transient slowing of heart rate may occur.

Absorption and excretion

1. The action of atropine occurs almost immediately with I.V. administration and peaks in 1 to 2 hours. Atropine stays in the serum up to 4 hours. It is well absorbed from all administration sites and is widely distributed in body tissues. Atropine crosses both the blood-brain and placental barriers.
2. Approximately 50% of the dose is rapidly excreted in the urine within 24 hours as an unchanged drug. Traces may appear in breast milk.[20,24,44]

Serum levels

Not established.

Side effects

1. Cardiac side effects include premature ventricular complexes, ventricular tachycardia, and/or fibrillation, especially in the presence of acute myocardial infarction. A rebound tachycardia may also occur.[35]

2. Other side effects include inability to void (more common in the elderly or in persons with prostatic hypertrophy), dryness of the mouth and skin, flushing, dilation of pupils, mental confusion, and acute glaucoma.
3. Toxic signs include rash on upper trunk and face, hypertension, restlessness, excitement, disorientation, delerium, hallucinations, hyperthermia, and respiratory depression. If these signs appear, simply withhold atropine.

Nursing management

1. Closely assess and monitor patients receiving atropine for changes in heart rate and rhythm, blood pressure, temperature, character of respirations, and neurovital signs
2. Maintain the patient on bedrest for a period of time after atropine administration to prevent postural hypotension
3. Observe for pulmonary complications that could develop as a result of a reduction in secretions.
4. Observe for urinary retention and visual changes, especially in the elderly; monitor intake and output every 8 hours
5. Assure adequate fluid intake to counteract the constipating effects of atropine; the effects of atropine are greatest in the younger person as vagal tone diminishes with age[20,24,44]

INVESTIGATIONAL DRUGS

The search for an ideal antidysrhythmic agent with minimal side effects is an ongoing process. Because of this, there will always be new pharmacological agents being introduced. The following drugs are currently listed as investigational in the United States and are not available for general use. However, Table 8-5 on pp. 214-215 gives a brief description of their actions, dosage, indications for use, and side effects.

The drugs included are tocainide,* flecainide, encainide, lorcainide, mexiletine, ethmozine, and cibenzoline. (See also amiodarone, p. 207.)

Electrolyte imbalances

Electrolytes play an important role in normal cardiac electrical and mechanical function. Abnormalities of any electrolyte will have some effects on cardiac function, and typically more than one electrolyte will be involved. Therefore the ECG effects of any one anion or cation is often masked. However, the ECG effects of potassium imbalances are often seen before the development of other

---

*Tocainide HCl is now available under the trade name, Tonocard, and is off investigational status.

TABLE 8-5. Comparison of investigational antidysrhythmic agents*

Drug	Class	Use	Form	Dosage	Serum levels	Half-life	Side effects
Tocainide†	IB	Premature ventricular complexes Symptomatic ventricular tachycardia Prevention of ventricular tachycardia/ ventricular fibrillation after myocardial infarction	p.o.	*Oral* 400-600 mg every 8 to 12 hours, taken with meals; daily dose total 1200-2400 mg	6-12 µg/ml	15 hours	*Lidocaine-like* Dizziness, nervousness, agitation, tremors, paresthesias, vertigo, diplopia, memory loss, confusion, seizures, pulmonary fibrosis, blood dyscrasias (rare) (symptoms may limit use)
Flecainide	IC	Premature atrial complexes and ventricular complexes	p.o. I.V.	*Oral* 200-400 mg/daily, given in divided doses every 12 hours	400-800 µg/ml	14-20 hours	*Negatively inotropic* Hypotension Prolongation of QRS/QT intervals
Encainide	I	Premature supraventricular and ventricular complexes	p.o. I.V.	*Oral* 25-75 mg every 6 to 8 hours (total dosage 75-240 mg/day); monitored to QRS widening up to limit of 50% *I.V.* 1 mg/kg for 15-20 minutes	16 µg/ml Higher for I.V.	3 hours	*May exacerbate dysrhythmias* Prolongation of PR, QRS, QT intervals; risk of *torsade de pointes*; may depress LV function; CHF nausea, headache, weakness, dizziness, and blurred vision
Lorcainide	IC	Premature ventricular complexes especially after myocardial infarction	p.o. I.V.	*Oral* 100-200 mg every 12 hours			Increased incidence of atrial flutter and fibrillations; sleep disturbances

Drug	Class	Indication	Route	Dose	Range	Half-life	Side effects
Mexiletine	IB	Premature ventricular complexes	p.o. I.V. (↑ incidence of side effects)	*Oral* 200-300 mg every 8 hours *Loading* 250 mg over 5 minutes, continuous infusion 60-90 mg/hr	Range 0.75-2 µg/ml (1.6 µg/ml)	9-13 hours	Tremors, seizures, dizziness, ataxia, nystagmus, paresthesias, diplopia, confusion, anorexia, nausea, dyspepsia, vomiting, hypotension, and bradycardia
Ethmozine	I	Premature ventricular complexes	p.o.	*Oral* 200-300 mg every 8 hours	3.5 µg/ml	5-7 hours	*Few side effects* Prolongation of QRS without QT, dizziness, vertigo, headache, nausea, G.I. distress palpitations with therapy, pruritis without rash
Cibenzoline	I	Supraventricular tachycardia in Wolff-Parkinson-White syndrome (WPW) Premature ventricular complexes/ventricular tachycardia	p.o.	*Oral* 65-100 mg every 6 hours or 130-160 mg every 12 hours			*Negatively inotropic and anticholinergic* Dry mouth and skin, urinary hesitancy, blurred vision, and epigastric distress

*See references 6, 22, 29, 32, 42, 52, and 60.
†Now off investigational status.

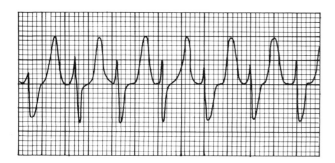

FIG. 8-9

Earliest sign of hyperkalemia: tall, peaked T wave.

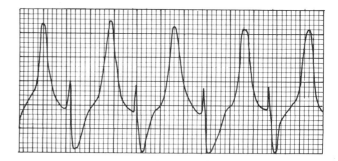

FIG. 8-10

Prolongation of PR interval with P buried in T, reflected as a notched T.

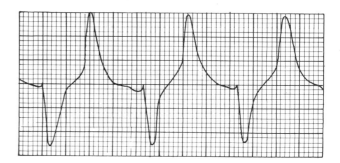

FIG. 8-11

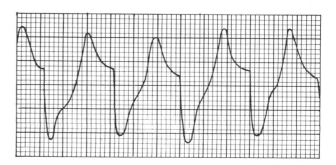

FIG. 8-12

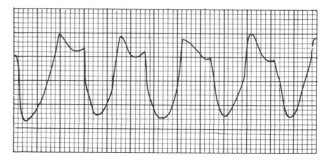

FIG. 8-13

symptoms. The nurse may be the first to discover these changes and can determine potassium excesses or deficiencies when serum levels may not be available. The following material discusses how increases or decreases of potassium, calcium, and magnesium affect cardiac function.

HYPERKALEMIA

With an elevated serum potassium (5.5 mEq/l) level, the earliest and most easily identifiable change on the ECG is a tall and peaked T wave (Fig. 8-9).

As the serum potassium continues to rise, there will be a flattening of the P wave and prolongation of the PR interval. Frequently the P wave gets buried in the T wave, and only a notch on the T wave is seen. These changes are usually seen with a potassium greater than 7.0 mEq/l (Fig. 8-10).

If the potassium is not controlled and continues to rise, there will be a disappearance of the P wave, the amplitude of the R wave will diminish, and the QRS will progressively widen. If this imbalance is not corrected immediately, the patient will develop intractable ventricular tachycardia, ventricular fibrillation, or asystole (Figs. 8-11 to 8-13).

See Table 8-6 for the causes, signs, and symptoms of hyperkalemia.

Since hyperkalemia is life threatening, prompt action must be taken. The following are methods for decreasing serum potassium:
1. Fluid challenge
2. Potassium-wasting diuretic therapy (Lasix, Edecrin)
3. Sodium bicarbonate I.V.
4. Glucose and insulin I.V.
5. Cation exchange resin (Kayexylate)
6. Peritoneal dialysis
7. Hemodialysis
8. Calcium chloride I.V. (does not lower potassium, only antagonizes its effects on the heart)

TABLE 8-6. Causes, signs, and symptoms of hyperkalemia (potassium over 5.5 mEq/l)[25,55]

Causes	Signs and symptoms
Renal failure	Muscle irritability
Excessive potassium in I.V. fluids	Weakness
	Malaise
Transfusion by large amounts of bank blood	Paresthesias of the scalp and face
Crushing injuries or other disorders involving lysis of cells	Flaccid paralysis
	Sinus node dysfunction resulting in bradycardia
Diabetic ketoacidosis	Nausea, vomiting, and abdominal distention
Addison's disease (decreased sodium and potassium exchange)	Intestinal colic
High doses of penicillin	Diarrhea
Use of potassium-sparing diuretics (triamterene, spironolactone)	Sudden cardiac death
Extracellular redistribution such as occurs in respiratory or metabolic acidosis	

HYPOKALEMIA

Hypokalemia is a more frequent clinical problem than hyperkalemia. Whereas an increase in serum potassium depresses the myocardium, a decrease in serum potassium increases the irritability. Other than its direct effect on the myocardium, a low serum potassium affects the action of many drugs, one of the more important being digoxin. Hypokalemia significantly enhances the effects of digoxin to the point of toxicity. Hypokalemia is manifested on the ECG by the presence of a U wave or TU fusion. The U wave signifies electrical instability. Along with the U wave, there is prolongation of the QT interval, T wave inversion, and sagging of the ST segment (Fig. 8-14).

Other common signs of hypokalemia seen on the ECG are premature atrial complexes and premature ventricular complexes because of increased irritability. These ectopics can lead to life-threatening dysrhythmias, especially in the known cardiac patient. Frequently a single dose of an antidysrhythmic agent may be given until the electrolyte imbalance can be corrected. For example, a postoperative coronary artery bypass patient who is experiencing excessive dizziness with resultant hypokalemia may receive a bolus of lidocaine to suppress the premature ventricular complexes while the hypokalemia is corrected. Correcting the hypokalemia is done by oral or I.V. supplements. Oral administration is the preferred route but when the deficit causes severe symptoms, parenteral replacement is necessary. When potassium is administered I.V., certain precautions must be taken:

1. Do not infuse potassium any faster than 0.5 mEq per minute since it may cause severe bradycardia or asystole
2. Watch for chemical phlebitis at the I.V. site, especially in critically ill patients or those unable to communicate pain; the phlebitis usually requires treatment with warm compresses
3. A central I.V. is the recommended route for I.V. potassium infusion; if potassium is to be given via a peripheral I.V. line, it is recommended that no more than 10 mEq be given diluted in 100 ml D_5W or in a normal saline solution infused over 1 hour. Table 8-7 on p. 218 lists the causes, signs, and symptoms of hypokalemia

HYPERCALCEMIA

The evident change in the ECG because of an increased serum calcium level—greater than 10.5 mEq/l—is

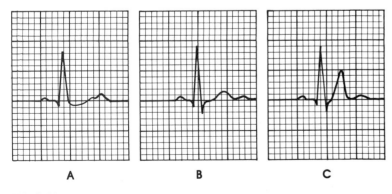

| A | B | C |

FIG. 8-14

ECG effects of potassium imbalances: **A,** hypokalemia: flattening of P wave, TU fusion, sagging of ST segment; **B,** normal P-QRS-T; and **C,** hyperkalemia: tall, peaked T wave.

TABLE 8-7. Causes, signs, and symptoms of hypokalemia (potassium less than 3.5 mEq/l)[25,55]

Causes	Signs and symptoms
Diuretic therapy	Decreased reflexes
Prolonged vomiting/diarrhea	Muscular irritability or weakness
Excessive sweating	
Excessive lactation	Anorexia, nausea, vomiting
Ulcerative colitis	Rapid, weak, irregular pulse
Laxative abuse	Abdominal distention
Prolonged gastric drainage	Flatulence
Steroid therapy	Decreased bowel sounds
Excessive licorice candy intake	Paralytic ileus
	Depressed mental state
Diabetic acidosis treated with insulin or sodium bicarbonate therapy	
Alkalosis	

a shortening of the QT interval. As levels increase, there may actually be a prolongation of the QT interval because of prolongation of the T wave (Fig. 8-15). Table 8-8 lists the common causes and signs and symptoms of calcium imbalances.

It is important to remember to always use the QT interval for evaluating whether an alteration is present. The treatment of hypercalcemia is two-fold with the more important factor being correction of the underlying cause. Modes of therapy to remove calcium ions include diuretics such as Lasix or ethacrynic acid, adequate hydration, frequent repositioning of the patient to avoid stasis of urine, careful attention to intake and output, and chelating agents that bind excessive calcium ions.[25] Hypercalcemia may predispose to digoxin toxicity, as it has additive effects with digoxin and may result in serious ventricular dysrhythmias.[25,54,55]

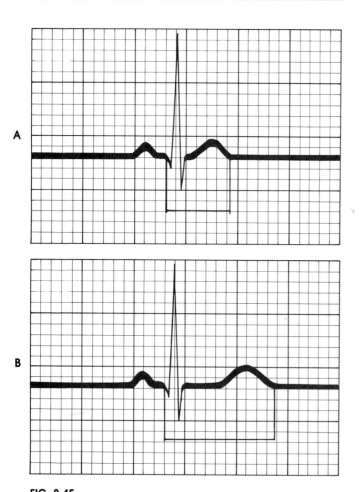

FIG. 8-15
A, Shortening of QT interval. **B,** Normal QT interval.

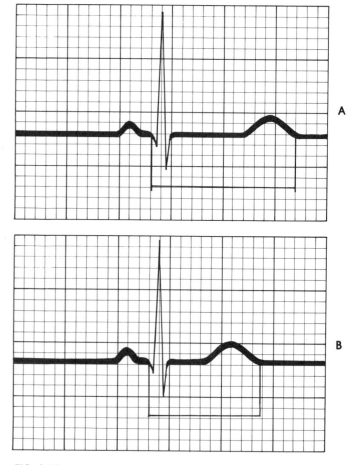

FIG. 8-16
A, Prolongation of QT interval. **B,** Normal QT interval.

TABLE 8-8. Causes, signs, and symptoms of calcium imbalances[25,55]

Causes	Signs and symptoms	Causes	Signs and symptoms
HYPERCALCEMIA (CALCIUM GREATER THAN 10.5 mEq/l)		**HYPOCALCEMIA (CALCIUM LESS THAN 8.5 mEq/l)**	
Prolonged immobilization	Depression	Chronic renal insufficiency	Muscle and abdominal cramps
Primary hyperparathyroidism	Lethargy	Hypoparathyroidism	
Parathyroid adenoma	Anorexia	Vitamin D deficiency	Perioral paresthesias
Multiple myeloma	Nausea	Pancreatitis	Twitching
Vitamin D overdose	Vomiting	Magnesium deficiency	Laryngospasm
Abuse of certain antacids	Constipation	Chronic laxative abuse	Tetany
Diuretic therapy	Dehydration	After parathyroidectomy or total thyroidectomy	Seizures
Serum phosphate depletion	Hallucinations	Prolonged suctioning (gastrointestinal)	
	Coma (extreme)	Hypoalbuminemia	

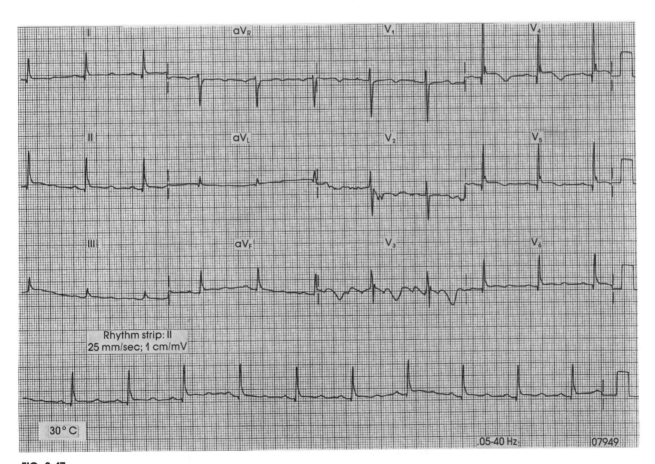

FIG. 8-17

Hypothermia and effects on the ECG: HR = 62, PR interval = 0.20 second, QT interval = 0.56 second, and QRS interval = 0.12 second.

HYPOCALCEMIA

When the serum calcium level is less than 8.5 mEg/l, hypocalcemia is present. It manifests itself as a prolongation of the QT interval. This lengthening occurs in the ST segment as opposed to QRS widening (Fig. 8-16, p. 218). Treatment of hypocalcemia requires the administration of calcium salts. When calcium is ordered in an intravenous form, it must be administered slowly, as rapid infusion may cause bradycardia or asystole. Table 8-8 gives the causes, signs, and symptoms of calcium imbalances.

MAGNESIUM ABNORMALITIES

Serum magnesium changes on the ECG follow those of potassium. Typically magnesium changes do not occur without the more prominent potassium changes. Hypermagnesemia may occur in renal insufficiency and after the ingestion of antacids such as Maalox or Gelusil, which contain absorbable magnesium. Hypomagnesemia may result from excessive diuretic therapy, diabetic acidosis, chronic alcoholism, malnutrition, and excessive gastric suctioning. Since hypomagnesemia promotes intracellular potassium loss, it predisposes to digoxin toxicity.[25,48]

HYPOTHERMIA

When the core temperature of the body is lowered, there are changes that occur on the ECG. When the temperature is less than 30 degrees C (87.8 degrees F), prolongation of all the ECG intervals, PR, PP, QRS, and QT occur (Fig. 8-17, p. 219). As the body continues to cool, atrial fibrillation may occur at 29 degrees C and ventricular fibrillation at 24 degrees C.

REFERENCES

1. Anderson, J.L.: Symposium on the management of ventricular dysrhythmias: antifibrillatory versus antiectopic therapy, Am. J. Cardiol. **54**(2):7A, 1984.
2. Andreoli, K.G., et al.: Comprehensive cardiac care, ed. 5, St. Louis, 1983, The C.V. Mosby Co.
3. Atkinson, A.J.: Lidocaine and procainamide therapy of ventricular arrhythmias—a clinical pharmacological perspective. In Melmon, K.L., editor: Drug therapeutics: concepts for physicians, New York, 1981, Elsevier Science Publishing Co. Inc.
4. Bassan, M.M., et al.: Improved prognosis during long-term treatment with beta blockers after myocardial infarction: analysis of randomized trials and pooling of results, Heart Lung **13**(2):164, 1984.
5. Bellet, S.: The electrocardiogram in electrolyte imbalances, Arch. Intern. Med. **96**:618, 1955.
6. Benchimol, A., and Desser, K.B.: New drugs for treating cardiac arrhythmias, Postgrad. Med. **69**(1):77, 1981.
7. Braunwald, E.: Management of cardiac arrhythmias. In Braunwald, E., editor: Heart disease—a textbook of cardio-vascular medicine, vol. 1, ed. 2, Philadelphia, 1984, W.B. Saunders Co.
8. Bussey, H.I., et al.: The influence of rifampin on quinidine and digoxin, Arch. Intern. Med. **144**(5):1021, 1984.
9. Castle, L.: Therapy of ventricular tachycardia, Am. J. Cardiol. **54**(2):26(A), 1984.
10. Conover, M.B.: Understanding electrocardiography: arrhythmias and the 12-lead ECG, ed. 4, St. Louis, 1984, The C.V. Mosby Co.
11. Counihan, T.B.: Clinical application of inotropic drugs, Eur. Heart J. **3**(D):143, 1982.
12. Danilo, F., and Rosen, M.R.: Cardiac effects of disopyramide, Am. Heart J. **92**:532, 1976.
13. DiMarco, J.P., et al.: Efficiency of quinidine in the treatment of ventricular arrhythmias: the role of electrophysiologic testing, Circulation **64**(IV):38, 1981.
14. Douste-Blazy, P.H., et al.: Influence of amiodarone on plasma and urine digoxin concentrations, Lancet, **1**:905, 1984.
15. Eddy, J.D., and Singh, S.P.: Treatment of cardiac arrhythmias with phenytoin, Brit. Med. J. **4**:240, 1976.
16. Fisch, C.: Electrocardiography and vectorcardiography. In Braunwald, E., editor: Heart disease—a textbook of cardiovascular medicine, vol. 1, ed. 2, Philadelphia, 1984, W.B. Saunders Co.
17. Gever, L.N.: Giving procainamide safely, Nursing **14**(5):116, 1984.
18. Gheorghiade, M., and Beller, G.A.: The role of digitalis in patients with coronary artery disease. In Roberts, R., editor: Cardiology clinics—symposium on prognosis after myocardial infarction **2**(1):135, Philadelphia, 1984, W.B. Saunders Co.
19. Gillis, R.D., et al.: Depression of the cardiac sympathetic nerve activity in diphenylhydantoin, J. Pharmacol. Exp. Ther. **179**:599, 1971.
20. Gilman, A.G., et al. editors: The pharmacologic basis of therapeutics, ed. 6, New York, 1980, Macmillan Publishing Co.
21. Heger, J., et al.: Clinical choice of antiarrhythmic drugs. In Josephson, M.E., editor: Ventricular tachycardia—mechanisms and management, Mt. Kisco, New York, 1982, Futura Publishing Co.
22. Heger, J.J., et al.: Drug therapy of cardiac arrhythmias. In Zipes, D.P., editor: Cardiology clinics—symposium on arrhythmias, II **1**(2):305, Philadelphia, 1983, W.B. Saunders Co.
23. Hillis, W.S., and Whiting, B.: Antiarrhythmic drugs, Brit. Med. J. **286**:1332, 1983.
24. Kastays, E., et al.: Facts and comparisons—drug information, St. Louis, 1984, J.B. Lippincott Co.
25. Kernicki, J.G., and Weiler, K.M.: Electrocardiography for nurses—physiological correlates, New York, 1981, John Wiley & Sons Inc.
26. Kligfield, P.: Calcium-blocking drugs: physiology and pharmacology, Primary Cardiol. **2**:40, 1983.
27. Koch-Weser, J., and Frishman, W.H.: Beta-adrenoreceptor antagonists: new drugs and new indications, N. Engl. J. Med. **305**:500, 1981.

28. Koren, G., et al.: Digoxin toxicity associated with amiodarone therapy in children, J. Pediatr. **104**(3):467, 1984.

29. Kvam, D.C., et al.: Antiarrhythmic and electrophysiologic actions of flecainide in animal models, Am. J. Cardiol. **53**(5):22B, 1984.

30. Latini, R., et al.: Clinical pharmacokinetics of amiodarone, Clin. Pharmacokinet. **9**(2):136, 1984.

31. Lee, D.C., et al.: Heart failure in outpatients—a randomized trial of digoxin versus placebo, N. Engl. J. Med. **306**:699, 1982.

32. Mann, D.E., et al.: Electrophysiologic effects of ethmozine in patients with ventricular tachycardia, Am. Heart J. **107**(4):674, 1984.

33. Marchlinski, F.E., et al.: Amiodarone pulmonary toxicity, Ann. Int. Med. **97**(6):839, 1982.

34. McEvoy, G., editor: American hospital formulary service—drug information 1984, Bethesda, Md., 1984, American Society of Hospital Pharmacists.

35. McIntyre, K.M., and Lewis, A.J., editors: Textbook of advanced cardiac life support, 1983, American Heart Association.

36. Myerburg, R.J., et al.: Relationships between plasma levels of procainamide, suppression of premature ventricular complexes, and prevention of recurrent ventricular tachycardia, Circulation **64**:280, 1981.

37. Nattel, S., and Zipes, D.P.: Clinical pharmacology of old and new antiarrhythmic drugs, Cardiovasc. Res. **11**:221, 1980.

38. Nikolic, G.: Lidocaine bradycardia, Heart Lung **13**(3):290, 1984.

39. Ochs, H.R., et al.: Disease-related alterations in cardiac glycoside disposition, Clin. Pharmacokinet. **7**:434, 1982.

40. Paton, D.M., et al.: A review of the clinical pharmacokinetics of amiodarone, Methods Find. Exp. Clin. Pharmacol. **1**:41, 1984.

41. Podrid, P.J., et al.: Congestive heart failure caused by oral disopyramide, N. Engl. J. Med. **302**(11):614, 1980.

42. Pratt, C.M., et al.: Investigational antiarrhythmic drugs for the treatment of ventricular rhythm disturbances. In Roberts, R., editor: Cardiology clinics—symposium on prognosis after myocardial infarction **2**(1):35, Philadelphia, 1984, W.B. Saunders Co.

43. Reimer, K.A., et al.: Effect of the calcium antagonist on necrosis following temporary coronary artery occlusion in dogs, Circulation **55**:581, 1977.

44. Reynolds, J.E., editor: Martindale: the extra pharmacopeia, ed. 28, London, 1982, Pharmaceutical Press.

45. Rosen, M.R., and Wit, A.L.: Electropharmacology of antiarrhythmic drugs, Am. Heart J. **106**(4):829, 1983.

46. Schenck-Gustafsson, K., et al.: Cardiac effects of treatment with quinidine and digoxin, alone and in combination, Am. J. Cardiol. **51**:777, 1983.

47. Schwartz, J.B., et al.: Acute and chronic pharmacodynamic interaction of verapamil and digoxin in atrial fibrillation, Circulation **65**:1163, 1982.

48. Smith, T.W., and Braunwald, E.: The management of heart failure. In Braunwald, E., editor: Heart disease—a textbook of cardiovascular medicine, vol. 1, ed. 2, Philadelphia, 1984, W.B. Saunders Co.

49. Smith, W.M. and Gallagher, J.J.: Les torsades de pointes: an unusual ventricular arrhythmia, Ann. Int. Med. **93**(4):578, 1980.

50. Smith, T.W., et al.: Treatment of life-threatening digitalis intoxication with digoxin-specific Fab fragments—experience in twenty-six patients, N. Engl. J. Med. **307**:1357, 1982.

51. Somberg, J.C., New directions in antiarrhythmic drug therapy, Am. J. Cardiol. **54**(4):8b, 1984.

52. Somberg, J.C., et al.: Evaluation of lorcainide in patients with symptomatic ventricular tachycardia, Am. J. Cardiol. **54**(4):43b, 1984.

53. Strasberg, B., et al.: Procainamide-induced polymorphous ventricular tachycardia, Am. J. Cardiol. **47**:1309, 1981.

54. Surawicz, B.: Electrolytes and the electrocardiogram, J. Cardiol. **12**:656, 1963.

55. Surawicz, B.: The interrelationship of electrolyte abnormalities and arrhythmias. In Mandel, W.J., editor: Cardiac arrhythmias—their mechanisms, diagnosis, and management, Philadelphia, 1980, J.B. Lippincott Co.

56. Vaughn Williams, E.M.: Classification of antiarrhythmic drugs. In Sandloe, E., et al., editors: Symposium on cardiac arrhythmias, Sodertalje, Sweden, 1970, A.B. Astra.

57. Walker, A.M., et al.: Drug toxicity in patients receiving digoxin and quinidine, Am. Heart J. **105**(6):1025, 1983.

58. Wellens, H.J.J., and Durrer, D.: Effect of digitalis on atrioventricular conduction and circus-movement tachycardias in patients with Wolff-Parkinson-White syndrome, Circulation **47**:1229, 1973.

59. Wellens, H.J.J., and Durrer, D.: Effect of procainamide, quinidine, and ajmaline in the Wolff-Parkinson-White syndrome, Circulation **50**:114, 1974.

60. Woosley, R.L., et al.: Pharmacology, electrophysiology, and pharmacokinetics of mexiletine, Am. Heart J. **107**(5):1058, 1984.

61. Wyman, M.G., and Gore, S.: Lidocaine prophylaxis in myocardial infarction—a concept whose time has come, Heart Lung **12**(4):358, 1983.

62. Wynne, J., and Braunwald, E.: The cardiomyopathies and myocarditides. In Braunwald, E., editor: Heart disease—a textbook of cardiovascular medicine, vol. 2, ed. 1, Philadelphia, 1984, W.B., Saunders Co.

63. Zipes, D.P., et al.: Amiodarone—electrophysiologic actions, pharmacokinetics, and clinical effects, J. Am. Coll. Cardiolog. **4**:1059, 1984.

SUGGESTED LEARNING ACTIVITIES AND EXPERIENCES

A. Locate patients in the special care areas who are receiving antidysrhythmic drug therapy. Do the following:

   1. Review the patient's record and identify the dysrhythmia history

2. Review the drug therapy and its effect on the patient's dysrhythmia
3. Examine the patient's ECGs and rhythm strips and identify the effect of the drug on:
   a. Controlling the dysrhythmia
   b. PR, QRS, and QT intervals
4. Identify any side effects of the drug
5. Review serum drug levels and determine if they are therapeutic, too low, or too high

B. Review all of your patient's drug therapy and be familiar with the rationale and appropriate dosages
C. Should an electrophysiology laboratory be available, ask permission to observe; identify the indications for the test, any antidysrhythmic drugs administered with dosages, and the plan for further treatment or follow-up
D. Locate patients in a trauma unit or medical intensive care unit who may be predisposed to electrolyte imbalances; review the serum electrolyte history, review the ECGs and rhythm strips for changes in the complexes and intervals, and review the treatment modalities
E. Participate in educating the patient and family members regarding drug therapy; seek assistance from peers who may be more experienced in patient and/or family education

POSTTEST (Answers on p. 229)

Directions: Circle one answer to each question unless otherwise indicated.

A. A trough serum procainamide level is drawn:
   1. 30 minutes before the next dose
   2. Immediately after the dose is given
   3. 30 minutes to 1 hour after the dose is given
   4. 6 hours after the dose is given

B. Which of the following are considered to be toxic effects of digoxin? (Circle all that apply.)
   1. Anorexia, nausea, vomiting
   2. Development of a slow, irregular heart rhythm, documented as second-degree AV block, type I, on the ECG
   3. Slurring of the ST segment on ECG
   4. Visual disturbances (seeing halos around objects)

C. Of the following antidysrhythmic drugs, which is not given as a continuous infusion?
   1. Lidocaine
   2. Phenytoin
   3. Procainamide
   4. Bretylium

D. The main concern about the digitalized patient who is receiving furosemide (Lasix) is:

1. Recording intake and output
2. Taking CVP readings
3. Observing for decreasing edema
4. Observing for dysrhythmias caused by hypokalemia

E. The usual total daily dose for disopyramide is:
   1. 1-2 gm
   2. 100-200 mg
   3. 200-400 mg
   4. 400-800 mg

F. Side effects of bretylium are (circle all that apply):
   1. Nausea and vomiting
   2. Orthostatic hypotension
   3. Diarrhea
   4. Severe headache

G. The drug of choice in the treatment of ventricular extrasystoles associated with digoxin toxicity is:
   1. Lidocaine
   2. Procainamide
   3. Phenytoin
   4. Quinidine

H. Which of the following beta blockers is considered to be cardioselective; that is, affecting beta$_1$ receptors only)? (Circle all that apply.)
   1. Propranolol
   2. Timolol
   3. Atenolol
   4. Nadolol
   5. Metoprolol

I. In administering an I.V. bolus of lidocaine prophylactically to a postmyocardial infarction patient, the *best* rate of infusion would be:
   1. 20 mg per minute
   2. 75 mg per minute
   3. 50 mg per minute
   4. 25 mg per minute

J. Isoproterenol is contraindicated in which of the following? (Circle all that apply.)
   1. Symptomatic bradycardia
   2. Tachydysrhythmias
   3. Acute myocardial infarction
   4. Asystole
   5. Hypovolemia

K. Which of the following may be side effects of amiodarone therapy? (Circle all that apply.)
   1. Anorexia
   2. Hyperthyroidism
   3. Pulmonary fibrosis
   4. Severe headache
   5. Corneal microdeposits
   6. Hypothyroidism

L.   Matching: Match the term in Column A with the
      definition in Column B.

Column A
Term

____ 1. Cation
____ 2. Excitation-contraction-coupling
____ 3. IHSS
____ 4. Steady state
____ 5. Bigeminy
____ 6. Reentry
____ 7. Cholinergic
____ 8. Systemic vascular resistance
____ 9. Antiadrenergic
____ 10. Wolff-Parkinson-White syndrome
____ 11. Cardioversion
____ 12. Preload
____ 13. Hyper-
____ 14. *Torsade de pointes*
____ 15. Absolute refractory period
____ 16. Serum levels
____ 17. Bioavailability
____ 18. Anion
____ 19. Inotropic
____ 20. Extrasystoles
____ 21. Accessory pathway
____ 22. Catecholamines
____ 23. Afterdepolarizations
____ 24. Hypo-
____ 25. Supraventricular dysrhythmias
____ 26. Chronotropic
____ 27. Excitability
____ 28. Half-life
____ 29. Conduction time
____ 30. Kilograms
____ 31. Dromotropic
____ 32. Beta-adrenergic receptor
____ 33. Cardiac output
____ 34. Adrenergic
____ 35. Third heart sound

Column B
Definition

a. Fibers that release and receptors that respond to catecholamines
b. An "extra" pathway that bypasses the AV node
c. A positively charged electrolyte
d. The ability of the heart to respond to a stimulus
e. The time it takes for one drug dose to be reduced in the serum by half
f. A premature impulse from a focus other than the SA node
g. A condition whereby the left ventricular wall and septum are hypertrophied and often cause obstruction to flow during systole
h. Refers to less than normal
i. A period whereby the cardiac cell is totally unexcited and cannot respond to a stimulus
j. A method of measuring drug serum levels to determine therapeutic effects
k. A weak cellular effort to depolarize just before or after normal repolarization is complete
l. A negatively charged electrolyte
m. Refers to nerve endings that, when stimulated, block epinephrine or norepinephrine at their sites
n. The amount of blood the heart pumps per minute
o. A group of neurohormones having a stimulating effect on the heart
p. The amount of drug available to the body after oral ingestion
q. Receptors found mainly in the heart and lungs
r. A rhythm composed of pairs of complexes
s. A term applied to nerve endings that release acetylcholine when stimulated
t. A direct electrical current that is synchronized to be delivered on the R wave of the ECG

u. Refers to greater than normal
v. The dosing frequency and amount of drug required to reach a therapeutic level
w. Resistance to the flow of blood from the left ventricle by the peripheral vasculature
x. Refers to speed of AV conduction
y. The complex mechanism involving calcium and muscle proteins whereby the myofibrils shorten in response to a stimulus
z. The amount of time it takes an impulse to travel through any part of the conduction system
aa. Abnormal impulse originating in any tissue above the ventricle
bb. Refers to heart rate
cc. A low pitched sound heard with the bell of the stethoscope, following the second heart sound, which indicates heart failure in the adult
dd. Refers to the volume of blood in the left ventricle before contraction
ee. A measurement of weight necessary to calculate drug dosages
ff. Refers to force of myocardial contractility
gg. The circus movement of an impulse traveling two pathways that have an imbalance in their response time to the impulse
hh. A paroxysmal type of ventricular fibrillation that is usually precipitated by prolongation of the QT interval
ii. The presence of an accessory pathway, formerly known as a Kent bundle, characterized on the ECG by a shortened PR interval and widened QRS

M. The major indication for use of verapamil is:
1. Hypertension
2. IHSS
3. Control of supraventricular tachycardias
4. Control of coronary artery spasm

N. Which of the following should be used with caution in the patient with myasthenia gravis?
1. Lidocaine
2. Procainamide
3. Phenytoin
4. Disopyramide

O. The usual dose of I.V. bolus lidocaine is:
1. 0.5 mg/kg of body weight
2. 1 mg/kg of body weight
3. 2 mg/kg of body weight
4. 5 mg/kg of body weight

P. T F Digoxin should be discontinued at least 1 week before elective exercise testing.

Q. T F Lidocaine is indicated for use in the treatment of tachydysrhythmias associated with accessory pathways.

R. T F Phenytoin may be given I.V. through a line containing D_5W.

S. T F Digoxin may precipitate atrial fibrillation from atrial flutter.

T. T F Caution must be used in all patients with liver disease who receive antidysrhythmic therapy.

U. T F Widening of the QT interval up to 25% in persons receiving quinidine is considered to be a toxic manifestation of the drug.

V. T F When bretylium I.V. is given to control ventricular tachycardia, initially the rate of ventricular tachycardia may increase.

W. T F A patient receiving verapamil or nifedipine must always be weaned because there is a rebound effect of vasoconstriction.

X. T F Amiodarone must be used with caution in persons with known iodine sensitivity.

Y. T F Isoproterenol is recommended for use in the treatment of asystole.

Z. T F It is safe to abruptly discontinue a patient from propranolol.

AA. T F Verapamil is recommended for treatment of Wolff-Parkinson-White syndrome.

BB. Which of the following may be ECG manifestations of hypokalemia? (Circle all that apply.)
1. Presence of TU fusion
2. Prolongation of QT interval
3. Shortening of QRS interval
4. Tall peaked T waves
5. Sagging of the ST segment

CC. The serum digoxin concentration may elevate with the addition of which of the following drugs? (Circle all that apply.)
1. Quinidine
2. Amiodarone
3. Disopyramide
4. Propranolol
5. Verapamil
6. Rifampin

DD. When giving procainamide I.V., the rate of infusion should be no faster than:
1. 25 mg per minute
2. 50 mg per minute
3. 75 mg per minute
4. 200 mg per hour

EE. Which of the following should not precipitate digoxin toxicity?
1. Hyperkalemia
2. Hypokalemia
3. Hypocalcemia
4. Hypomagnesemia
5. Altered renal function
6. Geriatric age group

FF. The usual initial dose of atropine I.V. to treat symptomatic bradycardia is:
1. 0.04 mg
2. 2 mg
3. 0.5-1 mg
4. 0.4 mg

SUPPLEMENTS

The supplement section includes a reference table (Table 8-9) of the antidysrhythmic drugs discussed in this module. This table may be used as a quick reference in the clinical setting. The key to the symbols used is as follows:

↑ = increase, lengthen
↓ = decrease, shorten
∅ = no change
GI = gastrointestinal
ng = nanograms
µg = micrograms

TABLE 8-9. Antidysrhythmic drugs

Generic Name	Trade Name	Indications for use	Dosage	Half-life	Therapeutic serum level	Major effect	Side effects	ECG effects	Observations
Digoxin	Lanoxin Novodigin	Paroxysmal supraventricular tachycardia Atrial flutter Atrial fibrillation Heart failure with associated S_3	*Loading* Oral 1.25-1.5 mg in divided doses > 12-24 hours I.V. 0.75-1 mg in divided doses > 12-24 hours *Maintainance* 0.125-0.5 mg daily, depending on clinical status	*Oral* 3-5 days I.V. 36-48 hours	0.6-2 ng/ml	↑ contractility ↓ heart rate ↓ automaticity → AV conduction ↑ diuresis ↓ edema	Premature atrial tachycardia with block Ventricular tachydysrhyth-mias Premature ventricular complexes Nonparoxysmal junctional tachycardia First-degree and second-degree, type I, AV block Anorexia, nausea and vomiting, halos around objects	↑ PR Ø QRS ↓ QT ↓ sinus rate ST-T changes "sagging"	Maintain normal K^+ Observe for digoxin toxicity with addition of: Quinidine Nifedipine Verapamil Amiodarone Rifampin
Quinidine	Quinidex Quiniglute Quinidine Sulfate or Gluconate	Atrial and ventricular dysrhythmias Wolff-Parkinson-White syndrome (WPW)	*Oral* 200-400 mg 4-6 times daily; total not to exceed 3-4 gm/day; less frequent dosing with sustained release *IM* 200 mg 4-6 times daily *I.V.* 300-750 mg; use only with extreme caution and review I.V. administration	4-8 hours	2-5 µg/ml	↓ automaticity → excitability → conductivity ↑ contractility ↑ AV conduction	Cinchonism: tinnitus, headache, blurred vision, diarrhea, nausea and vomiting, hypotension	↓ PR ↑ QRS ↑ QT ST-T changes U wave	Vagolytic effect; may ↑ heart rate Observe for: *Torsade de pointes* Anticholinergic effects
Procainamide	Pronestyl Procaine S.R.	Mainly ventricular dysrhythmias Some atrial dysrhythmias WPW	*Oral* 250-500 mg 4-8 times per day *Sustained release capsules* 500 mg 3-4 times a day	*Procainamide* 3-4 hours N = acetyl procain-amide 6-8 hours	*Procainamide* 4-10 µg/ml N = acetyl procain-amide 22 µg/ml	↓ atrial refractory time ↓ automaticity → excitability → conductivity ↓ contractility	Congestive heart failure (CHF) Thrombocytopenia Agranulocytosis Systemic lupus erythematosus ECG changes/ hypotension	↓ PR ↑ QRS ↑ QT ST-T changes	Monitor closely when giving I.V.; S.R. capsule passes through GI tract into stool (normal) ↓ dose with liver disease Observe for *torsade de pointes*

Continued.

TABLE 8-9. Antidysrhythmic drugs—cont'd

Generic Name	Trade Name	Indications for use	Dosage	Half-life	Therapeutic serum level	Major effect	Side effects	ECG effects	Observations
Disopyramide	Norpace Norpace CR (controlled release)	Ventricular dysrhythmias WPW	*Oral* 100-300 mg/ 4 times per day; controlled release 2 times per day	4-10 hours (7)	2-4 μg/ml	↓ automaticity ↓ excitability ↓ conductivity ↓ contractility	CHF Urinary retention Hypotension Nausea and vomiting	Ø PR Ø ↑ QRS ↑ QT	Anticholinergic effects Observe for *torsade de pointes*
Lidocaine	Xylocaine	Acute ventricular dysrhythmias Prophylactically to prevent ventricular fibrillation or ventricular tachycardia, especially in acute myocardial infarction Digoxin toxicity dysrhythmias	*I.V.* 1 mg/kg I.V. bolus; 25 mg/min every 5-10 minutes, up to 225 mg. continuous I.V. infusion 1-4 mg/min	*I.V.* 8 minutes after I.V. infusion Over 48 hours = 4 hours	2-5 μg/ml	↓ ventricular automaticity ↑ fibrillation threshold	Paresthesias Drowsiness Confusion Tremors Seizures Coma	No change (may in rare cases, ↓ sinus rate or ↑ AV conduction)	Follow initial bolus with continuous infusion; caution in elderly and in patients with renal or liver dysfunction No preservatives!
Phenytoin	Dilantin	Digoxin-induced dysrhythmias	*I.V.* 100 mg-1 gm I.V., no faster than 50 mg/min	7-42 hours	10-20 μg/ml	↓ refractory period ↓ automaticity of Purkinje fibers ↓ sympathetic activity in heart	Nystagmus Dizziness Confusion Hypotension Bradycardia	May cause sinus bradycardia or asystole; administer with caution	Administer *only* in normal saline solution Incompatible with dextrose solutions
Bretylium	Bretylol	Life-threatening ventricular dysrhythmias	*I.V.* 5 mg/kg I.V. bolus, may repeat up to 10 mg/kg if necessary	8-10 hours	Not correlated with effect	↓ automaticity ↓ contractility ↓ fibrillation threshold	Orthostatic hypotension Nausea and vomiting if given too rapidly to an alert patient	Ø ↑ PR Ø QRS ↓ sinus rate	Initial ↑ HR and hypertension, followed by hypotension Keep patient supine
Propranolol	Inderal	Supraventricular tachycardia Atrial flutter and fibrillation Digoxin-induced dysrhythmias Other effects: angina, hypertension, WPW	*Oral* Angina: 10-80 mg 3-4 times a day Hypertension: 160-480 mg/ day *I.V.* 0.5-3 mg I.V. in 1-mg increments	3.4-6 hours (4) 1-8 hours (4)	50-100 μg/ml	↓ heart rate ↓ automaticity ↓ excitability ↓ conductivity ↓ contractility ↓ AV conduction ↓ blood pressure ↓ myocardial oxygen demands ↑ bronchoconstriction	Hypotension Bradycardia Bronchospasm Heart block GI distress Fatigue and depression Impotence	Ø ↑ PR Ø QRS Ø ↓ QT ↓ Sinus rate	Caution in use with calcium blockers; do not stop abruptly, must wean

Generic	Trade	Uses	Dose/Route	Half-life	Therapeutic level	Action	Side effects	Nursing implications
Metoprolol	Lopressor	Angina Afterload reduction Hypertension	Oral Angina: 50-100 mg/day in divided doses every 8-12 hours Hypertension: 100-450 mg/day	3-4 hours	20-340 ng/ml	Less bronchospasm Inhibits beta$_1$ receptors only		
Atenolol	Tenormin	Angina Hypertension	Oral Angina: 100 mg/day Hypertension: 50-100 mg/day	16-27 hours	1-2 µg/ml	Inhibits beta$_1$ receptors only		Safe to use in patients with diabetes and lung disease
Nadolol	Corgard	Angina Hypertension Supraventricular tachycardia	Oral Angina: 40-240 mg/day Hypertension: 80-320 mg/day	10-24 hours	25-190 ng/ml	Inhibits both beta$_1$ and beta$_2$ receptors ↓ AV conduction		Less negative inotropic effects than propanolol Caution with renal failure
Timolol	Blockadren	Chronic Supraventricular tachycardia Angina Hypertension	Oral Angina: 15-45 mg/day in divided doses every 6-8 hours Hypertension: 20-40 mg/day	3-4 hours		Inhibits beta$_1$ and beta$_2$ receptors		
Pindolol	Visken	Hypertension Chronic angina	Oral Angina: 15-40 mg/day Hypertension: 5 mg 2 times a day	3-4 hours		Inhibits beta$_1$ and beta$_2$ receptors Intrinsic sympathetic agonist activity		
Amiodarone	Cordarone	Ventricular dysrhythmias Supraventricular tachycardia because of accessory pathway	Oral 200-800 mg/day until clinical response; then varies with clinical response I.V. 5-10 mg/kg over 10 minutes	13-100 days	0.5-2.5 ng/ml	↑ refractory period of atria and ventricles, AV junction, Purkinje fibers, and accessory pathways ↓ contractility	Pulmonary fibrosis Thyroid dysfunction Corneal microdeposits Bluish skin discoloration Anorexia, nausea, and vomiting ↓ PR ↑ QT ↓ sinus rate	Caution in use with digoxin and with beta blockers

Continued.

TABLE 8-9. Antidysrhythmic drugs—cont'd

Generic Name	Trade Name	Indications for use	Dosage	Half-life	Therapeutic serum level	Major effect	Side effects	ECG effects	Observations
Verapamil	Isoptin Calan	Supraventricular tachycardia Atrial flutter/fibrillation	*Oral* 80-120 mg 3-4 times a day *I.V.* 5-15 mg	*Oral* 3-7 hours *I.V.* 2-8 hours	30-120 mg/ml	↓ AV conduction ↓ contractility Vasodilation	Heart block, sinus arrest, ectopic dysrhythmias, CHF, GI upset	↑ PR Ø QRS Ø QT ↓ sinus rate	Observe for hypotension Caution when giving with digoxin and/or beta blockers
Nifedipine	Procardia	Angina Coronary artery spasm	*Oral* 10-30 mg 3-4 times a day *Sublingual* 10 mg PRN for angina			Vasodilation of coronary and cerebral vessels			May develop chest pain approximately 20 minutes after dose
Diltiazem	Cardizem	Angina	*Oral* 30-90 mg 4 times a day	1-4 hours	30-130 µg/ml	Vasodilation of coronary and cerebral vessels	GI upset Headache	↓ sinus rate	
Isoproterenol	Isuprel	Symptomatic bradycardia or sinoatrial block *Torsade de pointes* Asystole	*I.V.* 2-20 µg/min, titrated to clinical response		Not established	↑ contractility ↑ automaticity ↑ excitability ↑ conductivity Vasodilation	Anxiety Restlessness Sweating Flushing Nausea and vomiting Tachydysrhythmias, including ventricular tachycardia and/or fibrillation	↑ SR ↓ QT ↓ QRS	Monitor closely; caution with diabetes; monitor blood glucose
Atropine sulfate	Atropine	Symptomatic bradydysrhythmias Asystole	*I.V.* 0.5-1 mg; repeat up to 2.0 mg total		Not established	↑ sinus rate ↑ conduction ↑ blood pressure	Sinus or ventricular tachydysrhythmias Dryness of mouth, skin flushing, acute glaucoma, constipation		Caution in myocardial infarction patient Assure adequate hydration

ANSWERS TO PRETEST AND POSTTEST

Pretest

A. 1, 2, 4
B. 3
C. 2, 3
D. 1, 2, 3 and 4. Even though prolongation of the QRS with lidocaine therapy is rare, all intervals must be followed with antidysrhythmic drug therapy.
E. 4
F. 2
G. 3
H. 4
I. 2
J. 3
K. 3
L. 6
M. 3
N. 3
O. 3

Posttest

A. 1
B. 1, 2, 4
C. 2
D. 4
E. 4
F. 1, 2
G. 3
H. 3, 5
I. 4
J. 2, 3, 5
K. 1, 2, 3, 5, 6
L. Matching:
   1. c
   2. y
   3. g
   4. v
   5. r
   6. gg
   7. s
   8. w
   9. m
  10. ii
  11. t
  12. dd
  13. u
  14. hh
  15. i
  16. j
  17. p
  18. l
  19. ff
  20. f
  21. b
  22. o

23. k
24. h
25. aa
26. bb
27. d
28. e
29. z
30. ee
31. x
32. q
33. n
34. a
35. cc

M. 3
N. 2
O. 2
P. T
Q. F
R. F
S. T
T. T
U. F
V. T
W. F
X. T
Y. T
Z. F
AA. F
BB. 1, 2, 5
CC. 1, 2, 5, 6
DD. 2
EE. 3
FF. 3

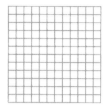

GLOSSARY

Aberrant conduction Because of a prolongation of the refractory period in the bundle branches, an impulse(s) is/are abnormally conducted through the ventricles, producing a change in the QRS morphology.

Absolute refractory period The interval of total unexcitability wherein a cell cannot respond to a stimulus. This correlates to the beginning of the QRS and the beginning of the T wave on the ECG, including the ST segment.

Accessory pathway An "extra" pathway through which impulses may be conducted to bypass the normal delay in the AV junction.

Acetylcholine Parasympathetic neurotransmitter substance.

Active rhythm A rhythm initiated by a premature complex (one that is early in the regular cycle), which continues at a rate faster than the normal pacemaker and usurps control of the heart rhythm.

Adrenergic A term used to describe the fibers that release and the receptors that respond to catecholamines.

Afterdepolarizations Rapid, repetitive, weak depolarizations that occur toward the end of normal repolarization or after normal repolarization is complete. Under normal conditions, the cells do not respond to these efforts to depolarize. However, if the cell environment is vulnerable because of hypoxia, catecholamines, etc., it can respond and set up a rapid tachycardia, either atrial, junctional, or ventricular. Also known as "triggered activity."

Afterload Term refers to resistance in the systemic vasculature. Vasoconstriction *increases* afterload (increases the workload of the myocardium) and vasodilation *decreases* afterload (decreases the workload of the myocardium).

Afterpotential The spread of the delivered electrical current from the pacemaker to the myocardial tissue. This can be of significant magnitude and may be sensed by the pacemaker to cause a lack of firing.

Anode The positive position of a pacer lead system.

Annulus A fibrous ring surrounding each atrioventricular valve orifice.

AN region The uppermost part of the AV node (atrionodal), thought to contain potential pacemaker fibers.

Anion A negatively charged electrolyte.

Antegrade conduction Impulse conduction that proceeds in a normal (foreward) direction.

Antiadrenergic A term applied to nerve fibers that at their endings, when stimulated, block epinephrine or other catecholamines.

Aortic semilunar valve A valve that consists of three pocket-like cusps through which blood ejected from the left ventricle passes into the aorta. The orifices (openings) of the two principal coronary arteries arise from two of these cusps.

Asynchronous A type of pacemaker that fires despite the heart's own intrinsic rate. It is also considered a fixed rate pacemaker. See Fixed rate pacemaker.

Asystole Lack of cardiac contraction and/or electrical cardiac activity, usually denoted as a straight line on the ECG.

Atrial appendage Irregularly shaped continuation of the atria.

Atrioventricular (AV) block Refers to atrioventricular block or the alteration of an impulse initiated in the sinoatrial (SA) node or atrium in conduction to the ventricles.

Atrioventricular junction An area of specialized conduction tissue that includes the AV node and the His bundle area.

Atrioventricular (AV) node A dense bundle of conduction fibers within the right side of the lower interatrial septum, the function of which is to delay impulse conduction from the atria to the ventricles.

Atrium One of two upper thin-walled receiving chambers of the heart.

Automaticity Electrical property of cells that permits spontaneous initiation of the cardiac impulse.

AV delay A constant pacemaker timing interval; it begins with an atrially paced or sensed event and ends with a ventricularly paced event. The usual AV delay is 200 ms (0.20 second).

Beta-adrenergic receptor Beta receptors are found mainly in the heart (beta$_1$) and lungs (beta$_2$).
1. Stimulation of these receptors results in:
   a. ↑ heart rate
   b. ↑ AV conduction (velocity/time)
   c. ↑ myocardial contractility
   d. ↑ bronchial dilation
2. Blocking of these receptors results in:
   a. ↓ heart rate
   b. ↓ AV conduction
   c. ↓ myocardial contractility
   d. ↑ bronchial constriction

Bigeminy A rhythm composed of pairs of complexes.

Bioavailability A means of expressing the overall efficiency of drug absorption. It is the amount of drug available systemically after oral ingestion divided by the amount of drug available following I.V. administration.

Bradycardia A heart rate below 60 beats per minute.

Bundle of His Compact conduction tissue fibers through which the impulse passes from the AV node into the ventricles. It divides into the right and left bundle branches.

Cadence The flow or beat of a rhythm as in music or dancing.

Cardiac output The volume of blood pumped by the heart per minute. The normal amount is 4 to 8 liters per minute.

Cardioversion A direct electrical current synchronized to be delivered on the R wave of the ECG via paddles applied to the chest in order to terminate a tachycardia.

Carotid sinus massage Unilateral pressure over the carotid artery bifurcation in the carotid sinus region, causing increased vagal nervous discharge. An ectopic atrial pacemaker may abruptly cease firing while a sinus pacemaker often slows gradually.

Carotid sinus sensitivity An exaggerated vagal response to slight pressure on the carotid sinus (a point on the neck where the internal and external carotid arteries divide). The SA and AV nodes are richly endowed with parasympathetic nerve fibers and a mild pressure on the carotid sinus can result in profound slowing of the sinus node impulse and may even result in sinus arrest.

Catecholamines A group of neurohormones (epinephrine and norepinephrine) produced largely by the adrenal medulla and ·adrenergic nerve endings, which have a stimulating (sympathetic) effect on the autonomic nervous system, resulting in:
1. ↑ heart rate
2. ↑ AV conduction
3. ↑ myocardial contractility

Cathode The negative portion of a pacer lead system.

Cation A positively charged electrolyte.

Cholinergic A term applied to nerve endings that liberate acetylcholine, such as the vagus nerve.

Chordae tendineae Fine fibrous threads anchoring the AV valve leaflets to their respective papillary muscles.

Chronotropic Refers to automaticity from the SA node; may be positive (↑ heart rate) or negative (↓ heart rate).

Cinchonism The toxic effects produced from overingestion of cinchona bark from which quinidine is extracted. Effects are usually headache, tinnitus, deafness, and blurred vision.

Committed sequential pacing The DVI (dual chamber–paced, ventricular chamber–sensed, mode of response is inhibited) pacing modality in which ventricular output is obligated after atrial output.

Compensatory pause (complete) A type of pause that occurs after a premature complex. If the interval measured between the R wave of the beat preceding the premature beat and the R wave of the beat following it is equal to twice that of the RR interval between two normal beats, the pause is fully compensatory. This occurs when the premature beat does not interrupt the sinus node cycle.

Conduction time Refers to the amount of time it takes for an impulse to travel through any part of the conduction system.

Conductivity The spread of electrical activity from one specialized cell to another.

Contractility A mechanical property characterized by the coordinated shortening of cardiac muscle fibers, resulting in a pumping effect.

Coronary arteries The vessels that feed the myocardium with blood. They consist of the left main, left anterior descending, circumflex, diagonals, obtuse marginals, right, and posterior descending arteries.

Coronary sinus An opening into the right atrium, draining venous blood from the myocardium into the general circulation.

Crux The point on the posterobasal surface of the heart that is the junction at which all four chambers meet.

Defibrillation A direct unsynchronized electrical current delivered via paddles applied to the chest in order to terminate ventricular fibrillation.

Demand pacemaker A type of pacemaker that fires only when necessary; that is, when the heart's own intrinsic rate becomes slower than the rate at which the pacemaker is set. It is synchronized to the patient's intrinsic rate.

Depolarization The process of activation of automatic, conductile, and contractile elements from the resting or polarized state.

Diastole Relaxation phase of the cardiac cycle during which the ventricles and coronary arteries are filling.

Dromotropic Refers to AV conduction that may be positive (accelerates AV conduction) or negative (slows AV conduction).

Ectopic Refers to an impulse that originates outside the sinus node.

Einthoven's triangle An equilateral triangle, which, when drawn on the chest, plots the axes of the bipolar standard limb leads.

Electrical axis The mean direction of current flow within the heart.

Electrical potential The energy possessed by a cell relative to ionic imbalance across its membrane.

Electrocardiogram (ECG) A graphic recording of the electrical activity of the heart plotted against time.

Electrophysiology study A procedure performed with intracardiac catheters to measure impulse formation and the speed of conduction at various sites in the conduction system.

Endocardium The smooth inner lining of the cardiac chambers, including the papillary muscles which is composed of epithelial cells.

Epicardium The outer layer of the heart, which is continuous with the visceral portion of the pericardium overlying the heart and the proximal segments of the great vessels.

Escape complex/rhythm A complex/rhythm that is initiated by a lower pacemaker when the sinus node fails or slows. Usually preceded by a pause in the normal heart rhythm, it is also termed "passive rhythm" or "rhythm by default."

Escape interval The interval in milliseconds, between an intrinsic complex and the subsequent paced complex.

Excitability The ability of the heart to respond to a stimulus.

Excitation-contraction-coupling A complex mechanism involving calcium and muscle proteins whereby the myofibrils in the myocardium shorten and contract in response to a stimulus.

Extrasystole A premature impulse from a focus other than the SA node.

Fibrillation Rapid, chaotic, unsynchronized quivering or twitching in the myocardium during which no effective pumping occurs.

Fixed-rate pacemaker A type of pacemaker that fires constantly despite the patient's intrinsic rate. It is said to be asynchronous as it does not synchronize its firing with the patient's own intrinsic rate.

Fossa ovalis A shallow, ovoid depression in the interatrial septum; a trace of the embryological interatrial opening.

Frank-Starling law of the heart The force of contraction is directly proportional to the stretch of myocardial fibrils, up to a point of physiological limits.

"f" waves Fine, undulating fibrillatory waves seen on the ECG in atrial fibrillation.

"F" waves Coarse flutter waves with a distinct sawtooth configuration seen on the ECG in atrial flutter.

Half-life The time it takes for an amount of drug dose in the blood to be reduced by one half.

Heart sound (third) (S_3) A low-pitched sound heard with the bell of the stethoscope, occurring immediately after the second heart sound (S_2) or the "dub" of the "lub-dub" sequence. It indicates heart failure in the adult.

Hyper- Refers to greater than normal.

Hypo- Refers to less than normal.

Hysteresis The extended time interval after an intrinsic beat and before the next paced beat.

Idiojunctional rhythm A rhythm arising from the branching area of the bundle of His at its own inherent rate of 40 to 50 beats per minute and producing a normal QRS complex. It is also known as an escape or passive rhythm.

Idiopathic hypertrophic subaortic stenosis (IHSS) A congenital heart defect characterized by enlargement (hypertrophy) of the muscle of the left ventricular wall and ventricular septum. During systole, obstruction occurs beneath the aortic valve, which may decrease stroke volume and cardiac output. Also known as hypertrophic obstructive cardiomyopathy (HOCM).

Idioventricular rhythm A rhythm arising in and controlling only the ventricles at their slow inherent rate. Also known as an escape or passive rhythm.

Inotropic Refers to contractility of the myocardium that may be positive (increased force of contractility) or negative (decreased force of contractility).

Interatrial septum Fibromuscular wall separating the atria.

Interventricular septum A wall separating the right and left ventricles:
  1. *Membranous:* thinner, upper portion of the septum between the aortic valve cusps and the tricuspid valve.
  2. *Muscular:* major part of the septum that participates in left ventricular contraction.

Junctional Area of conduction tissue that includes the AV node and the bundle of His.

Lead Arrangement of electrical conductors through which electrical activity from the body is brought to a recording device.

Lead axis The direct line between the negative and positive poles of a bipolar lead or between the positive pole and reference point of a unipolar lead.

Lead systems Reference systems that look at the heart's electrical activity. Made up of frontal leads, standard limb leads (I, II, III), augmented vector leads (aV_R, aV_L, aV_F), and horizontal (chest) leads (V_1, V_2, V_3, V_4, V_5, V_6).

Left bundle branch Fibers in the subendocardial layer of the left interventricular septum that conduct the impulse from the bundle of His to the Purkinje fibers. There are two divisions: anterior-superior division or fascicle and posterior-inferior division or fascicle.

Microshock Stray electrical current that may result from static electricity or current from a short-circuited electrical device. The current enters the pacer leads and elicits myocardial depolarization during the vulnerable period, thereby producing tachydysrhythmias.

Mitral valve Atrioventricular (AV) valve composed of two leaflets (bicuspid) through which blood passes from the left atrium to the left ventricle.

Multifocal A term referring to ectopic impulses that originate from different foci.

Myocardium Thick muscular contractile portion of the heart wall.

Myopotential The electrical current of muscle contraction resembling cardiac potentials that can cause sensitive pulse generators to inhibit or trigger with the muscle activity.

NH region Lowermost part of the AV node (AV node–His bundle area) thought to contain potential pacemaker fibers.

Noncommitted sequential pacing The DVI (dual chamber–paced, ventricular chamber–sensed, mode of response is inhibited) pacing modality in which ventricular output is optional after atrial output.

Noncompensatory pause A delay in ventricular systole following a premature complex that resets the sinus cadence. If the interval measured between the R wave of the beat preceding the premature beat and the R wave of the beat following it is less than twice that of the RR interval between two normal beats, the pause is noncompensatory. This occurs when the premature beat interrupts the sinus node cycle.

Norepinephrine Neurotransmitter substance of the sympathetic nervous system.

N region Midnodal region whose main function is to slow the transmission of the impulse from the atria to the ventricles. It is thought to be void of pacemaking capabilities.

Overdrive pacing The use of an artificial pacemaker to stimulate the heart's own intrinsic rate in order to suppress an abnormal tachydysrhythmia.

Papillary muscle Located in the endocardium of the right and left ventricles, these muscles anchor the AV valves via the chordae tendineae and prevent eversion of the valve leaflets into the atria during ventricular systole. There is one papillary muscle for each valve cusp.

Parasympathetic A division of the autonomic nervous system. Stimulation decreases cardiac impulse formation and conduction.

Paroxysmal A term referring to a dysrhythmia with sudden onset and termination that recurs periodically.

Passive complex/rhythm A term referring to escape complex/rhythm.

P cells Specialized cells located in the center of the SA node, which possess the property of automaticity.

Pericarditis Inflammation of the pericardium.

Pericardium Conical-shaped serous cavity covering the heart and proximal portions of the great vessels.

Polarity Refers to the location of the positive and negative poles of a lead axis or the difference in electrical potential between the inner and outer surface of the cell membrane.

PP interval The interval of distance between two sinus P waves, measured from the beginning of one P wave to the beginning of the next P wave. The PP interval is normally regular in rhythm.

P¹ (P prime) wave A term used to describe a P wave that differs in shape from the sinus P wave because the impulse originates outside the sinus node.

Precordium Refers to the anterior surface of the lower thorax.

Preload Refers to the volume of blood in the left ventricle before contraction.

Pressoreceptors Receptors found in the superior vena cavae, right atrium, aortic arch, and carotid sinus, which sense stretch and increase or decrease heart rate and blood pressure accordingly.

Programmability The ability to change an implantable pacemaker's mode (rate, impulse amplitude, etc.) by noninvasive means. An example of simple programmability is the placement of a magnet over an implanted synchronous pacemaker to change it to the asynchronous mode.

Pulmonary artery The vessel transporting venous blood from the right ventricle to the lungs.

Pulmonary veins There are usually two veins from each lung transporting arterial blood from the lungs to the left atrium.

Pulmonic semilunar valve A valve consisting of three pocket-like cusps through which blood is ejected from the right ventricle to the pulmonary artery.

Purkinje cells Cells located at the junction of the SA node and atrial muscle tissue. The cells conduct impulses from the transitional cells to the atrial myocardial cells to depolarize the atria.

Purkinje fibers Terminal branches of the right and left bundles that bring the impulse rapidly and directly to the myocardial cells of the septum, ventricular walls, and papillary muscles, depolarizing the ventricles and allowing the mechanical event of ventricular contraction to occur.

Reentry The circus movement of an impulse traveling two pathways that have a disparity (imbalance) in their response time to the impulse. This sets up a rapid tachycardia that may originate in the atrium, AV junction, Purkinje fibers, ventricular muscle, or accessory pathways.

Refractory The period during which fibers are unresponsive to a stimulus.

Refractory period (absolute or effective) See Absolute refractory period.

Relative refractory period A period corresponding from the beginning of the T wave to almost the end of the T wave on the ECG in which a stronger than normal stimulus may excite and depolarize the cells.

Repolarization The process of restoration of a cell to its normal resting electrical state following depolarization.

Retrograde conduction Impulse conduction that occurs in a backward direction.

Right bundle branch (RBB) A long, thin bundle of fibers within the subendocardial layer of the right interventricular septum that conduct impulses from the bundle of His to the Purkinje fibers in the right ventricle.

Sensitivity The minimum signal that consistently activates the pacemaker pulse generator. This is also known as the sensing threshold.

Serum levels A method that assays drug levels in the serum. There is a standard that indicates whether a drug level is "therapeutic" (whether enough drug is in the serum to be beneficial to the patient) or the drug level is too high and may produce toxic effects.

Sine wave A smooth biphasic wave representing end-stage hyperkalemia and ventricular tachycardia. A disparity in the depolarization process in the myocardium widens the QRS complex, which merges with the T wave, producing the sine wave.

Sinoatrial (SA) node The node located at the junction of the superior vena cava and right atrium, consisting of specialized automatic cells and known as the natural pacemaker of the heart.

Sinus of Valsalva Pocket-like pouches of the aortic valve cusps in which the openings of the coronary arteries are located.

Steady state The timing and dosage required for a drug to reach a therapeutic serum level in a patient. It takes approximately five dosing intervals or five "half-lives" of a drug for this to occur.

Stokes-Adams syndrome Episodes characterized by sudden syncope or seizures resulting from intermittent severe bradycardia, third-degree AV block, or ventricular tachycardia, fibrillation, or standstill.

Sulcus A groove.

Supernormal period A period at the end of the T wave during which depolarization may be initiated by a lesser stimulus than is normally required. Also known as the vulnerable period.

Supraventricular dysrhythmias Refers to abnormal impulse formation originating above the ventricle, which may be from the SA node, atrial muscle, or AV node. This also refers to abnormal impulse conduction such as occurs in the circus-type reentry movement in atrial tissue, the AV junction, or in accessory pathways.

Surface ECG The usual 12-lead ECG that is performed with electrodes placed on the skin. This differs from an electrode wire that is placed inside the heart to obtain a more precise picture of electrical activity.

Sympathetic A division of the autonomic nervous system which, when stimulated, increases impulse formation (automaticity), speed of conduction, and force of myocardial contraction.

Sympathomimetic Mimicking the effects of sympathetic nerve stimulation.

Synchronous Refers to having the same period or phase. See Demand pacemaker.

Systemic vascular resistance (SVR) Resistance to the flow of blood from the left ventricle, which is determined by vascular muscle tone and the diameter of the vessel, usually the arterioles. Also known as "peripheral vascular resistance."

Systole The contraction phase of the cardiac cycle, related to expelling blood from chambers.

Threshold The lowest amount of electrical energy necessary to cause the heart to contract from a pacemaker stimulus.

Torsade de pointes A term used to describe a paroxysmal type of ventricular fibrillation and/or tachycardia, characterized by alterations in voltage that appear to be twisting around an isoelectric line. It is usually precipitated by lengthening of the QT interval.

Transitional cells Specialized cells that lie in the periphery of the SA note that conduct impulses from the P cells to the Purkinje cells and then to the atrial myocardium.

Tricuspid valve Atrioventricular (AV) valve composed of three leaflets through which blood passes from the right atrium to the right ventricle.

Trigeminy A term used to describe three successive complexes, normal and ectopic, which repetitively occur in triplets.

Unifocal A term referring to ectopic impulses that originate in the same pacemaker site.

U wave A small wave on the ECG following the T wave, which may represent repolarization of the Purkinje fibers.

Vagus The major nerve of the parasympathetic nervous system, the tenth cranial nerve.

Valsalva maneuver A maneuver whereby an individual takes a quick inspiratory breath followed by forced expiratory straining against a closed glottis. An example would be straining at stool. This maneuver elevates venous pressure by obstructing blood flow into the chest, which results from stimulation of the parasympathetic nervous system. It may decrease heart rate.

Vasovagal reaction A reaction resulting in slowing of heart rate and lowering of blood pressure. Any large volume of blood or mechanical or chemical stimulation of pressure sensors or receptors located in the carotid artery and arch of the aorta convey impulses to the vagus (parasympathetic) nerve at its origin in the medulla of the brain. This stimulates receptors that affect parasympathetic fibers in the heart, which reflexively slow heart rate and decrease contractility of the myocardium. This is known as the vasovagal reflex and can occur from strong emotional stress as well.

Vector A force with direction and magnitude, representing electrical current flow by use of an arrow.

Ventricle One of two lower muscular pumping chambers of the heart.

Ventricular escape rhythm See Idioventricular rhythm.

Weight Most drug dosages are based on a patient's weight in kilograms (kg), (2.2 pounds = 1 kg).

Wolff-Parkinson-White syndrome The presence of an accessory pathway, formerly known as a Kent bundle, which allows impulses to prematurely activate a portion of the ventricle before the normal impulse has time to arrive. This is characterized on the ECG by a short PR interval and a widened QRS interval. This may also precipitate a circus reentry through the dual pathways.

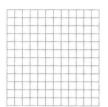

Index